Clinics in Developmental Medicine No. 164 - 165
THE TREATMENT OF GAIT PROBLEMS IN
CEREBRAL PALSY

© 2004 Mac Keith Press
Mac Keith Press, 30 Furnival Street, London, EC4A 1JQ

Senior Editor: Martin CO Bax
Editor: Hilary M Hart
Managing Editor: Michael Pountney

First published in this edition 2004

British Library Cataloguing-in-Publication data:
A catalogue record for this book is available from the British Library

ISSN: 0069 4835
ISBN: 1 898683 37 9

Printed by The Lavenham Press Ltd, Water Street, Lavenham, Suffolk
Mac Keith Press is supported by Scope

Clinics in Developmental Medicine No. 164 - 165

The Treatment of Gait Problems in Cerebral Palsy

Edited by

JAMES R GAGE
Medical Director Emeritus
Gillette Children's Specialty Healthcare
St Paul, Minnesota;
Professor of Orthopaedics
University of Minnesota, USA

2004
Mac Keith Press

Distributed by 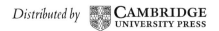 **CAMBRIDGE** UNIVERSITY PRESS

CONTENTS

AUTHORS' APPOINTMENTS

Leland Albright, M.D.   Professor of Neurosurgery, Children's Hospital of Pittsburgh; Professor and Chief, Department of Pediatric Neurosurgery, University of Pittsburgh, Pennsylvania, USA

Allison S. Arnold, Ph.D.   Research Associate, Biomechanics Engineering Division, Mechanical Engineering Department, Stanford University, California, USA

Henry G. Chambers, M.D.   Chief of Staff, Medical Director of Motion Analysis Laboratory, San Diego Children's Hospital and Health Center; Clinical Associate Professor of Orthopedic Surgery, University of California at San Diego, California, USA

Lynn Christianson, M.D.   Director of Anesthesiology, Department of Anesthesiology, Gillette Children's Specialty Healthcare, St Paul, Minneapolis, USA

Roy B. Davis, Ph.D.   Director of Engineering, Motion Analysis Laboratory, Shriners Hospitals for Children, Greenville, South Carolina, USA

Scott L. Delp, Ph.D.   Chairman, Bioengineering Department, Stanford University, Stanford, California, USA

Adré J. du Plessis, M.D.   Director, Neonatal Neurology Program, Neuromotor Therapy Program, Children's Hospital, Boston, Massachusetts; Associate Professor in Neurology, Harvard Medical School, Harvard, USA

James R. Gage, M.D.   Medical Director Emeritus, Gillette Children's Specialty Healthcare, St Paul, Minnesota; Professor of Orthopaedics, University of Minnesota, Minneapolis, Minnesota, USA

Mark E. Gormley, M.D.

Staff Physiatrist, Gillette Children's Specialty Healthcare, St Paul, Minnesota; Clinical Assistant Professor, Department of Physical Medicine and Rehabilitation, University of Minnesota, Minneapolis, Minnesota, USA

Steven Koop, M.D.

Medical Director, Gillette Children's Specialty Healthcare, St Paul, Minnesota; Associate Professor of Orthopaedics, University of Minnesota, Minneapolis, Minnesota, USA

Linda E. Krach, M.D.

Director, Research Administration, Gillette Children's Specialty Healthcare, St Paul, Minnesota; Clinical Assistant Professor, Department of Physical Medicine and Rehabilitation, University of Minnesota, Minneapolis, Minnesota, USA

Sue Murr, P.T.

Supervisor of Programs in Rehabilitation Therapies, Gillette Children's Specialty Healthcare, St Paul, Minnesota, USA

Tom F. Novacheck, M.D.

Director, Center for Gait and Motion Analysis, Gillette Children's Specialty Healthcare, St Paul, Minnesota; Associate Professor of Orthopaedics, University of Minnesota, Minneapolis, Minnesota, USA

Sylvia Õunpuu, M.Sc.

Director/Kinesiologist, Center for Motion Analysis, Hartford, Connecticut; Assistant Professor, School of Medicine, University of Connecticut, USA

Warwick J. Peacock, M.D.

Professor Emeritus, Department of Neurological Surgery, University of California, San Francisco, USA

Jessica Rose, Ph.D.

Assistant Professor, Department of Orthopaedic Surgery, Stanford University School of Medicine; Director, Motion and Gait Analysis Laboratory, Lucile Packard Children's Hospital, Stanford University Medical Center, USA

Deborah S. Quanbeck, M.D.   Director of Medical Education, Gillette Children's Specialty Healthcare, St Paul, Minnesota; Assistant Professor, Orthopaedic Surgery, University of Minnesota, Minneapolis, Minnesota, USA

Michael Schwartz, Ph.D.   Director of Bioengineering Research, Gillette Children's Specialty Healthcare, St Paul, Minnesota; Assistant Professor, Orthopaedic Surgery Graduate Faculty, Biomedical Engineering, University of Minnesota, Minneapolis, Minnesota, USA

Jean Stout, M.S., P.T.   Research Physical Therapist, Center for Gait and Motion Analysis, Gillette Children's Specialty Healthcare, St Paul, Minnesota, USA

Joyce Trost, P.T.   Research Physical Therapist, Center for Gait and Motion Analysis, Gillette Children's Specialty Healthcare, St Paul, Minnesota, USA

Ann E. Van Heest, M.D.   Associate Professor, Department of Orthopaedic Surgery, University of Minnesota, Minneapolis, Minnesota, USA

INTRODUCTION

When I wrote my first book, *Gait Analysis in Cerebral Palsy*, automated gait analysis for the treatment of children with walking disorders was just starting to come into widespread use. That book, a monograph/handbook of treatment principles that I had gleaned from 10 years of clinical experience with gait analysis at Newington and Gillette Children's Hospitals, was intended for those who were just starting to use clinical gait analysis in the treatment of children with neuromuscular gait problems.

In the preface of that book, I quoted the words of A. Bruce Gill: "Study principles not methods. If one understands the principle, he can devise his own methods." Reviewing the book now, 10 years after its publication, it is interesting to note that while the principles of treatment have changed very little, the methods of treatment have changed a great deal; furthermore, there has been tremendous growth in the number of health-care professionals eagerly at work in a field that we once had pretty much to ourselves. As such, I felt it was time for another attempt to summarize the gains that have been made in the treatment of gait disorders in cerebral palsy in the intervening years. It quickly became apparent, however, that I was not capable of writing such a book alone, since the field is now far too broad and diverse for one individual to adequately cover it.

Progress has been made in every aspect of cerebral palsy diagnosis and treatment. Computer advances have made gait analysis laboratories better, cheaper, and almost ubiquitous. Diagnostic imaging and other new investigative techniques have provided much greater insight into the causes and prevention of brain injuries in newborns. General progress in the understanding of brain function has helped us to create a better picture of how the brain controls locomotion. Increased understanding of the biomechanics of human locomotion has yielded essential information about how muscles produce movement and greater appreciation of the role of the skeletal lever-arms on which they act.

Neurosurgical techniques such as selective dorsal rhizotomy and the intrathecal baclofen pump have allowed us to reduce the primary spasticity as well as some of its secondary effects. Pharmaceutical advances such as intramuscular botulinum toxin have enabled us to block the local effects of spasticity and so minimize fixed muscle contracture. And we have learned that when these newer treatments are combined with other modalities such as physical therapy, stretching casts and appropriate night splinting, muscle-lengthening surgeries can often be minimized or avoided altogether.

To ensure that this new book would have sufficient breadth and depth of scope to do justice to all these developments, I assembled a group of people whom I view as authorities in their respective disciplines to write its component chapters. Contact or collaboration with each person involved has taught me a great deal over the past 20 years, and has contributed to the better results of treatment that we are now experiencing.

My sincere thanks go out to all of the individuals who have contributed to this book. Most of them are credited in the headings of the chapters they contributed. Some, however, are not and deserve special mention here. One such individual is Jean-Pierre Lin, a clinical neurologist at Guy's Hospital in London, who provided me with his invaluable help editing the chapters which fall within his area of expertise, but outside of mine. His contributions have greatly enriched the content and bibliography of the chapters dealing with spasticity and the control of locomotion. In addition, I want to thank him personally, for I have gained valuable additional insight from the process. Two others who should be mentioned by name are Roy Wervy, one of the engineers who works in our motion analysis laboratory here at Gillette Children's Hospital, and Chad Halvorson, who works in Interactive Development at Meditech Communications, Inc. in St Paul, Minnesota. It is difficult to discuss problems relating to gait without showing pre- and post-treatment outcomes of affected individuals in motion. Roy and Chad are responsible for the excellent CD-Rom at the back of this book that makes this possible.

Thanks are also in order to those individuals who helped with the illustrations. Illustrating a text by multiple authors is always a problem and this book was no exception. For example, Warwick Peacock hand-sketched the particular illustrations he wanted to see used in his chapters dealing with control of locomotion and spasticity. I owe a great debt of gratitude to Jenny Dahl, a very talented graphic artist, who was able to convert Dr Peacock's sketches into the excellent illustrations that can now be found in Chapters 1 and 3. I also wish to thank Derek Petersen, who used his artistic ability and knowledge of Photoshop to create several of the illustrations in this book and enhance others. Anna Bitner and Jim Strobel, who work in the media department at Gillette Children's Specialty Healthcare, have also contributed a great deal of time and effort to the preparation of the final illustrations. I am indebted to them as well.

Locomotion begins in the brain with the thought to re-locate, to move from one place to another. So we must begin our study of gait problems in cerebral palsy with the brain, because that is where things have gone wrong. Once one has some concept of what has occurred in the brain, the next thing that is needed is knowledge of how normal locomotion occurs and how it is measured. Upon this basis, one can begin to understand how cerebral palsy affects the musculoskeletal system in a growing child. Next, if children with the condition are to be treated thoughtfully and well, one must review the available treatments in the context of the pathologies they address. Only with this knowledge as a background can one comfortably target and treat the various types of locomotor pathology cerebral palsy produces. And finally, once the treatment has been completed, it becomes imperative, if we wish to "raise the bar" for future treatments, to accurately assess its outcome.

The book has been divided into five sections that correspond to the philosophy of treatment I have sketched above: (1) Clinical Background, (2) Patient Assessment, (3) Gait Pathology in Cerebral Palsy, (4) Treatment, and (5) Assessment of Outcome. Because of the depth of knowledge and expertise of the various authors involved in this project, I eagerly looked forward to reading the final text, and I have learned a great deal from it. I sincerely hope that you will find it as enjoyable and rewarding to your practice as I have to mine.

JAMES R. GAGE, M.D.
Medical Director Emeritus, Gillette Children's Specialty Healthcare
Professor of Orthopaedics, University of Minnesota

1
THE NEUROLOGICAL CONTROL SYSTEM FOR LOCOMOTION

Warwick J. Peacock

The only action that a human can bring about is muscular contraction. This muscular contraction will cause movement that may in turn produce actions such as locomotion or speech. However, any action must start as a thought. Thoughts arise in certain areas of the brain which, through their connections, stimulate cortical motor centers. This initiation of motor actions has been recorded as an electrical potential known as the "readiness potential", and it is located in the supplementary motor area, just anterior to the motor strip (Deecke et al. 1969). This readiness potential occurs up to 1 second before the onset of movement, whether the movement occurs in the hand, toe, mouth, tongue or eye, and irrespective of whether the movements are complex and programmed (as in speech) or simple (Brinkman and Porter 1979, 1983, Schreiber et al. 1983, Kornhuber and Deecke 1985, Porter and Lemon 1993). Large, fast-firing neurons in the cortex, which are known as Betz cells, contribute axons to motor tracts which descend from the cortex to the brainstem (corticobulbar fibers) and spinal cord (corticospinal tracts) to connect with motor nerves that innervate muscles. The muscles, when stimulated by these motor tracts, then contract to bring about the desired purposeful movement and action.

The structural unit of the nervous system is the nerve cell or neuron, each of which is made up of a nerve cell body and a number of impulse conducting processes (Fig. 1.1). Gray matter is comprised of nerve cell bodies and white matter of nerve processes.

The various parts of the central nervous system are made up only of gray and white matter (Fig. 1.2). Gray matter is discrete and easily recognizable. In the cerebral hemispheres it forms the outer cerebral cortex and the deep nuclei of the corpus striatum. The nuclei of the brainstem are made up of gray matter. In the cerebellum the cortex and the deep dentate nucleus is gray matter. The spinal cord has centrally placed H-shaped gray matter.

The motor system

The motor system is hierarchical, and is made up of a chain of command from the cortical centers down to the motor nerves that connect with the muscles (Fig. 1.3). An upper motor neuron runs down from the motor cortex to connect with either a bulbar or a spinal lower motor neuron, which in turn leaves the central nervous system via a peripheral nerve to innervate a muscle. The components of the system are as follows.

Cortical motor control centers (Fig.1.3) constitute the supreme command of motor activity.

The basal ganglia (Fig. 1.4) play an important role in previewing and planning movement

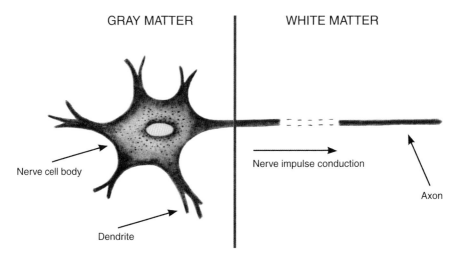

GRAY MATTER   WHITE MATTER

Nerve cell body

Nerve impulse conduction

Axon

Dendrite

Fig. 1.1. A neuron: the basic unit of the central nervous system. Impulses enter the nerve cell through the dendrites and exit via the axon. Gray matter is composed of nerve cell bodies, while white matter is made up of nerve processes.

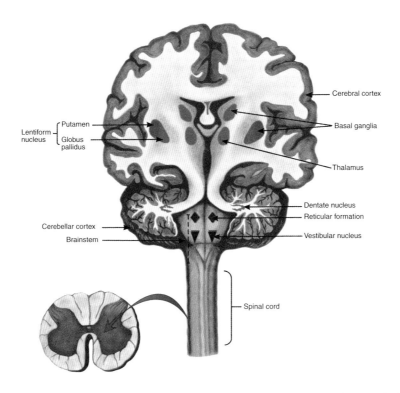

Cerebral cortex

Putamen
Lentiform
nucleus
Globus
pallidus

Basal ganglia

Thalamus

Dentate nucleus
Reticular formation

Cerebellar cortex
Brainstem

Vestibular nucleus

Spinal cord

Fig. 1.2. Diagrammatic representation of a coronal section taken through the brain and spinal cord, showing some of the major control centers.

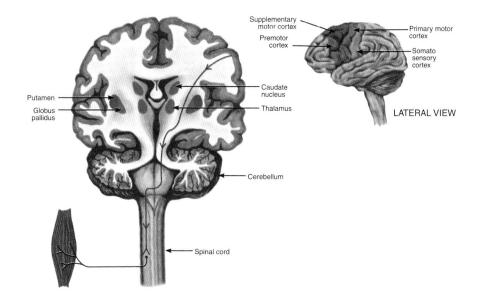

Fig. 1.3. Coronal and lateral diagrams of the brain showing the relative locations of the primary, premotor and supplementary motor cortices. Axons from neurons in the pyramidal system run uninterrupted from the motor cortex to synapse on lower motor neurons. Pyramidal neurons in the cortex can initiate a muscle movement since they synapse directly with lower motor neurons. However, for coordinated movement to occur, many other circuits between the motor cortex and other brain centers are required.

patterns willed by the cerebral cortex, and are made up of a number of deep-seated gray-matter nuclei including the putamen, globus pallidus and caudate nucleus (comprising the corpus striatum) with the substantia nigra and subthalamic nucleus. All these structures are directly or indirectly connected to the thalamus, which in turn is connected to the frontal lobe cortex.

The cerebellum (Fig. 1.5) is involved in assessing the degree to which a movement conforms to the order issued by the cortical motor centers in relation to information from peripheral sense organs for muscle length and velocity of contraction (muscle spindles) and rate of change of contraction force (Golgi tendon organs).

The *brainstem motor nuclei* (see below, Fig. 1.11) provide a background of posture and tone against which specific voluntary movements can be executed.

The *spinal cord* (Fig. 1.6) provides the motor neurons that connect with muscles to bring about contraction and movement. Important motor reflexes are also a feature of the cord's connections.

1. CORTICAL MOTOR-CONTROL CENTERS

A thought, which will lead to a movement, may arise in any part of the cerebral cortex, and an impulse is then relayed to the supplementary motor area in the anterior part of the frontal lobe (Fig 1.3). Dynamic studies show that if a person simply thinks about an intended

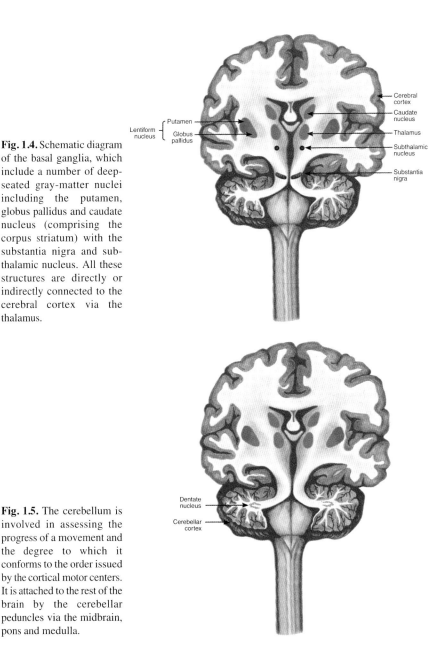

Fig. 1.4. Schematic diagram of the basal ganglia, which include a number of deep-seated gray-matter nuclei including the putamen, globus pallidus and caudate nucleus (comprising the corpus striatum) with the substantia nigra and subthalamic nucleus. All these structures are directly or indirectly connected to the cerebral cortex via the thalamus.

Fig. 1.5. The cerebellum is involved in assessing the progress of a movement and the degree to which it conforms to the order issued by the cortical motor centers. It is attached to the rest of the brain by the cerebellar peduncles via the midbrain, pons and medulla.

movement the supplementary motor area becomes active (Deecke et al. 1969, Roland et al. 1980). If the supplementary motor area is stimulated during awake neurosurgical procedures, subjects experience an urge to move, or feel that a movement is about to occur (Fried et al. 1991). The command is then passed on to the premotor cortex (Fig 1.3), which is involved in the preparation for movement. The next relay is to the primary motor cortex

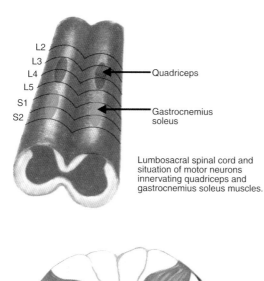

L2
L3
L4 — Quadriceps
L5
S1
S2 — Gastrocnemius soleus

Lumbosacral spinal cord and
situation of motor neurons
innervating quadriceps and
gastrocnemius soleus muscles.

Distal
muscles
Proximal
muscles

Fig. 1.6. Longitudinal and cross-sectional views of the lumbosacral spinal cord. The longitudinal view shows the situation of the motor neurons innervating the quadriceps and the gastrocsoleus muscles. The horizontal cross-section shows the relative position of motor neurons innervating proximal- and distal-limb muscles.

in the precentral gyrus (Fig. 1.3), from where the corticospinal or pyramidal tract arises. The corticospinal fibers, which account for only one million of the 30 million fibers running through the internal capsule, are found in the posterior third of the posterior limb of the internal capsule (Brodal 1981). These fibers become the pyramidal tracts of the medulla. The opposite half of the body is arranged in the precentral gyrus as an inverted homunculus, with the leg represented superiorly near the midline with the trunk, arm and face found lower down and more laterally (Fig. 1.7). The corticospinal tract then passes downwards as part of the deep hemispheral white matter and through the internal capsule, before forming the cerebral peduncles and then entering the brainstem (Fig. 1.7). At the level of the medulla the corticospinal tract crosses over to become the "pyramid" and descends in the opposite side of the lower medulla before coursing in the spinal cord in the lateral corticospinal tracts to synapse with a motor neuron in the lateral part of the anterior horn (Fig. 1.7). The anterior corticospinal tracts contain uncrossed motor fibers (i.e. from the ipsilateral hemisphere). The motor neurons in the lateral part of the anterior horn control distal muscles in the limbs, whereas the medially situated motor neurons, which are under different upper motor-neuron influence, control proximal limb and trunk muscles. The axon of the motor neuron then exits from the spinal cord, becoming a peripheral nerve that travels out to its specific muscle and brings about a contraction, which in turn leads to the intended movement.

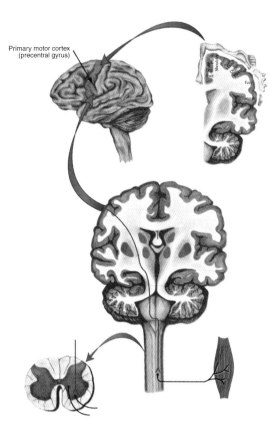

Fig. 1.7. Coronal and lateral diagrams of the precentral gyrus. The opposite half of the body is arranged in the precentral gyrus as an inverted homunculus (diagrammatic representation of a "little man"). The corticospinal tract, which arises from the precentral gyrus, crosses over to the opposite side at the level of the medulla and then descends in the spinal cord to synapse with a motor neuron.

2. THE BASAL GANGLIA

The basal ganglia are large gray-matter nuclei found in the basal part of the cerebral hemispheres. The basal ganglia are involved in the appropriate planning and initiation of voluntary movement. They receive a large cortical input and, after processing all of the relevant information, relay back to the motor cortex. The basal ganglia form a closed loop with the cerebral cortex and have no direct contact with lower motor neurons that are connected to the muscles and bring about the desired movement. The caudate nucleus and putamen are known as the corpus striatum, and work in conjunction with the globus pallidus (Fig. 1.8). Also included in the basal ganglia are the subthalamic nucleus and the substantia nigra. The basal ganglia store information about previously performed movements. When the cortex intends to bring about a purposeful movement the basal ganglia are called upon to provide the memory for that particular movement in relationship to the body's posture and position in space at that moment. The integrated information about the purpose and sequence of the movement is then relayed back to the cortex so that appropriate instructions can be sent down the upper motor neurons to the lower motor neurons, and finally out to the group of muscles which will be involved in performing the movement and achieving the intended goal.

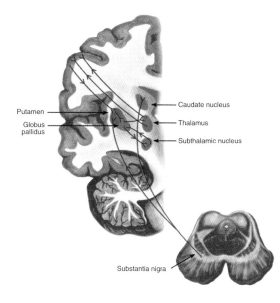

Putamen
Globus pallidus
Caudate nucleus
Thalamus
Subthalamic nucleus
Substantia nigra

Fig. 1.8. Diagrammatic representation of the anatomy and connections of the basal ganglia. The basal ganglia form a closed loop with the cerebral cortex and are involved in the planning and initiation of voluntary movement. The basal ganglia store motor engram (memories) which the cortex draws upon when deciding which movement will be most effective in achieving the desired goal. Neurons dive down from the cortex to connect with neurons in the putamen and caudate nucleus. The circuitry then involves the globus pallidus, the subthalamic nucleus and the substantia nigra before heading back to the cortex via the thalamus. The cortex now chooses the most appropriate motor engram to perform the desired movement.

Almost all cortical areas project to the caudate nucleus and the putamen. These two structures then project to the globus pallidus and on to the thalamus, which completes the circuit back to the cortex. Also hooked into the loop are the substantia nigra and the subthalamic nucleus.

The main functions of the basal ganglia are the initiation and smooth performance of voluntary movements. The two common neurological disorders that are caused by pathology in the basal ganglia are Parkinson's disease, in which the substantia nigra is destroyed, and Huntington's disease, in which there is marked atrophy of the caudate nucleus and putamen. In Parkinson's disease there is difficulty with the initiation of movement and spontaneous movement is diminished. With Huntington's disease entire motor programs are inappropriately released, as manifested by jerky, random and repetitive writhing movements, which are referred to as chorea or athetosis.

3. THE CEREBELLUM

The cerebellum is made up of two lateral hemispheres and the midline vermis (Fig. 1.9). There is a folded cortex overlying central white matter with deep nuclei, the main one being called the dentate nucleus. The cerebellum is extensively connected to the rest of the central nervous system via the cerebellar peduncles and is involved with the smooth execution and completion of movements and with truncal balance. There are three broad anatomical and physiological divisions to the cerebellum, which follow the stages of evolution of this organ (Brodal 1981):

1. The oldest part of the cerebellum, the *vestibulocerebellum* or *archicerebellum*, is the small floculonodular lobe which receives ipsilateral vestibular input, essential for the sense of balance, via the inferior cerebellar peduncles.

2. The *midline vermis*, also known as the *spinocerebellum* or *paleocerebellum*, receives

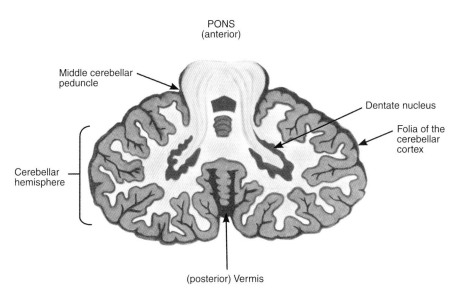

PONS
(anterior)

Middle cerebellar peduncle

Dentate nucleus

Folia of the cerebellar cortex

Cerebellar hemisphere

(posterior) Vermis

Fig. 1.9. Cross-section of the cerebellum at the level of the pons showing the connections via the middle cerebellar peduncle to the pons. The gray matter of the cortex and the dentate nucleus are shown. It is involved with the smooth execution and completion of movements and with truncal balance.

sensory input via the inferior cerebellar peduncles from the muscle spindles (which detect muscle length and velocity) and Golgi tendon organs (sensing changes in tendon force) which in turn course up the spinal cord in the spinocerebellar tracts.

3. The lateral parts of the cerebellum, the *cerebellar hemispheres*, are recent additions and are known as the *neocerebellum* or *pontocerebellum* because of the huge input from the pontine nuclei via the middle cerebellar peduncle. Some 20 million afferent fibers are carried from pontine nuclei via the middle cerebellar peduncle to the cerebellar hemispheres.

The inferior cerebellar peduncle contains almost exclusively afferent fibers from the inferior olive (approximately 0.5 million in all) and from these other vital peripheral sense organs. The superior cerebellar peduncle, which contains approximately 0.8 million efferent fibers, carries information from the cerebellar nuclei to the brainstem, red nucleus and thalamus.

At the same time that the cortical motor centers send an instruction to a group of muscles to bring about a purposeful movement, they also send a message to the cerebellum informing it of the desired movement pattern (Fig. 1.10a). With the onset of muscular contraction, information about the pattern of the contraction is conducted back from the muscles to the cerebellum (Fig. 1.10b). In the cerebellar cortex the error between what was instructed and what is being carried out is computed, and this information is sent to the dentate nucleus in the cerebellar hemisphere. The necessary correction is then relayed to the cortical motor centers (Fig. 1.10c). This is followed by an adjusted command to the muscles so that the movement is carried out as originally intended. This monitoring and correcting is carried out throughout every tiny fraction of the movement until the objective is achieved.

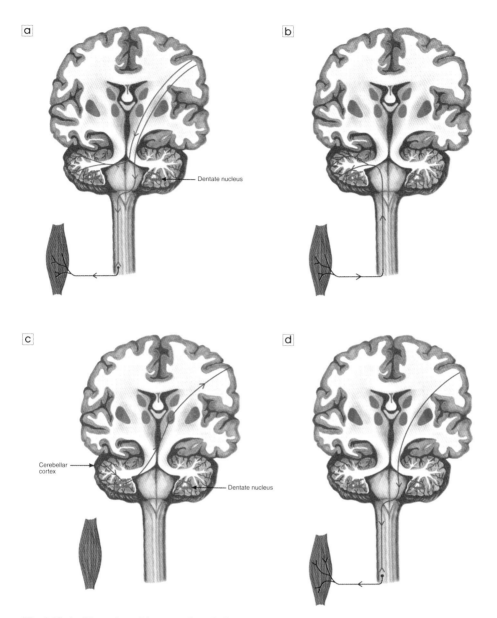

Fig. 1.10. An illustration of the steps of cerebellar motor control. (a) When the cortex decides to perform a movement an impulse is sent via the pyramidal tract to the spinal motor neuron but, at the same time, this instruction is also sent to the cerebellum. (b) As soon as the movement begins, receptors in the involved muscles and joints relay back to the cerebellum information concerning the rate and direction of the movement. (c) The cerebellar cortex now computes the error between the instruction and the information received about the first few milliseconds of the movement. A correction is calculated and relayed back to the cortex via the cerebellar dentate nucleus and thalamus. (d) A revised instruction is now sent from the motor cortex down the pyramidal tract to the motor neurons of the spinal cord. This monitoring and correcting is carried out throughout every tiny fraction of the movement until the objective is achieved

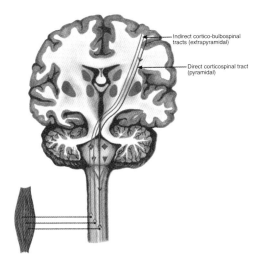

Indirect cortico-bulbospinal tracts (extrapyramidal)

Direct corticospinal tract (pyramidal)

Fig. 1.11. The brainstem motor nuclei. Whereas the pyramidal (direct corticospinal) tract reaches the spinal motor neurons without interruption, the extrapyramidal (indirect cortico-bulbospinal) tracts relay in the brainstem in the reticular and vestibular nuclei. The vestibular and reticular tracts then descend to the spinal motor neurons and provide a background of posture and tone against which specific voluntary movements can be executed.

Damage to the cerebellum causes symptoms on the ipsilateral side. Lesions of the cerebellum cause a loss of coordination with ongoing movements. Dysmetria is a common problem with cerebellar pathology; difficulty picking up a pencil is one example of how it may be manifested. The hand tends to overshoot the pencil and then rebounds back too far, and only after a number of movements of decreasing amplitude does the hand achieve its goal.

4. THE BRAINSTEM MOTOR NUCLEI

Apart from the cranial-nerve motor nuclei there are a number of nuclei in the brainstem that are involved in providing a background of posture and tone in the trunk and proximal limbs so that fine distal movements can be executed efficiently. These nuclei are the vestibular nucleus and the reticular formation (Fig. 1.11). These two structures are under the control of the cortical motor centers and the tracts can be described as the cortico-bulbospinal tracts. The vestibular nucleus is also connected to the vestibular apparatus in the inner ear and is involved with balance. The reticular formation is a cluster of gray matter scattered throughout the brainstem and is involved with rhythmic activity such as heart beat, respiration and sleep–wake cycles. The direct corticospinal (pyramidal) tracts and the indirect cortico-bulbospinal (extrapyramidal) tracts make up the upper motor neurons, which control muscular activity. Both the vestibulospinal and reticulospinal tracts synapse with motor neurons that lie in the medial part of the anterior horns of the spinal cord and innervate trunk and proximal-limb muscles. The corticospinal (pyramidal) tracts synapse with motor neurons found in the lateral part of the anterior horn that innervate distal limb muscles used for finely adjusted movements.

5. SPINAL-CORD MOTOR CONTROL

The majority of the neurons that control the body's skeletal muscles are to be found in the anterior horn of the spinal cord. We will not be discussing the motor neurons found in the

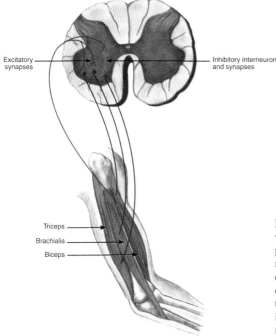

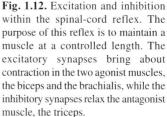

Fig. 1.12. Excitation and inhibition within the spinal-cord reflex. The purpose of this reflex is to maintain a muscle at a controlled length. The excitatory synapses bring about contraction in the two agonist muscles, the biceps and the brachialis, while the inhibitory synapses relax the antagonist muscle, the triceps.

cranial nerve nuclei, which mainly innervate the muscles of the head and neck. The motor neurons in the spinal cord are also known as lower motor neurons. Their nerve fibers, which exit the spinal cord to innervate muscles, are referred to as the final common pathway. Each of these motor neurons innervates one or more muscle fibers within the same muscle, and a given neuron and the group of muscle fibers it supplies are collectively known as a motor unit. All the motor neurons that innervate a specific muscle lie within a longitudinal column within the anterior horn. This column usually spans more than one spinal-cord segment. For example, the longitudinal column of motor neurons innervating the quadriceps muscle extends through the L3, L4 spinal-cord segments and those for the gastrocnemii are in the L5, S1 segments. The medial groups innervate axial and proximal limb muscles while the lateral groups innervate distal limb muscles.

The spinal cord has its own intrinsic circuitry, which is best illustrated by the spinal reflex arc, also known as the stretch reflex (Fig. 1.12). The purpose of this reflex is to maintain a muscle at a given length. The muscle length is set for specific function and any stretch will set up a reflex to bring the muscle back to the desired length. Stretch is detected by muscle spindles within the skeletal muscle, and an impulse is then generated which travels to the spinal cord in the afferent or posterior nerve root. This afferent nerve fiber enters the spinal cord where it synapses with the motor neuron, and an efferent impulse then travels out of the spinal cord via the motor or anterior root and the spinal nerve to the muscle. The muscle now contracts to return to the appropriate length. The muscle-spindle afferent impulse is thus excitatory. Although this stretch reflex is somewhat autonomous, it is under the inhibitory influence of the upper motor neurons. Normal muscle tone is maintained by the balanced interaction between the excitatory muscle-spindle afferent and the descending inhibitory influences. This balance is referred to as presynaptic inhibition. If the upper motor-neuron inhibition is reduced, velocity-dependent increases in the stretch reflex (spasticity) occur along with abnormal postures, abnormal motor sequencing, loss of fine-motor dexterity, and weakness of voluntary muscle contraction. Changes in posture are also associated with a rise in background muscle tone and, if sustained over time, may be a prelude to fixed contractures.

During a movement at a joint, one or more muscles (known as agonists, and opposed by one or more antagonists) assist the primary muscle. With flexion at the elbow, for example, when biceps is the primary muscle, brachialis would be the agonist assisting biceps while the triceps would be the antagonist. Muscle afferents (neurons returning from the muscle) also make connections with motor neurons that innervate agonist and antagonist muscles. Excitatory synapses are found on neurons that bring about contraction in agonistic muscles facilitating the movement brought about by the primary muscle and this is known as reciprocal excitation. Reciprocal inhibition occurs when the muscle-spindle afferent neuron has an inhibitory influence on neurons that activate an antagonist muscle.

Apart from the spinal reflex discussed above, which is based on afferent input from the muscle spindle, there is another reflex in which the afferent input is from the skin. This flexion reflex is produced by a painful cutaneous stimulus. The flexor muscles are activated to produce a withdrawal while the extensor muscles are inhibited. In the case of a painful stimulus to the foot, the hamstring muscles of the affected leg contract while the quadriceps relaxes and the foot is lifted from the offending object. At the same time the reverse occurs in the opposite limb to maintain the upright posture.

The spinal cord also contains circuitry for certain intrinsic movement patterns (Pearson 1976, 2000). During walking and running a single limb passes through two phases: a stance phase, during which the body is supported and propelled forward, and a swing phase, during which the limb is advanced in order to repeat the propulsive part of the cycle. As the hindlimbs move faster the timing of stance phase is decreased. In cats, if the spinal cord is transected in the thoracic region, rhythmic movements can be elicited in the absence of corticospinal influence. If the animal is placed on a moving treadmill, the hindlimbs will begin moving with a characteristic walking pattern, which can be accelerated by increasing the speed of the treadmill. This indicates that there are central pattern generators in the spinal cord that control these basic motions (Grillner 1996).

Overview
Let us now put all these pieces together and follow the steps in the neural pathways that bring about a purposeful movement. Imagine that you are about to pick up a cup of coffee and take a sip. Subconsciously your brain will quickly assess such variables as the size of the cup, how full it is, and whether or not it has a handle. The size of the cup will determine how powerful the contraction will be. If it is very full, the lifting movement will have to be performed smoothly in order to avoid spillage. If the cup does not have a handle, the

outside temperature will influence how careful the initial contact will be. How far away is the cup and at what angle? Sight, smell, taste, temperature and weight assessment will be important to achieve your goal. All of these subconscious assessments of the nature of the task contribute to what is referred to as *anticipatory control*. Studies have shown that, for children with hemiplegia, use of the "unimpaired hand" provides information about anticipatory control to the damaged hemisphere and hence to the "impaired hand". To this extent, practice with the "good" hand contributes to improved use of the impaired hand (Gordon et al. 1999, Gordon and Duff 1999a, b).

The thoughts about drinking coffee occur in your frontal and parietal lobes, from where they are transferred to your supplementary motor area where the overall desire to pick up and drink from the cup is converted to a motor plan. The plan is refined in the premotor area in the frontal lobe, and finally the specific motor neurons in the primary motor area in the precentral gyrus are activated. During the preparation of this movement the basal ganglia are brought into the planning. They look at the intended goal and refer to memories of previous similar actions. They also take into account time and space factors like the position of your trunk and arm and the exact site of the cup; will you need to turn, and how much will your shoulder need to be braced? Once all this information has been computed, the motor cortex is informed of the most efficient movement pattern to achieve the goal. The cortical motor-control center initially sends an order to the brainstem motor nuclei (vestibular and reticular) to set up the appropriate background of posture and tone in the truncal and proximal limb muscles. This is done through the cortico-bulbospinal (extrapyramidal) tracts. The next step is to send instructions via the corticospinal (pyramidal) tracts to the spinal motor neurons (anterior horn cells). Simultaneously, this exact set of instructions is relayed to the cerebellum where the muscles' performance are carefully monitored. As soon as the muscles begin their contraction, information is sent back to the cerebellum where the ongoing movement is compared with what was intended. The error is calculated and a proposed correction is forwarded to the cortical motor-control centers. A revised command is now sent to the muscles via the upper and lower motor neurons. This constant shuttling of plans, commands, corrections and revised commands continues until the goal is achieved. Experience of movement produces movement engrams that are immediately adaptable to most environments. It is only when conscious correction of those movements is required that the motor task is poorly performed and looks clumsy.

REFERENCES

Brinkman C, Porter R. (1979) Supplementary motor area in the monkey: activity of neurons during performance of a learned motor task. *J Neurophysiol* **42:** 681–709.
Brinkman C, Porter R. (1983) Supplementary motor area and premotor area of monkey cerebral cortex: functional organization and activities of single neurons during performance of a learned movement. *Adv Neurol* **39:** 393–420.
Brodal A. (1981) *Neurological Anatomy in Relation to Clinical Medicine*, 3rd edn. Oxford: Oxford University Press. p 212, 294–297.
Deecke L, Scheid P, Kornhuber HH. (1969) Distribution of the readiness potential, pre-motion positivity, and motor potential inhuman cerebral cortex preceding voluntary finger movements. *Exp Brain Res* **7:** 158–168.

Fried IKA, McCarthy G, Sass KJ, Williamson P. (1991) Functional organization of human supplementary cortex studied by electrical stimulation. *J Neurosci* **11:** 3656–3666.

Gordon AM, Duff SV. (1999a) Fingertip forces during object manipulation in children with hemiplegic cerebral palsy. I: Anticipatory scaling. *Dev Med Child Neurol* **41:** 166–175.

Gordon AM, Duff SV. (1999b) Relation between clinical measures and fine manipulative control in children with hemiplegic cerebral palsy. *Dev Med Child Neurol* **41:** 586-591.

Gordon AM, Charles J, Duff SV. (1999) Fingertip forces during object manipulation in children with hemiplegic cerebral palsy. II: Bilateral coordination. *Dev Med Child Neurol* **41:** 176–185.

Grillner S. (1996) Neural networks for vertebrate locomotion. *Sci Am* **247:** 64–69.

Kornhuber HH, Deecke L. (1985) The starting function of the supplementary motor area. *Behav Brain Sci* **8:** 591–592.

Pearson K. (1976) The control of walking. *Scientific American* **235:** 72–86.

Pearson K. (2000) Motor systems. *Curr Opin Neurobiol* **10:** 649–654.

Porter R, Lemon R. (1993) *Corticospinal Function and Voluntary Movement*. Oxford: Clarendon Press. p 96–100, 289–290.

Roland P, Lassen N, Skinhof E. (1980) Supplementary motor area and other cortical areas in organization of voluntary movements in man. *J Neurophysiol* **43:** 118–136.

Schreiber H, Lang M, Lang W, Kornhuber A, Heise B, Keidel M, Deecke L, Kornhuber HH. (1983) Frontal hemispheric differences in the Bereitschaftspotential associated with writing and drawing. *Hum Neurobiol* **2:** 197–202..

2
MECHANISMS AND MANIFESTATIONS OF PRENATAL AND PERINATAL BRAIN INJURY

Adré J. du Plessis

Cerebral palsy is caused by a wide spectrum of developmental and acquired abnormalities of the immature brain. Until comparatively recently, the cause of cerebral palsy remained unknown in more than half of all cases (Hagberg et al. 1989a). In 1862, William Little associated cerebral palsy with "abnormal parturition" and "difficult labours" (Little 1862). Subsequent epidemiologic studies challenged the importance of intrapartum asphyxia in the overall prevalence of cerebral palsy (Nelson and Ellenberg 1986, Blair and Stanley 1988), and emphasized instead the role of antenatal factors. In these reports, perinatal factors such as intrapartum asphyxia were implicated in only 8%–30% (Blair and Stanley 1988, Hagberg et al. 1989a, 1996, 2001) of cases of cerebral palsy. However, even at these lower rates, the absolute number of children afflicted is high and the debilitating consequences are lifelong.

In recent years, major developments in basic neuroscience, medical care and neurodiagnostic technology have advanced our understanding of the mechanisms of early-life brain injury and their clinical manifestations. Sophisticated neuroimaging techniques such as magnetic resonance imaging (MRI), with its superb tissue resolution, have facilitated the accurate early-life diagnosis of the etiologies, mechanisms and timing of the cerebral abnormalities underlying cerebral palsy (Volpe 1992, Huppi and Barnes 1997, Inder et al. 1999a, b). Improved obstetric and neonatal care have influenced the rate, the etiologic spectrum and the clinical subtypes of cerebral palsy. In spite of, or perhaps because of, the decreased mortality of sick newborn infants, the overall incidence of cerebral palsy has remained unchanged or has even increased in recent decades (Hagberg et al. 1989a, b). This is particularly true of preterm infants whose risk of cerebral palsy is up to 30 times greater than that of full-term infants (Stanley 1992, Pharoah et al. 1996). The increased survival of infants born before full term has translated into an increase in the clinical subtypes of cerebral palsy more commonly seen in ex-preterm infants, e.g. spastic diplegia (Dale and Stanley 1980, Volpe 1994).

Experimental neuroscience has elucidated many of the fundamental mechanisms of perinatal and neonatal brain injury, and in so doing has stimulated the development of experimental agents that prevent or arrest brain injury in animal models. These developments have fueled expectations for future effective neuroprotection in the human newborn at-risk for cerebral palsy. Thus the importance of intrapartum and neonatal causes of cerebral

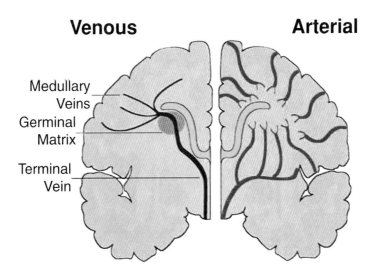

Venous   **Arterial**

Medullary
Veins
Germinal
Matrix

Terminal
Vein

Fig. 2.1. Diagrammatic representation of the cerebral venous and arterial circulation in preterm infants.

palsy goes far beyond medicolegal culpability, and lies in the exciting possibility that some of these injuries may be preventable in future.

For all of the above reasons, the current chapter will focus on the mechanisms and manifestations of brain injury in preterm and term infants acquired during the perinatal and early neonatal periods.

Mechanisms of brain injury associated with cerebral palsy

Cerebrovascular injury is the leading cause of acquired brain injury in both the preterm and term newborn infant. Although there is overlap in the brain lesions affecting infants at these two ends of the gestational spectrum, they are sufficiently different to warrant separate discussion.

Brain injury in the preterm infant

The intrinsic vulnerability of the preterm brain to ischemic and hemorrhagic injury is related to both the anatomic-structural and functional immaturity of the cerebral vessels.

VULNERABILITY OF THE PRETERM CEREBRAL VASCULATURE

The *anatomic underdevelopment* of the cerebral arterial and venous systems of the preterm infant is illustrated in Figure 2.1. Between mid-gestation and term, arterial branches of the surface vessels penetrate the cerebral wall and grow toward the ventricles. Since the extent of arterial growth into the white matter is proportional to the gestational age, the periventricular white matter of the preterm infant lies in an end-zone relatively deficient in arterial supply. Immature vessels may be extremely thin in certain regions (e.g. the involuting germinal matrix) and are easily ruptured. Consequently, germinal matrix hemorrhage (GMH, previously called grade I intraventricular hemorrhage) is common in the preterm infant. Since this structure

16

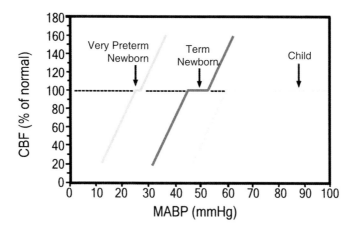

Fig. 2.2. Pressure-flow autoregulation at different ages. Compared with term infants and adults, the autoregulatory plateau in the preterm infant is narrow and shifted to the left. Normal blood pressure (arrows) in preterm infants approaches the lower limit of the autoregulatory plateau.

is situated adjacent to the lateral ventricles, extension of the hemorrhage through the ependymal lining results in *intraventricular hemorrhage* (IVH). Two grades of GMH–IVH are distinguished depending on whether the intraventricular *blood* (not CSF) causes distention of the ventricle (grade III) or not (grade II). The terminal vein is a major venous conduit draining large areas of the cerebral hemisphere. This vessel courses along the lateral margin of the lateral ventricle and through the germinal matrix, an anatomic relationship that predisposes to obstruction of venous drainage. When the terminal vein is compressed by hemorrhagic distention of the germinal matrix or lateral ventricle, widespread venous ischemia may develop in the cerebral hemisphere.

The *physiologic immaturity* of the cerebral vasculature in preterm infants manifests as defective intrinsic regulation of cerebral bloodflow, with the tenuous pressure-flow autoregulation being particularly important. In the mature brain, pressure-flow autoregulation maintains steady cerebral bloodflow over a wide range of blood pressure changes, i.e. the autoregulatory plateau (Fig. 2.2). In the preterm infant the autoregulatory plateau is narrow and shifted to the left. Furthermore, the normal blood pressure in preterm infants may be perilously close to the lower limit of this autoregulatory plateau. Finally, the already narrow autoregulatory plateau is particularly vulnerable to insults such as hypoxia–ischemia, which render the cerebral vasculature "pressure-passive". In this condition, fluctuations in systemic blood pressure are transmitted directly into the immature cerebral microvasculature.

VULNERABILITY OF THE IMMATURE OLIGODENDROCYTE
Superimposed on this vascular predisposition to injury is a developmental vulnerability of the immature oligodendrocyte (Back et al. 1998, 2001, Kadhim et al. 2001). The ultimate responsibility of the oligodendrocyte lineage is myelination of the developing central nervous system. During the critical period of high risk for injury to the immature white matter (i.e. 24–32 gestational weeks), the developing oligodendrocyte is particularly vulnerable

to oxidative stress (Oka et al. 1993, Yonezawa et al. 1996). This vulnerability is in part due to a mismatch between development of critical anti-oxidant enzymes (e.g. catalase, superoxide dismutase and glutathione peroxidase) and development of pro-oxidant pathways (e.g. accumulation of iron for oligodendrocyte differentiation) (Ozawa et al. 1994, Iida et al. 1995, Back and Volpe 1997). The propensity of the immature white matter to hypoxia–ischemia during this phase of development provides a potent trigger for the generation of particularly noxious free radicals. Although most oligodendrocytes are in a premyelination phase of development between 24 and 32 weeks of gestation, injury at this stage will disrupt subsequent myelination and result in abnormal and incomplete white-matter development.

CEREBRAL INSULTS IN THE PRETERM INFANT
In the sick preterm infant, instability of the immature cardiorespiratory system is common, causing fluctuations in systemic blood pressure and circulating oxygenation. Even minor routine handling of these infants (e.g. a diaper change or positioning for X-ray studies) may precipitate sharp fluctuations in blood pressure. If the cerebral circulation is pressure-passive, increases in pressure may rupture small vessels, the most fragile of which are in the germinal matrix. Conversely, fluctuations in perfusion pressure may cause repeated ischemia in the arterial end-zones of the periventricular white matter. The immature oligodendrocytes in these areas may be poorly equipped to deal with the free radicals generated by such ischemia-reperfusion events. Taken together, these features of the immature systemic and cerebral vasculature and the immature cerebral parenchyma underlie the occurrence and topography of brain injury in the preterm infant.

CEREBRAL INJURY IN THE PRETERM INFANT
1. Primary arterial ischemic injury to the white matter (periventricular leukomalacia)
During hypotensive episodes, hypoxic–ischemic insults in the arterial end-zones may cause the classic lesion of immature white matter, i.e. periventricular leukomalacia (PVL). The pathology of this lesion is infarction with necrosis of all cell types and of axonal pathways coursing adjacent to the ventricles in these regions. These foci of infarction are usually bilateral and situated dorsolateral to the external angle of the lateral ventricle (Banker and Larroche 1962). The two most common locations for PVL (Fig. 2.3) along the length of the ventricle are (1) the peritrigonal area of the parietal white matter, and (2) the white matter adjacent to the frontal horns. These two foci have different clinical manifestations (see below) but in severe cases may occur together. If large enough, the ultrasound features of PVL evolve through a focal echodense phase and a later cystic phase. Surrounding the areas of focal infarction, more diffuse and relatively selective oligodendrocyte loss occurs. This selective oligodendrocyte injury may occur without the focal infarction, in which case the long-term picture at autopsy shows diffuse hypomyelination, while the long-term imaging findings show an "ex vacuo" form of ventriculomegaly.

2. Parenchymal complications of intraventricular hemorrhage
Periventricular hemorrhagic infarction develops when GMH–IVH impairs drainage through the terminal vein, causing venous stasis and ischemia through large areas of the hemisphere.

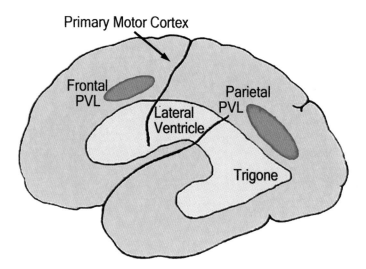

Fig. 2.3. Common locations for PVL in the parietal and frontal white matter of the preterm infant. Lesions in these locations have different clinical sequelae described in the text. In severe cases these lesions become confluent along the periventricular white matter. By brain ultrasound these lesions evolve through an initial echodense phase and a later cystic phase.

Characteristic of venous ischemia, this lesion typically undergoes hemorrhagic transformation. Cerebral perfusion studies (Volpe et al. 1983) suggest that the area of ischemia may be far more extensive than the lesion shown using ultrasound. Periventricular hemorrhagic infarction tends to be unilateral or obviously asymmetric, which influences the clinical manifestations of this lesion.

Posthemorrhagic hydrocephalus is another major complication of IVH that results when extravasated blood obstructs the cerebrospinal fluid pathways. The onset of posthemorrhagic hydrocephalus is usually after one or more weeks of life, with later-onset ventricular distention likely to be mediated by an inflammatory arachnoid response in the posterior fossa. With progressive ventricular distention, there is distortion and compression of periventricular white-matter structures (Quinn et al. 1992, Guzzetta et al. 1995, Del Bigio and Kanfer 1996, Del Bigio et al. 1997). In addition to injuring axonal tracts coursing alongside the distending ventricles, compression of the immature arterial and venous structures (see above) may cause ischemic injury to the white matter (Shirane et al. 1992, Chumas et al. 1994, Da Silva et al. 1994, 1995).

3. Inflammatory cytokines and injury to the immature brain
Although this discussion is focused almost exclusively on the cerebrovascular mechanisms of brain injury in the newborn, recent data suggesting a role for pro-inflammatory substances warrant brief review. In recent years a number of epidemiologic (Alexander et al. 1998, Nelson et al. 1998, Grether et al. 1999) and animal studies (Yoon et al. 1996, 1997, 2000, Cai et al. 2000) have demonstrated an association between maternal, fetal and neonatal

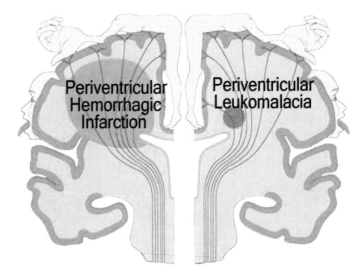

Fig. 2.4. Location of common brain lesions in the preterm infant and their motor sequelae. Diagram of cerebral hemispheres (coronal view) with superimposed homunculus to demonstrate the cortical origin and white-matter pathways of motor fibers to the face, trunk and extremities. PVL in the frontal regions (shown on the right, but typically bilateral) involves pathways to the lower extremities and results in the typical clinical picture of spastic diplegia. PVHI (shown on the left and usually unilateral) affects pathways to the arms, legs and even the face, producing the typical form of hemiparesis seen in surviving preterm infants (contrast with arterial stroke in term infants, Fig. 2.6).

infection (Yoon et al. 1996, 1997, 2000, Dammann and Leviton 1997, Baud et al. 1999) and injury (Martinez et al. 1998) to the immature brain. One postulated mechanism of injury is the toxic effect of inflammatory cytokines on the immature oligodendrocyte (Selmaj and Raine 1988). However, circulating cytokines may also have important effects on the systemic and cerebral circulations that predispose to cerebral ischemia. Furthermore, cerebral ischemia may trigger the release of cytokines from certain cell types as part of the cascade of injury. In summary, the precise relationship or causal pathway(s) (Stanley et al. 2000) between infection, cytokines, ischemia and brain injury in the newborn is extremely complex, and its understanding awaits further study.

CLINICAL–PATHOLOGIC CORRELATION OF BRAIN INJURY IN THE PRETERM INFANT
The relationship between the topography of the various brain lesions in the preterm infant and their long-term clinical sequelae is depicted in Figures 2.4 and 2.5. The superimposed homunculus cartoon in Figure 2.4 shows the cortical origin and white-matter pathways of motor fibers to the face, trunk and extremities. Periventricular leukomalacia is typically bilateral and occurs most frequently toward the posterior aspects of the ventricles in the peritrigonal white matter, as well as in the white matter adjacent to the frontal horns of the lateral ventricles (Figs 2.3, 2.4). In severe cases these regions of injury may be confluent. Since the axons conducting input to the lower extremities course through the frontal regions, injury in this location produces the typical clinical picture of spastic diplegia, in which the

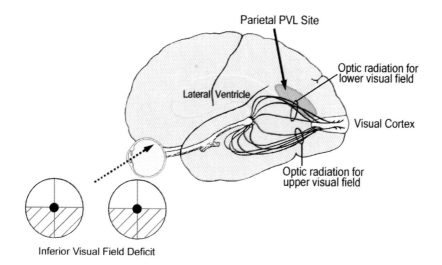

Parietal PVL Site

Optic radiation for
lower visual field

Lateral Ventricle

Visual Cortex

Optic radiation for
upper visual field

Inferior Visual Field Deficit

Fig. 2.5. Visual-field deficits in the preterm infant. Diagram of cerebral hemispheres (sagittal view) showing the course of the optic radiations for the lower visual field through the white matter superolateral to the occipital horns of the lateral ventricles. As shown in Figure 2.3, this is a high-risk region for PVL, which may result in lower visual-field deficits.

most prominent motor impairment is in the legs, but may also involve the trunk, arms, and face to a lesser extent. Periventricular leukomalacia, confined to the parietal white matter, is associated with cognitive and visual deficits (described below) but tends to cause less severe motor dysfunction. *Periventricular hemorrhagic infarction* (PVHI) is usually unilateral but may involve extensive areas of the hemisphere. This lesion has a poor prognosis, being associated in the long term with a 90% prevalence of neurodevelopmental impairment that is often severe. The diffuse lesion of periventricular hemorrhagic infarction affects fibers supplying the upper and lower extremities, and possibly also the face. This topography of injury underlies the typical picture of preterm infants who survive periventricular hemorrhagic infarction, i.e. *hemiparesis* involving the upper and lower extremity more or less equally. The clinical picture of hemiparesis in ex-preterm infants differs from that in (usually term) infants with middle cerebral artery stroke (see below). *Post-hemorrhagic hydrocephalus* manifests as progressive ventricular distention that may distort or compress the adjacent axonal tracts directly, or cause regional periventricular ischemia and secondary injury to these pathways. Similar to the primary arterial ischemic lesion of periventricular leukomalacia, this lesion tends to affect pathways to the lower extremities earlier and more severely, although in advanced cases the arms and face may also be affected.

The clinical correlates of these different lesions in the preterm brain have been discussed separately. However, the clinical picture is often difficult to ascribe to one mechanism alone, and in these cases more than one lesion type is likely to be present. For example, coexisting PVL (usually bilateral) and periventricular hemorrhagic infarction (usually unilateral) will result in combined hemiparesis and spastic diplegia, a picture sometimes called *spastic triplegia*.

21

A number of other, *non-motor manifestations* of brain injury in preterm infants may indirectly impact motor function and management strategies. Cognitive and learning deficits become evident in 25%–50% of ex-preterm infants after school entry (Msall et al. 1991, McCormick et al. 1993, Robertson et al. 1994, Botting et al. 1998, Saigal et al. 2000). Not surprisingly, these deficits are more prevalent among children who suffer severe bilateral lesions, in which case there is also marked motor impairment of the upper extremities. These cognitive and learning deficits may be related to injury of the visual and auditory association pathways in the parietal white matter. As discussed above, these areas are particularly prone to injury in periventricular leukomalacia and posthemorrhagic hydrocephalus. In addition, these intellectual deficits as well as later epilepsy may also reflect disturbances in later cortical development following earlier white matter injury (Volpe 1996, Inder et al. 1999c). Fortunately, later epilepsy in this population is uncommon (Amess et al. 1998) and in general relatively easily controlled (Kwong et al. 1998).

Visual deficits in survivors of preterm birth may result from a variety of causes (e.g. so-called "retinopathy of prematurity"). Here we consider cerebral visual dysfunction due to injury in the posterior visual pathways (Cioni et al. 1996, Jacobson et al. 1996), specifically the optic radiations. As shown in Figure 2.5, the optic radiations for the lower visual field course through the peritrigonal white matter around the superolateral aspects of the occipital horns of the lateral ventricles. As discussed above, this is a particularly high-risk area for PVL, and injury in these regions may thus result in cerebral visual dysfunction, particularly in the lower visual fields. Since spastic diplegia is the most common motor abnormality in preterm infants with PVL, such inferior field defects may compound the already compromised gait. Since the motor dysfunction usually dominates the clinical picture, cerebral visual impairment may go unrecognized unless specific testing is performed. Visual function in the preterm infant differs from that in term infants, as discussed below.

Brain injury in the term infant
VULNERABILITY TO BRAIN INJURY IN THE TERM INFANT
The cerebrovascular system
By term gestation, the *anatomic maturation* of the cerebrovascular system approximates that of the adult. In the term infant with systemic hypotension, the brain regions most vulnerable to ischemia are those situated in the watershed areas of the three main cerebral artery (anterior, middle and posterior) territories. The most prominent watershed areas (Fig. 2.6) are in the parasagittal cortex and subcortical white matter along the superior convexity of the cerebral hemispheres. Parasagittal cerebral injury is usually bilateral and most intense in the parieto-occipital regions, i.e. an end-zone for all three major cerebral arteries.

At term the *functional maturation* of the cerebral vasculature has advanced the efficacy and robustness of cerebral pressure-flow autoregulation. Compared to the tenuous plateau of the preterm infant, the autoregulatory plateau is wider and shifted rightward. However, although autoregulatory function has improved in the term infant, the cerebral vasculature may still be rendered pressure-passive by even moderate hypoxic–ischemic insults. In the asphyxiated term infant, the loss of autoregulatory function in combination with compromised myocardial function predisposes to cerebral injury (see below).

Vulnerability of the developing neuron

By term gestation, the oligodendrocyte lineage has passed through its most vulnerable developmental phases. In the term infant, the most intense cellular and regional maturation events in the brain involve the developing neuron. Synaptogenesis and organizational events are occurring most rapidly in specific regions of cortex, deep gray matter and brainstem (see below). The rapid developmental activity in these areas is highly demanding of constant glucose and oxygen supply; if this supply becomes inadequate, the developmental demands render these regions particularly susceptible to ischemic insults. At a cellular level, a critical feature of neuronal vulnerability in these rapidly developing regions is the high density of neuronal glutamate receptors, particularly NMDA receptors (Johnston 1995). When activated by glutamate, these NMDA ionophores allow calcium influx into the cytoplasm for the activation of enzymes critical for neuronal development. Activity of these NMDA receptors is highly regulated and very dependent on consistent energy supply. During cerebral hypoxia–ischemia, control of calcium influx through these receptors is lost, allowing sustained calcium influx to toxic levels in the neuronal cytoplasm. In so doing, cerebral hypoxia–ischemia transforms glutamate receptors from important mediators of normal brain development into potentially lethal mediators of neuronal cytotoxicity. During hypoxia–ischemia, this form of neuronal toxicity is maximally expressed in areas of greatest glutamate-receptor density, i.e. the basal ganglia (especially the caudate and putamen), thalamus, brainstem nuclei, and specific areas of cerebral cortex (e.g. hippocampus, sensorimotor cortex). To summarize, it is the confluence of the above vascular, cellular and regional factors that determine the severity and distribution of cerebral injury in the term infant.

CEREBRAL INSULTS IN THE TERM INFANT

The principal cerebrovascular lesions in the term infant result from global hypoxia-hypoperfusion insults to the entire brain (e.g. perinatal asphyxia) and focal infarction following embolic occlusion of a cerebral artery.

Global cerebral hypoxic–ischemic insults

During the development of intrauterine asphyxia, the impaired oxygen and glucose supply triggers certain compensatory hemodynamic responses in the systemic and cerebral circulations of the fetus. These responses are aimed at so-called "brain sparing". Specifically, these adaptive mechanisms redirect fetal blood supply to the brain at the expense of organs such as the kidney, liver, and heart. Within the brain, blood supply is redirected toward the most actively developing areas, which at term include the basal ganglia-thalamus, brainstem and sensorimotor cortex. Decompensation of these adaptive mechanisms can occur in two broad ways, each with its characteristic topography of injury. If the impairment in fetal oxygenation is brief, these adaptive responses may effectively preserve cerebral integrity with little detriment to other organs. However, when the insult is either too prolonged or too severe, these intrinsic attempts at brain protection fail. With prolonged but incomplete asphyxia, end-organ damage develops in the liver, kidney and heart, while in the brain the areas most affected are the watershed areas of the parasagittal cortex (Fig. 2.6) and white

23

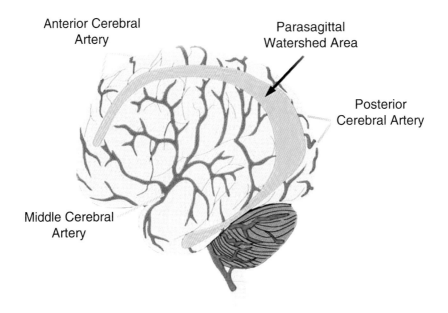

Fig. 2.6. Diagram of cerebral hemisphere (sagittal view) showing watershed areas between the supply territories of the anterior, middle and posterior cerebral arteries.

matter. Conversely, when asphyxia is severe (e.g. with placental abruption, maternal cardiac arrest or uterine rupture) but rapidly reversed, the hemodynamic compensatory mechanisms fail from the outset. In these situations, the severe disruption of cerebral oxygen and substrate supply results in injury that is most marked in regions with the greatest metabolic demand, i.e. the basal ganglia-thalamus, brainstem (see Fig. 2.7, left side) and the primary sensorimotor cortex. With rapid delivery and effective resuscitation, these infants may show minimal injury to other end organs and other less demanding brain regions.

Arterio-occlusive stroke in the term newborn infant
Cerebral infarction, or stroke, due to embolic occlusion of one or more cerebral arteries is another important cause of cerebral palsy that originates in most cases during the perinatal or early neonatal period, (see Fig. 2.7, right side). A definite etiology is seldom identified, and the assumption is that emboli generated by involuting placental or fetal vessels enter the cerebral circulation through fetal vascular pathways such as the foramen ovale and ductus arteriosus, prior to their closure in early life. Rarely, a hypercoagulable state or congenital heart defect is identified. Focal strokes may also complicate perinatal asphyxia and occur in twin-to-twin transfusion syndromes.

Clinical–pathologic correlation of brain injury in the term infant
For the purposes of this discussion, the long-term clinical correlates will be considered in the context of the distinct mechanisms and topographies of injury outlined above.

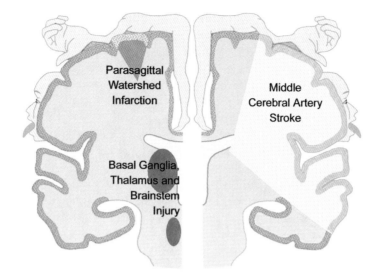

Fig. 2.7. Location of brain lesions in the term infant and their motor sequelae. Diagram of cerebral hemispheres (coronal view) with superimposed homunculus to demonstrate the cortical origin of motor fibers to the face, trunk and extremities. The left side of the figure shows parasagittal watershed infarction and regions of selective neuronal necrosis. The right side of the figure shows the distribution of injury in the most common vaso-occlusive lesion, i.e. middle cerebral artery stroke

Parasagittal cerebral injury resulting from watershed ischemia between the anterior and middle cerebral arteries affects the motor cortex, particularly regions innervating the upper extremities (especially proximal muscles) and trunk (Figs 2.6, 2.7, left side), usually with lesser involvement of areas representing the pelvic girdle and leg muscles. This topography of injury results in a characteristic type of spastic quadriparesis involving the arms more than the legs, i.e. the reverse of spastic diparesis in the preterm infant (see above). The *gradient* of weakness (i.e. arm more than leg), which resembles that in hemiplegia following middle cerebral artery stroke, has led to the use of the term "bilateral hemiplegia", which is a confusing and inappropriate way of referring to the motor deficits after parasagittal injury. Because the parasagittal watershed area is particularly broad in the important association areas of the parietal cortex, cognitive/intellectual deficits are common after this form of injury, as are distinct learning disabilities (Yokochi 1998). Visual function following parasagittal cerebral injury in infants is not well described. However, in adults watershed injury in this area causes visual neglect, disordered tracking and difficulties interpreting complex diagrams (Balint's syndrome). Because of the cortical involvement, epilepsy is particularly common following this form of brain injury.

Basal ganglia-thalamic injury (Fig. 2.7, left side) typically occurs during severe but brief insults (see above). Following more severe insults, injury may extend to include the tegmental brainstem nuclei. The typical long-term clinical picture is one of fluctuating but predominantly rigid muscle tone, with varying degrees of underlying spasticity. Superimposed

25

on this fluctuating tone are different types of involuntary movements, presumably reflecting the predominant basal ganglia nuclei injured in each case (Rutherford et al. 1992). For reasons that are poorly understood, increasing rigidity and dyskinetic features may emerge after years of predominant spasticity (Burke et al. 1980, Saint Hilaire et al. 1991). This form of injury is associated with prominent oromotor dysfunction especially if brainstem nuclei are also involved. As a consequence, speech is often markedly dysarthric and the common feeding difficulties often require gastrostomy tube placement (Roland et al. 1988, Pasternak et al. 1991). Cognitive function in these children spans a wide range but many appear to have cognitive function that is *relatively* preserved (Kyllerman et al. 1982, Rosenbloom 1994), compared to the motor dysfunction. Specific learning disabilities may occur (Lou et al. 1989). In cases with cognitive impairment, these deficits may be due to thalamic injury. Another cause of extrapyramidal cerebral palsy results from the acute bilirubin toxicity (or kernicterus) in severe neonatal jaundice (Connolly and Volpe 1990). After decades of steady decline in the incidence of this condition, kernicterus appears to be resurfacing (Ebbesen 2000). In this condition neuronal injury is widespread but is particularly prominent in the basal ganglia, brainstem and cerebellum (Ahdab-Barmada and Moossy 1984, Connolly and Volpe 1990). The long-term features of chronic bilirubin encephalopathy include often severe retrocollis and opisthotonus, athetosis, and gaze abnormalities (Connolly and Volpe 1990). The athetosis in this condition often fluctuates (Hayashi et al. 1991), and may be triggered by attempted skilled movements. In addition, neuronal injury in the cochlear nuclei and auditory nerve result in high-frequency hearing-loss (Byers et al. 1955). More than half of affected children have cognitive function in the normal range (Byers et al. 1955).

Focal arterio-occlusive injury or stroke has long-term sequelae that are influenced by the particular arterial territory involved. The acute presentation of the vast majority of strokes is with focal neonatal seizures in the first days of life (Clancy et al. 1985, Levy et al. 1985), while motor deficits may remain relatively subtle over the first 6 months or more. In fact, imaging studies suggest that hemiparesis may develop in only one-quarter of infants with unilateral strokes (Bouza et al. 1994a, b, Dall'Oglio et al. 1994, de Vries et al. 1997, Estan and Hope 1997, Rutherford et al. 1998, Mercuri et al. 1999). Since strokes most commonly involve the left middle cerebral artery, right hemiparesis is more common (Volpe 2001). Unlike the hemiparesis that follows PVHI in the preterm infant, hemiparesis in the term infant tends to affect the arm and face more than the leg (Fig. 2.7, right side); unlike the upper-extremity weakness in parasagittal injury which is predominantly proximal, in focal stroke the distal upper extremities are more impaired. Hemiparesis is virtually assured when occlusion of the proximal middle cerebral artery segment causes injury of the entire territory including the basal ganglia, white matter, posterior limb of the internal capsule and cortex (de Vries et al. 1997). Conversely, when injury is confined to the proximal penetrating branches or more distal branches, functionally significant hemiparesis is rare (de Vries et al. 1997). Even when motor deficits become manifest, their functional severity is often less than would be expected for the volume of cerebral injury on imaging studies. This has been ascribed to the incompletely understood phenomenon of "plasticity" in the immature brain (Stiles 2000). Cognitive function in neonatal stroke survivors is normal in

50%, and 18% have an IQ of more than 100 (Fennell and Dikel 2001). Lesions of either hemisphere may impair non-verbal function, often with dissociation of verbal and performance IQs. Children with a left-hemisphere lesion are at greater risk for impairment of syntactic awareness and sentence repetition, while receptive vocabulary appears to be intact. Conversely, right-hemisphere lesions are associated with decreased mathematical ability, possibly due to the associated visuospatial dysfunction (Fennell and Dikel 2001). Later epilepsy has been reported in 10%–60% of children after unilateral neonatal strokes (Sran and Baumann 1988, Wulfeck et al. 1991, Koelfen et al. 1995, Sreenan et al. 2000). The presence of epilepsy may be a more powerful predictor of impaired cognitive function than the laterality of the lesion.

Visual dysfunction in unilateral lesions, e.g. PVHI and unilateral stroke, may cause contralateral homonymous hemianopia, which impair the child's ability to appreciate both learning material and obstacles in the affected field. Fortunately, this complication appears to be relatively rare (Black 1980, 1982).

Summary

The mechanisms and manifestations of brain injury leading to cerebral palsy have been presented as discrete entities for the purposes of this discussion. More often than not, however, varying degrees of more than one mechanism may be operative in a causal pathway (Stanley et al. 2000). Likewise, the long-term manifestations of injury to the immature brain may reflect the combined effects of more than one lesion. Furthermore, although the ultimate manifestations of each injury type are generally those discussed above, it is important to note that although the injury underlying cerebral palsy is static, the manifestations may evolve over time. For example, infants who ultimately develop spastic diplegia may initially evolve through phases of hypotonia and dystonia (Bax 1992). Likewise, infants destined for an extrapyramidal form of cerebral palsy may initially evolve through hypotonic or spastic phases before manifesting extrapyramidal features as late as the second decade of life (Burke et al. 1980, Saint Hilaire et al. 1991). The reasons for this changing clinical picture after a static insult remain poorly understood but raise intriguing questions about the interaction between brain injury and development, and potential avenues for future intervention.

REFERENCES

Ahdab-Barmada M, Moossy J. (1984) The neuropathology of kernicterus in the premature neonate: diagnostic problems. *J Neuropathol Exp Neurol* **43:** 45–56.
Alexander JM, Gilstrap LC, Cox SM, McIntire DM, Leveno KJ. (1998) Clinical chorioamnionitis and the prognosis for very low birth weight infants. *Obstet Gynecol* **91:** 725–729.
Amess PN, Baudin J, Townsend J, Meek J, Roth SC, Neville BG, Wyatt JS, Stewart A. (1998) Epilepsy in very preterm infants: neonatal cranial ultrasound reveals a high-risk subcategory. *Dev Med Child Neurol* **40:** 724–730.
Back S, Volpe J. (1997) Cellular and molecular pathogenesis of periventricular white matter injury. *Ment Retard Dev Disabil Res Rev* **3:** 96–107.
Back SA, Gan X, Li Y, Rosenberg PA, Volpe JJ. (1998) Maturation-dependent vulnerability of oligodendrocytes to oxidative stress-induced death caused by glutathione depletion. *J Neurosci* **18:** 6241–6253.
Back SA, Luo NL, Borenstein NS, Levine JM, Volpe JJ, Kinney HC. (2001) Late oligodendrocyte progenitors

coincide with the developmental window of vulnerability for human perinatal white matter injury. *J Neurosci* **21:** 1302–1312.

Banker B, Larroche J. (1962) Periventricular leukomalacia in infancy. *Arch Neurol* **7:** 386–410.

Baud O, Emilie D, Pelletier E, Lacaze-Masmonteil T, Zupan V, Fernandez H, Dehan M, Frydman R, Ville Y. (1999) Amniotic fluid concentrations of interleukin-1beta, interleukin-6 and TNF-alpha in chorioamnionitis before 32 weeks of gestation: histological associations and neonatal outcome. *Br J Obstet Gynaecol* **106:** 72–77.

Bax M. (1992) Cerebral palsy. In: Aicardi J, editor. *Diseases of the Nervous System in Childhood,* vol. 115–118. London: Mac Keith Press. p 330–374.

Black PD. (1980) Ocular defects in children with cerebral palsy. *Br Med J* **281:** 487–488.

Black P. (1982) Visual disorders associated with cerebral palsy. *Br J Ophthalmol* **66:** 46– 52.

Blair E, Stanley FJ. (1988) Intrapartum asphyxia: a rare cause of cerebral palsy. *J Pediatr* **112:** 515–519.

Botting N, Powls A, Cooke RW, Marlow N. (1998) Cognitive and educational outcome of very-low-birthweight children in early adolescence. *Dev Med Child Neurol* **40:** 652–660.

Bouza H, Dubowitz LM, Rutherford M, Pennock JM. (1994a) Prediction of outcome in children with congenital hemiplegia: a magnetic resonance imaging study. *Neuropediatrics* **25:** 60–66.

Bouza H, Rutherford M, Acolet D, Pennock JM, Dubowitz LM. (1994b) Evolution of early hemiplegic signs in full-term infants with unilateral brain lesions in the neonatal period: a prospective study. *Neuropediatrics* **25:** 201–207.

Burke RE, Fahn S, Gold AP. (1980) Delayed-onset dystonia in patients with "static" encephalopathy. *J Neurol Neurosurg Psychiatry* **43:** 789–797.

Byers R, Payne R, Crothers B. (1955) Extrapyramidal cerebral palsy with hearing loss following erythroblastosis. *Pediatrics* **15:** 248.

Cai Z, Pan ZL, Pang Y, Evans OB, Rhodes PG. (2000) Cytokine induction in fetal rat brains and brain injury in neonatal rats after maternal lipopolysaccharide administration. *Pediatr Res* **47:** 64–72.

Chumas P, Drake J, Del Bigio M, da Silva M, Tuor U. (1994) Anaerobic glycolysis preceding white-matter destruction in experimental neonatal hydrocephalus. *J Neurosurg* **80:** 491–501.

Cioni G, Fazzi B, Ipata AE, Canapicchi R, van Hof-van Duin J. (1996) Correlation between cerebral visual impairment and magnetic resonance imaging in children with neonatal encephalopathy. *Dev Med Child Neurol* **38:** 120–132.

Clancy R, Malin S, Laraque D, Baumgart S, Younkin D. (1985) Focal motor seizures heralding stroke in full-term neonates. *Am J Dis Child* **139:** 601–606.

Connolly AM, Volpe JJ. (1990) Clinical features of bilirubin encephalopathy. *Clin Perinatol* **17:** 371–379.

Dale A, Stanley FJ. (1980) An epidemiological study of cerebral palsy in Western Australia, 1956-1975. II: Spastic cerebral palsy and perinatal factors. *Dev Med Child Neurol* **22:** 13–25.

Dall'Oglio AM, Bates E, Volterra V, Di Capua M, Pezzini G. (1994) Early cognition, communication and language in children with focal brain injury. *Dev Med Child Neurol* **36:** 1076–1098.

Dammann O, Leviton A. (1997) Maternal intrauterine infection, cytokines, and brain damage in the preterm newborn. *Pediatr Neurol* **42:** 1–8.

Da Silva MC, Drake JM, Lemaire C, Cross A, Tuor UI. (1994) High-energy phosphate metabolism in a neonatal model of hydrocephalus before and after shunting. *J Neurosurg* **81:** 544–553.

Da Silva MC, Michowicz S, Drake JM, Chumas PD, Tuor UI. (1995) Reduced local cerebral blood flow in periventricular white matter in experimental neonatal hydrocephalus: restoration with CSF shunting. *J Cereb Blood Flow Metab* **15:** 1057–1065.

Del Bigio MR, Kanfer JN. (1996) Oligodendrocyte-related enzymes in hydrocephalic rat brains. *Soc Neurosci* **22:** 482.

Del Bigio MR, Kanfer JN, Zhang YW. (1997) Myelination delay in the cerebral white matter of immature rats with kaolin-induced hydrocephalus is reversible. *J Neuropathol Exp Neurol* **56:** 1053–1066.

de Vries LS, Groenendaal F, Eken P, van Haastert IC, Rademaker KJ, Meiners LC. (1997) Infarcts in the vascular distribution of the middle cerebral artery in preterm and fullterm infants. *Neuropediatrics* **28:** 88–96.

Ebbesen F. (2000) Recurrence of kernicterus in term and near-term infants in Denmark. *Acta Paediatr* **89:** 1213–1217.

Estan J, Hope P. (1997) Unilateral neonatal cerebral infarction in full term infants. *Arch Dis Child Fetal Neonatal Ed* **76:** F88–93.

Fennell EB, Dikel TN. (2001) Cognitive and neuropsychological functioning in children with cerebral palsy.

J Child Neurol **16:** 58–63.

Grether JK, Nelson KB, Dambrosia JM, Phillips TM. (1999) Interferons and cerebral palsy. *J Pediatr* **134:** 324–332.

Guzzetta F, Mercuri E, Spano M. (1995) Mechanisms and evolution of the brain damage in neonatal post-hemorrhagic hydrocephalus. *Childs Nerv Syst* **11:** 293–296.

Hagberg B, Hagberg G, Olow I, von Wendt L. (1989a) The changing panorama of cerebral palsy in Sweden. V. The birth year period 1979-82. *Acta Paediatr Scand* **78:** 283–290.

Hagberg B, Hagberg G, Zetterstrom R. (1989b) Decreasing perinatal mortality—increase in cerebral palsy morbidity. *Acta Paediatr Scand* **78:** 664–670.

Hagberg B, Hagberg G, Olow I, van Wendt L. (1996) The changing panorama of cerebral palsy in Sweden. VII. Prevalence and origin in the birth year period 1987-90. *Acta Paediatr* **85:** 954–960.

Hagberg B, Hagberg G, Beckung E, Uvebrant P. (2001) Changing panorama of cerebral palsy in Sweden. VIII. Prevalence and origin in the birth year period 1991–94. *Acta Paediatr* **90:** 271–277.

Hayashi M, Satoh J, Sakamoto K, Morimatsu Y. (1991) Clinical and neuropathological findings in severe athetoid cerebral palsy: a comparative study of globo-luysian and thalamo-putaminal groups. *Brain Dev* **13:** 47–51.

Huppi PS, Barnes PD. (1997) Magnetic resonance techniques in the evaluation of the newborn brain. *Clin Perinatol* **24:** 693–723.

Iida K, Takashima S, Ueda K. (1995) Immunohistochemical study of myelination and oligodendrocyte in infants with periventricular leukomalacia. *Pediatr Neurol* **13:** 296–304.

Inder T, Huppi PS, Zientara GP, Maier SE, Jolesz FA, di Salvo D, Robertson R, Barnes PD, Volpe JJ. (1999a) Early detection of periventricular leukomalacia by diffusion-weighted magnetic resonance imaging techniques. *J Pediatr* **134:** 631–634.

Inder TE, Huppi PS, Warfield S, Kikinis R, Zientara GP, Barnes PD, Jolesz F, Volpe JJ. (1999b) Periventricular white matter injury in the premature infant is followed by reduced cerebral cortical gray matter volume at term. *Ann Neurol* **46:** 755–760.

Inder TE, Huppi PS, Zientara GP, Jolesz FA, Holling EE, Robertson R, Barnes PD, Volpe JJ. (1999c) The postmigrational development of polymicrogyria documented by magnetic resonance imaging from 31 weeks' postconceptional age. *Ann Neurol* **45:** 798–801.

Jacobson L, Ek U, Fernell E, Flodmark O, Broberger U. (1996) Visual impairment in preterm children with periventricular leukomalacia—visual, cognitive and neuropaediatric characteristics related to cerebral imaging. *Dev Med Child Neurol* **38:** 724–735.

Johnston M. (1995) Developmental aspects of NMDA receptor agonists and antagonists in the central nervous system . *Psychopharmacol Bull* **30:** 567–575.

Kadhim H, Tabarki B, Verellen G, De Prez C, Rona AM, Sebire G. (2001) Inflammatory cytokines in the pathogenesis of periventricular leukomalacia. *Neurology* **56:** 1278–1284.

Koelfen W, Freund M, Varnholt V. (1995) Neonatal stroke involving the middle cerebral artery in term infants: clinical presentation, EEG and imaging studies, and outcome. *Dev Med Child Neurol* **37:** 204–212.

Kwong KL, Wong SN, So KT. (1998) Epilepsy in children with cerebral palsy. *Pediatr Neurol* **19:** 31–36.

Kyllerman M, Bager B, Bensch J, Bille B, Olow I, Voss H. (1982) Dyskinetic cerebral palsy. I. Clinical categories, associated neurological abnormalities and incidences. *Acta Paediatr Scand* **71:** 543–550.

Levy SR, Abroms IF, Marshall PC, Rosquete EE. (1985) Seizures and cerebral infarction in the full-term newborn. *Ann Neurol* **17:** 366–370.

Little W (1862) On the influence of abnormal parturition, difficult labour, premature birth and asphyxia neonatorum on mental and physical conditions of the child, especially in relation to deformities. *Trans Obstet Soc London* **3:** 293–344.

Lou HC, Henriksen L, Bruhn P, Borner H, Nielsen JB. (1989) Striatal dysfunction in attention deficit and hyperkinetic disorder. *Arch Neurol* **46:** 48–52.

Martinez E, Figueroa R, Garry D, Visintainer P, Patel K, Verma U, Sehgal PB, Tejani N. (1998) Elevated amniotic fluid interleukin-6 as a predictor of neonatal periventricular leukomalacia and intraventricular hemorrhage. *J Matern Fetal Investig* **8:** 101–107.

McCormick MC, McCarton C, Tonascia J, Brooks-Gunn J. (1993) Early educational intervention for very low birth weight infants: results from the Infant Health and Development Program. *J Pediatr* **123:** 527–533.

Mercuri E, Rutherford M, Cowan F, Pennock J, Counsell S, Papadimitriou M, Azzopardi D, Bydder G, Dubowitz L. (1999) Early prognostic indicators of outcome in infants with neonatal cerebral infarction: a clinical, electroencephalogram, and magnetic resonance imaging study. *Pediatrics* **103:** 39–46.

29

Msall ME, Buck GM, Rogers BT, Merke D, Catanzaro NL, Zorn WA. (1991) Risk factors for major neurodevelopmental impairments and need for special education resources in extremely premature infants. *J Pediatr* **119:** 606–614.

Nelson KB, Ellenberg JH. (1986) Antecedents of cerebral palsy. Multivariate analysis of risk. *N Engl J Med* **315:** 81–86.

Nelson KB, Dambrosia JM, Grether JK, Phillips TM. (1998) Neonatal cytokines and coagulation factors in children with cerebral palsy. *Ann Neurol* **44:** 665–675.

Oka A, Belliveau MJ, Rosenberg PA, Volpe JJ. (1993) Vulnerability of oligodendroglia to glutamate: pharmacology, mechanisms, and prevention. *J Neurosci* **13:** 1441–1453.

Ozawa H, Nishida A, Mito T, Takashima S. (1994) Development of ferritin-positive cells in cerebrum of human brain. *Pediatr Neurol* **10:** 44–48.

Pasternak JF, Predey TA, Mikhael MA. (1991) Neonatal asphyxia: vulnerability of basal ganglia, thalamus, and brainstem. *Pediatr Neurol* **7:** 147–149.

Pharoah PO, Platt MJ, Cooke T. (1996) The changing epidemiology of cerebral palsy. *Arch Dis Child Fetal Neonatal Ed* **75:** F169–173.

Quinn M, Ando Y, Levene M. (1992) Cerebral arterial and venous flow-velocity measurements in post-hemorrhagic ventricular dilation and hydrocephalus. *Dev Med Child Neurol* **34:** 863–869.

Robertson C, Sauve RS, Christianson HE. (1994) Province-based study of neurologic disability among survivors weighing 500 through 1249 grams at birth. *Pediatrics* **93:** 636–640.

Roland E, Hill A, Norman M, Flodmark O, MacNab A. (1988) Selective brainstem injury in an asphyxiated newborn. *Ann Neurol* **23:** 89–92.

Rosenbloom L. (1994) Dyskinetic cerebral palsy and birth asphyxia. *Dev Med Child Neurol* **36:** 285–289.

Rutherford MA, Pennock JM, Murdoch-Eaton DM, Cowan FM, Dubowitz LM. (1992) Athetoid cerebral palsy with cysts in the putamen after hypoxic–ischaemic encephalopathy. *Arch Dis Child* **67:** 846–850.

Rutherford MA, Pennock JM, Counsell SJ, Mercuri E, Cowan FM, Dubowitz LMS, Edwards AD. (1998) Abnormal magnetic resonance signal in the internal capsule predicts poor neurodevelopmental outcome in infants with hypoxic–ischemic encephalopathy. *Pediatrics* **102:** 323–328.

Saigal S, Burrows E, Stoskopf BL, Rosenbaum PL, Streiner D. (2000) Impact of extreme prematurity on families of adolescent children. *J Pediatr* **137:** 701–706.

Saint Hilaire MH, Burke RE, Bressman SB, Brin MF, Fahn S. (1991) Delayed-onset dystonia due to perinatal or early childhood asphyxia. *Neurology* **41:** 216–222.

Selmaj KW, Raine CS. (1988) Tumor necrosis factor mediates myelin and oligodendrocyte damage in vitro. *Ann Neurol* **23:** 339–346.

Shirane R, Sato S, Sato K, Kameyama M, Ogawa A, Yoshimoto T, Hatazawa J, Ito M. (1992) Cerebral blood flow and oxygen metabolism in infants with hydrocephalus. *Childs Nerv Syst* **8:** 118–123.

Sran SK, Baumann RJ. (1988) Outcome of neonatal strokes. *Am J Dis Child* **142:** 1086-8.

Sreenan C, Bhargava R, Robertson CM. (2000) Cerebral infarction in the term newborn: clinical presentation and long-term outcome. *J Pediatr* **137:** 351–355.

Stanley FJ. (1992) Survival and cerebral palsy in low birthweight infants: implications for perinatal care. *Paediatr Perinat Epidemiol* **6:** 298–310.

Stanley F, Blair E, Alberman E. (2000) *Cerebral Palsies: Epidemiology and Causal Pathways*. London: Mac Keith Press.

Stiles J. (2000) Neural plasticity and cognitive development. *Dev Neuropsychol* **18:** 237–272.

Volpe JJ. (1992) Value of MR in definition of the neuropathology of cerebral palsy in vivo. *Am J Neuroradiol* **13:** 79–83.

Volpe JJ. (1994) Brain injury in the premature infant—current concepts. *Prev Med* **23:** 638-645.

Volpe J. (1996) Subplate neurons—missing link in brain injury of the premature infant? *Pediatrics* **97:** 112–113.

Volpe JJ. (2001) *Neurology of the Newborn*. Philadelphia: W.B. Saunders. p 217–276.

Volpe JJ, Herscovitch P, Perlman JM, Raichle ME. (1983) Positron emission tomography in the newborn: extensive impairment of regional cerebral blood flow with intraventricular hemorrhage and hemorrhagic intracerebral involvement. *Pediatrics* **72:** 589–601.

Wulfeck BB, Trauner DA, Tallal PA. (1991) Neurologic, cognitive, and linguistic features of infants after early stroke. *Pediatr Neurol* **7:** 266–269.

Yokochi K. (1998) Clinical profiles of subjects with subcortical leukomalacia and border-zone infarction revealed by MR. *Acta Paediatr* **87:** 879–883.

Yonezawa M, Back S, Gan X, Rosenberg P, Volpe J. (1996) Cystine deprivation induces oligodendroglial death: rescue by free radical scavengers and by a diffusible glial factor. *J Neurochem* **67:** 566–573.

Yoon BH, Romero R, Yang SH, Jun JK, Kim IO, Choi JH, Syn HC. (1996) Interleukin-6 concentrations in umbilical cord plasma are elevated in neonates with white matter lesions associated with periventricular leukomalacia. *Am J Obstet Gynecol* **174:** 1433–1440.

Yoon BH, Jun JK, Romero R, Park KH, Gomez R, Choi JH, Kim IO. (1997) Amniotic fluid inflammatory cytokines (interleukin-6, interleukin-1beta, and tumor necrosis factor-alpha), neonatal brain white matter lesions, and cerebral palsy. *Am J Obstet Gynecol* **177:** 19–26.

Yoon B, Romero R, Park J, Kim C, Kim S, Choi J, Han T. (2000) Fetal exposure to an intra-amniotic inflammation and the development of cerebral palsy at the age of three years. *Am J Obstet Gynecol* **182:** 675–681.

.

3
THE PATHOPHYSIOLOGY OF SPASTICITY

Warwick J. Peacock

Spasticity is one of the most serious problems in patients who have an upper motor lesion in the brain or spinal cord. Pathology in the nervous system produces negative features such as loss of power, decreased fine motor control and sensory deficit, but it also produces positive features. These positive or release effects manifest as spasticity, involuntary movements or epileptic seizures. The site of the lesion rather than the pathology determines the combination of positive and negative features that produce the characteristic clinical picture. For example, a lesion in the cervical spinal cord produces negative effects such as weakness and loss of fine-motor control as well as the positive feature of increased muscle tone (spasticity) in all four limbs frequently associated with muscle spasms, whereas a lesion in the left cerebral hemisphere in an adult causes weakness in the right face, arm and leg with loss of speech (negative features). The right-sided weakness is associated with spasticity (positive feature). The spasticity in this case is not accompanied with muscle spasms and, in addition, right-sided focal motor seizures (positive feature) may appear some time later. Children born with a congenital hemiplegia (acquired in utero or perinatally) seldom have facial weakness or loss of speech.

Spasticity is difficult to define, but one humorous definition may be helpful:

> *Spasticity is like love,*
> *You know it when you feel it,*
> *It is all embracing.*
> *It is centrally mediated*
> *And has important peripheral manifestations.*
>
> (J. Oppenheim, personal communication)

Lance (1980) offers us a more clinical and practical definition:

> *Spasticity is a motor disorder characterized by a velocity-dependent increase in tonic stretch reflexes, with exaggerated tendon jerks resulting from hyperexcitability of the stretch reflex, as one component of the upper motoneuron syndrome.*

In a healthy individual at rest, "background tone" is electrically silent. However, in individuals with upper motor-neuron disorders, an "electrically active" excessive "background muscle tone" may be observed, to the extent that the individual may have great difficulty in resting. It follows from the above definition of spasticity given by Lance, that posture

32

is not spastic. Burke (1988) points out that postures are conditioned by motor acts and are necessary for their proper execution. They are also conditioned by vestibular stimuli which in turn are governed by the alignment of the head in relation to gravity and by rotational movements of the head. In addition, damage to the extrapyramidal inputs to the vestibular nuclei may result in the loss of central nervous system inhibition, so that changes in the state of arousal of the patient such as excitement, hunger, pain (particularly reflux esophagitis) and even intellectual tasks such as mental arithmetic may cause alterations in background tone.

Although spasticity could be considered to be a compensation for weakness, the increased muscle tone it produces may interfere with a movement pattern, once that movement program is being executed.

It is well recognized that spasticity in a growing child frequently leads to deformities such as muscle contractures and joint dislocations. The mechanisms by which this occurs will be discussed in Chapter 12.

Does a lesion at any site in the nervous system produce spasticity, or are there very specific sites where a lesion will lead to spasticity? To answer this question, we will review the different areas of the central nervous system involved in movement and see which one of these, when damaged, will lead to spasticity.

There are five different areas in the central nervous system that are involved in the control of movement: (1) the pyramidal and extrapyramidal systems, (2) the corpus striatum, (3) the cerebellum, (4) the brainstem motor nuclei, and (5) the spinal cord.

The pyramidal and extrapyramidal systems

All movements start as a thought or desire in a remote area of the cerebral cortex and are then relayed to the supplementary motor area and other cortical control centers. An order is then issued to initiate appropriate muscular contraction to achieve the desired goal (Fig. 3.1). The basal ganglia are consulted for advice about the best strategy to achieve this goal based on memory of previous similar movements and the position of the body at that time (Fig. 3.2). The cerebellum is informed of the motor plan and asked to monitor it throughout its course (Fig. 3.3). The brainstem motor nuclei are instructed to provide the correct background posture and tone to enable the movement to be carried out (Fig. 3.4). The cortical motor-control centers then issue their order to the spinal cord and muscles to bring about the appropriate sequence of muscle contractions. The final order is delivered via the corticospinal (pyramidal) tract. This recently evolved and highly specialized tract mainly controls the distal limb muscles, and would be involved in such discrete movements such as writing, using a knife and fork, and for speaking.

The spasticity seen in a patient with a stroke or in a child with cerebral palsy is often attributed to damage to the corticospinal tract. This is incorrect. Damage to the corticospinal tract alone only produces loss of fine-motor control in distal limb muscles without spasticity (Hepp-Reymond et al. 1974, Kuypers and Martin 1981). However, it is uncommon for the corticospinal tract to be injured in isolation. Many other motor tracts such as the cortico-bulbospinal (extrapyramidal) tract, which are also damaged, surround this tract along its course. It is the involvement of these other tracts that lead to the increase in muscle tone. Which tracts these are we will have to work out by a process of elimination. What we can

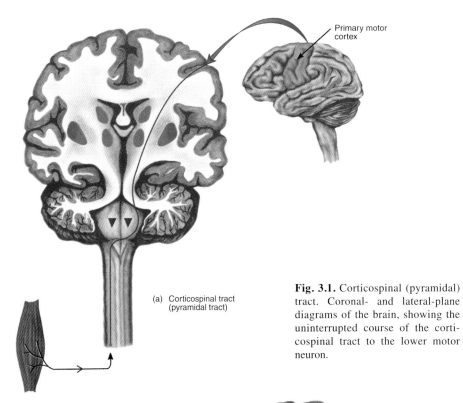

Primary motor cortex

(a) Corticospinal tract
(pyramidal tract)

Fig. 3.1. Corticospinal (pyramidal) tract. Coronal- and lateral-plane diagrams of the brain, showing the uninterrupted course of the corticospinal tract to the lower motor neuron.

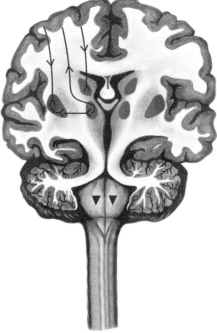

Fig. 3.2. Basal ganglia (corpus striatum). Coronal-plane diagram of the basal ganglia and connections to the motor cortex.

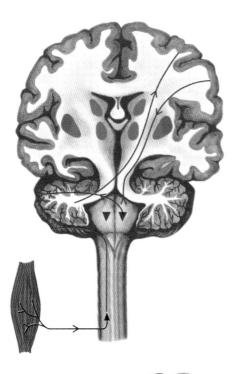

Fig. 3.3. Cerebellar system. Coronal-plane diagram of the cerebellum, showing its afferent connections to the muscle and its afferent and efferent connections to the motor cortex.

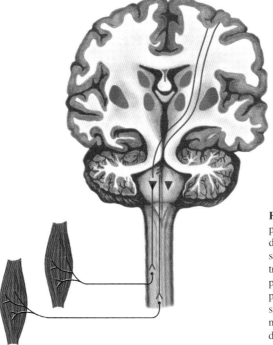

Fig. 3.4. Cortico-bulbospinal (extra-pyramidal) tract. Coronal-plane diagram of the brain and spinal cord showing the course of the corticobulbar tract. Note the fact that, unlike the direct pyramidal tract, the indirect extra-pyramidal (corticobulbospinal) tract synapses in the vestibular and reticular nuclei in the brainstem and continues down as the vestibulospinal and reticulospinal tracts.

say with certainty is that isolated injury to the corticospinal (pyramidal) tract does not produce spasticity.

We will first review the other possibilities before returning to the cortico-bulbospinal tract.

Corpus striatum

The corpus striatum is made up of large clusters of gray matter (nuclei) situated deep within the cerebral hemispheres. The caudate nucleus, the putamen and the globus pallidus can be seen by the naked eye on a cross-section through the cerebral hemisphere, while the substantia nigra can similarly be seen when the midbrain has been sectioned. These structures play a role in the planning and initiation of any movement. What happens to muscle tone when they are damaged? Is spasticity found in Huntington's and Parkinson's diseases, the most well-known neurological disorders associated with pathology in the corpus striatum?

Huntington's disease is inherited in an autosomal dominant pattern with the pathological substrate being atrophy of the caudate nucleus and putamen (Fig. 3.5). The characteristic clinical feature is a movement disorder involving choreiform movements that are purposeless, involuntary and jerky. They are almost imperceptible at first but slowly increase in amplitude until the patient becomes incapacitated. What is thought to be happening is that somehow the movement patterns stored in the corpus striatum are inappropriately released, so that they are no longer under voluntary control. As far as muscle tone is concerned, it fluctuates but does not have the characteristic features of spasticity.

With Parkinson's disease there is loss of neurons in the substantia nigra in the midbrain. Individuals experience a tremor at rest and have difficulty initiating movement. They have an expressionless face and a short, stepping gait. Muscle tone in extremities is described as rigid. Rigidity is often considered to be the same as spasticity. It is not. In rigidity the tone is elevated but does not have a clasp-knife quality to it. Rather, when a limb is moved against this rigidity, a resistance is encountered which is the same throughout the range of the movement and is likened to the feel of bending a lead pipe. Rigidity is not muscle-spindle-dependent and is therefore not relieved by cutting the posterior roots.

In Huntington's disease the involuntary movement patterns are released whereas in Parkinson's disease involuntary movements are lost. However, spasticity does not result in either case. Thus we can conclude that spasticity is not a feature of pathology in the corpus striatum.

Cerebellum

The cerebellum is made up of the two cerebellar hemispheres and the midline vermis. The cerebellum is attached to the brainstem via three peduncles on each side. It has a highly folded cortex and deep-seated nuclei of which the dentate is the most important.

When the midline vermis is damaged the main clinical feature is an ataxic gait with loss of balance. If the lateral lobes are affected the patient loses the ability to perform rapidly repetitive alternating movements in the ipsilateral limbs. With involvement of either the vermis or the lateral lobes there is no increase in muscle tone; instead, muscle hypotonia may be noted. Consequently, spasticity does not reside in the cerebellum.

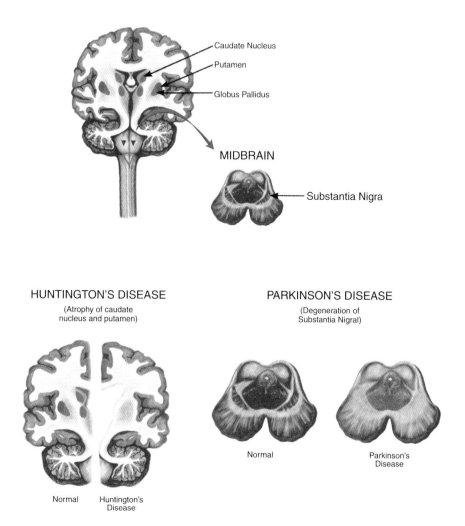

Fig. 3.5. Corpus striatum. Schematic drawings of (a) the healthy basal ganglia, (b) atrophy of the caudate nucleus and putamen in Huntington's disease, and (c) degeneration of the substantia nigra in Parkinson's disease.

Spinal cord

Although damage to the spinal cord can produce spasticity, it occurs because the spinal cord motor neurons are disconnected from the higher centers in the brain. Poliomyelitis (the myelitis referring to the spinal cord), which is characterized by destruction of the anterior horn cells (the nerve cell body of the spinal motor neurons), does not produce spasticity. Rather, it causes a flaccid paralysis of the affected muscles leading to marked wasting. Thus, although spasticity can arise from spinal-cord injury, the cause of that spasticity is really the severing of connections between the brain and spinal cord. Nevertheless, it is these spinal lesions that produce the most intractable, disabling and painful spasticity.

37

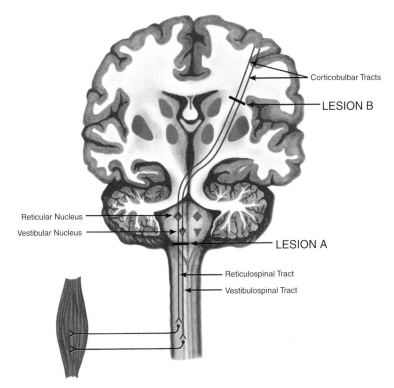

Fig. 3.6. Coronal-plane diagram showing two different lesions producing different types of spasticity. Note lesion A in the brainstem or spinal cord is distal to the brainstem nuclei, and lesion B in the cerebral hemisphere is proximal to the brainstem nuclei. (See text for explanation.)

The brainstem motor nuclei

Muscle tone, especially in the lower limbs, is controlled by brainstem nuclei, especially the reticular and vestibular nuclei. (Although there are subdivisions of these nuclei and other centers in the brainstem that are involved with the maintenance of posture and tone, for the purpose of this chapter only the major parts of these two nuclei will be discussed.) The reticular nucleus sends the reticulospinal tract down the spinal cord where its fibers synapse with motor neurons that innervate muscles. The effect of this tract is to inhibit muscle tone (Houk and Rymer 1981). In addition, the cerebral cortex is connected to the reticulospinal tract via a bundle of fibers, which excite the nucleus, increasing its inhibitory influence on the motor neurons in the cord. When the reticular nucleus or the reticulospinal tract is damaged the inhibitory influence is lost and muscle tone rises. The vestibular nucleus, via the vestibulospinal tract, is connected to and excites the motor neurons in the spinal cord. The vestibular nucleus is involved with balance and antigravity support and brings about contraction in the antigravity or extensor muscles in the lower limbs. The cortical connections with the vestibular nucleus inhibit its activity and thus reduce antigravity or extensor activity in the lower limbs.

When the spinal cord or lower brainstem is damaged, both the reticulospinal and vestibulospinal nuclei are disconnected from the spinal motor neurons (Fig. 3.6, lesion A). The loss of reticulospinal inhibition leads to increased firing of the spinal motor neurons with resultant increased muscle tone or spasticity. The loss of vestibulospinal excitation leads to decreased firing of the motor neurons responsible for lower-limb extensor-muscle contraction so the patient tends to develop a flexed posture and flexor spasms.

When the cerebral hemisphere is damaged (Fig. 3.6, lesion B), there is loss of excitation of the reticular nucleus by the cerebral cortex so that its inhibitory influence on the spinal motor neurons is reduced. Muscle tone rises because the reticular nucleus fires less enthusiastically. At the same time, the inhibitory influence of the cortex on the vestibular nucleus is lost so that the vestibular nucleus fires more vigorously, resulting in increased antigravity or extensor activity in the lower limbs.

Natural history of spasticity
Acute cerebral injury is often accompanied by an initial flaccid weakness with the advent of increased reflex excitability reaching a maximum over the ensuing few months. Over the next few years, this reflex excitability may subside as intramuscular changes such as muscle wasting and contracture develop at which time postural and reflex stiffness are replaced by intramuscular stiffness and the absence of clonus. These features were carefully documented by the American physician/physiologist Richard Herman, in his detailed studies of adult stroke patients (Herman 1970), and by Thilman et al. (1991). Hufschmidt and Mauritz (1985) demonstrated an increase in the "viscoelastic" resistance to passive muscle stretch as the time from the stroke elapsed. This was accompanied by an increase in the work done to stretch the muscle passively. In gait analysis, this would be seen as absorption of energy in the power graphs (Davis and DeLuca, 1996).

Importantly, viscous resistance is also velocity-dependent but, naturally, is electromyographically silent. A typical example of viscous resistance to motion can be experienced in the swimming-pool. If the observer walks slowly through the water, relatively little resistance is experienced. As the subject attempts to walk faster through the water the resistance to motion increases until a point is reached at which motion becomes impossible. Consequently, the trick is to walk through the water slowly to minimize viscous drag. Another example of viscous resistance to motion is that of the spoon being dragged through honey. Examples of increased viscoelastic stiffness in children were first demonstrated by Dietz et al. (1981), this increased mechanical resistance being accompanied by little or no electromyographic (EMG) activity. The reader may also see Dietz and Berger (1995) for a more complete review of this topic.

Co-contraction
When dealing with spastic gait, it is important to ask whether the disturbance is pathologically abnormal, due to developmental delay, or altered by the physiological task. An interesting study by Leonard et al. (1991) compared the EMG and joint patterns of infants and toddlers with and without cerebral palsy. Initially, both groups had similar patterns of co-contraction during supported walking, accompanied by joint synchronies (e.g. simultaneous flexion of

the hip, knee and ankle joints). Children without cerebral palsy eventually developed fluid patterns of unsupported walking (characterized by less co-contraction and associated with physiological joint asynchrony, e.g. hip flexion, knee extension and ankle dorsiflexion), which are typical of mature gait patterns; whereas children with cerebral palsy retained the co-contraction pattern of unsupported walking.

An additional problem is the fact that the faster one walks, the greater the duration of EMG in both the stance and swing phases of gait (Detrembleur et al. 1997). That is, the faster the speed of walking, the greater the degree of physiological "wrap-around" of EMG activity that occurs. Since gait is usually assessed at a self-selected speed, care must be taken to ensure that EMG patterns are not interpreted as pathological on the basis of the speed of walking. Many diplegic children have a tendency to rush or run when intending to walk, which would favor a "wrap-around" pattern of EMG discharge. This phenomenon could be termed "task-dependent co-contraction". A fundamental stimulus to walking fast is the combination of weakness and instability of the stance limb. However, it is clear that the diplegic child has active co-contraction of the leg muscles both the in supine and vertical positions, and even on waking up. In other words, the spasticity is there before the first step is taken.

It is thus possible to have excessive electromyographic activity associated with co-contraction from a variety of causes: (1) as the result of delayed maturation in healthy children (Sutherland et al. 1988); (2) as a consequence of increasing the speed of walking, which induces wrap-around EMG and co-contraction (Detrembleur et al. 1997); or (3) pathologic co-contraction as a feature of abnormal motor planning (Leonard et al. 1991).

Summary

To summarize, a lesion below the reticular and vestibular nuclei produces spinal spasticity, which is characterized by increased tone, or spasticity (reticulospinal tract damage), with a tendency to flexor spasms and a flexed posture (damage to the vestibulospinal tract). A cerebral lesion, i.e. above the reticular and vestibular nuclei tends to produce a lesser degree of spasticity (there is less excitatory cortical influence on the reticular nucleus which is itself intact), but extensor posturing in the lower limbs is commonly seen as a result of the loss of the inhibitory influence of the cortex on the vestibular nucleus (which tends to produce extension in the antigravity muscles).

REFERENCES

Burke D. (1988) Spasticity as an adaptation to pyramidal tract injury. In: Waxman SG, editor. *Functional Recovery in Neurological Disease*. New York: Raven Press. p 401–423.
Davis RB, DeLuca PA. (1996) Gait characterization via dynamic joint stiffness. *Gait Posture* **4**: 224–231.
Detrembleur C, Willems P, Plaghki L. (1997) Does walking speed influence the time pattern of muscle activation in normal children? *Dev Med Child Neurol* **39**: 803–807.
Dietz V, Berger W. (1995) Cerebral palsy and muscle transformation. *Dev Med Child Neurol* **37**: 180–184.
Dietz V, Quintern J, Berger W. (1981) Electrophysiological studies of gait in spasticity and rigidity. Evidence that altered mechanical properties of muscle contribute to hypertonia. *Brain* **104**: 431–449.
Hepp-Reymond M, Trouche E, Wiesendanger M. (1974) Effects of unilateral and bilateral pyramidotomy on a conditioned rapid precision grip in monkeys (*Macaca fascicularis*). *Exp Brain Res* **21**: 519–527.
Herman R. (1970) The myotatic reflex. Clinico-physiological aspects of spasticity and contracture. *Brain* **93**:

273–312.

Houk J, Rymer JC. (1981) Neural control of muscle length and tension. In: Brookhart JM, Mountcastle VB, editors. *Handbook of Physiology—The Nervous System*, vol. 2. Bethesda, Maryland: American Physiological Society. p 623–634.

Hufschmidt A, Mauritz KH (1985) Chronic transformation of muscle in spasticity: a peripheral contribution to increased tone. *J Neurol Neurosurg Psychiatry* **48:** 676–685.

Kuypers HGJM, Martin GF. (1981) *Anatomy of the Descending Pathways to the Spinal Cord*, vol. 2. Amsterdam and New York: Elsevier.

Lance JW. (1980) Pathophysiology of spasticity and clinical experience with baclofen. In: Feldman RG, Young RR, Koella WP, editors. *Spasticity: Disordered Motor Control*. Chicago: Year Book Medical. p 185–203.

Leonard CT, Hirschfeld H, Forssberg H. (1991) The development of independent walking in children with cerebral palsy. *Dev Med Child Neurol* **33:** 567–577.

Sutherland D, Olshen R, Biden EN, Wyatt MP. (1988) Dynamic electromyography by age. In: Sutherland D, editor. *The Development of Mature Walking*. London: Mac Keith Press. p 154–162.

Thilmann AF, Fellows SJ, Garms E. (1991) The mechanism of spastic muscle hypertonus. Variation in reflex gain over the time course of spasticity. *Brain* **114:** 233–244.

4
A QUALITATIVE DESCRIPTION OF NORMAL GAIT

James R. Gage

Locomotion is a feature of all animals. Quadrupeds are inherently fast and stable. Their center of mass is located just under the trunk, inside the base of support. A long stride is possible, because the body is interposed between the front and back limbs. In fast-running animals such as cougars, the flexors and extensors of the vertebral column are actually used to augment stride length and power. Thus, when galloping, the back is rolled into flexion as the animal brings the hindlimbs past the planted forelimbs. Once weight is transferred to the hindlimbs, the spine and hips are powerfully extended as the shoulders flex to swing the forelimbs far forward in preparation for contact (Fig. 4.1).

Humans employ bipedal gait that is less efficient and less stable than quadrupedal gait. Bipeds are unstable because their center of mass is located above their base of support. In the human, the center of mass is located just in front of the S2 vertebra. In order to remain upright, the center of mass must be maintained in balance over the base of support. Since this is more easily obtained in quadrupeds, it maybe one of the reasons why ambulation is delayed for a significant period after birth in bipeds as opposed to quadrupeds. In addition, speed and stride length are constrained by the fact that the trunk musculature is not used as extensively in gait and the body is not interposed between the limbs in the line of progression. In fact, however, pelvic rotation is used to partially interpose the pelvic width into the line of progression during gait. Bipedal gait does have the significant advantage of freeing the upper extremities for other use (Fig. 4.2).

Gait is a complex activity. It requires a control system, an energy source, levers to provide movement, and forces to move the levers.

The control system
Central nervous system control of locomotion has been covered in detail in Chapter 1. Control of locomotion is initiated from the pyramidal region of the motor cortex, and the controlling system needs to have complete integration of sensory and motor function if it is to perform properly. Furthermore, the complexity of the central locomotor control system requires interaction between several other brain regions and the spinal cord in what could best be described as a pyramidal hierarchy. This hierarchical system of motor control begins with the cerebral cortex and ends with the final common pathway (the motor neuron) (Fig. 4.3). The components of this system include (1) the motor cortex, (2) the basal ganglia, (3) the thalamus and hypothalamus, (4) the midbrain, (5) the cerebellum, and (6) the brainstem and spinal cord.

The energy source

Energy is required for walking. Since this ultimately depends on the delivery of metabolic fuel and oxygen to the muscles by the cardiovascular system and the oxidation of that fuel in the muscles, energy production and utilization have a finite limit. We measure that limit by a parameter known as the VO_2 max. This is defined as the rate of oxygen usage (liters/minute) under maximal aerobic metabolism. For short-term metabolic debt we can depend on anaerobic glycolysis, but for sustained activity locomotion must be carried out aerobically, i.e. without oxygen debt. As such, energy conservation is critical to normal performance. Therefore speed and distance traveled are dependent upon (1) the rate of energy production and transport to the muscles (VO_2 max), and (2) the extent to which energy is conserved.

The levers

Movement of the body is generated by moments. A moment is a force couple, which is defined as force acting at a distance about an axis of rotation that produces an angular acceleration about that axis. As such moments are made up of two components: (1) a force, and (2) a lever arm. Mathematically, moments are equal to the magnitude of the force times the length of the lever arm. Since the Newton is the metric unit used to measure the magnitude of the force and the length of the lever arm is measured in meters, moments are measured in units of Newton meters. In the body, motion occurs through skeletal joints. The skeleton itself provides the levers needed for the movement. Moments and their components will be discussed in more detail when we come to "lever-arm dysfunction" in Chapter 13.

The forces

Our muscles are the physiologic motors that generate the forces that allow us to move. In so doing they produce internal moments around the joint centers. However, when we stand or perform any activity in which our muscles resist the force of gravity, ground reaction and/or inertial forces are created. These forces, which are external to the body, also act on skeletal levers to produce external joint moments. Walking then is a trade-off between the internal moments generated by the muscles and the external moments generated by the ground reaction and inertial forces (Fig. 4.4).

Muscles are well designed for function with respect to their shape, internal architecture, power, endurance, speed, and type of contraction. Muscle contraction requires energy. In the muscle, a contraction is produced by cross-bridging between the two major muscle proteins actin and myosin. Adenosine triphosphate binds to the myosin head and supplies energy for cross-bridging through the reaction:

$$ATP \geq ADP + P + Energy$$

The reaction is refreshed by one of three mechanisms: (1) enzymatic breakdown of phosphocreatine to produce ATP and creatinine, (2) anaerobic glycolysis of glucose which produces ATP and lactic acid, or (3) aerobic glycolysis of glucose which produces ATP plus carbon dioxide and water. Thus lactic acid and creatinine are end-products of muscle energy production.

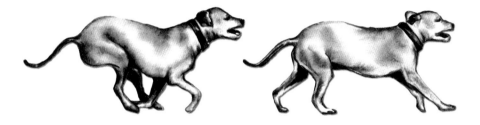

Fig. 4.1. A dog uses the power of its spinal extensors when running, and its center of gravity is located inside its base of support.

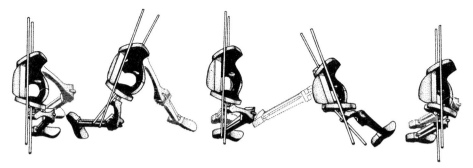

Fig. 4.2. Pelvic rotation in human gait. Although not as efficient as quadrupedal gait, bipedal gait does have the significant advantage of freeing the upper extremities for other use. This is an illustration of the transverse rotations of the pelvis, lower extremities and feet. Small sticks have been attached to the pelvis and femurs and the actual rotations amplified threefold to emphasize that the lower extremities rotate through a greater range than the pelvis. Notice that the pelvis rotates with and acts to elongate the swinging limb, thus allowing a longer stride than would otherwise be possible. (Reproduced from Inman VT, Ralston HJ, Todd F, 1981, Human walking. In: Libermann JC, editor *Human Walking*. Baltimore: Williams and Wilkins, p85–117, by permission.)

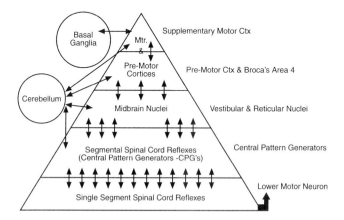

Fig. 4.3. The hierarchical system of motor control. Motor control is extremely complex. Motion is initiated in the pyramidal cortex, but in order for a coordinated movement to occur many other circuits in the basal ganglia, cerebellum and spinal cord need to be involved (see Chapter 1).

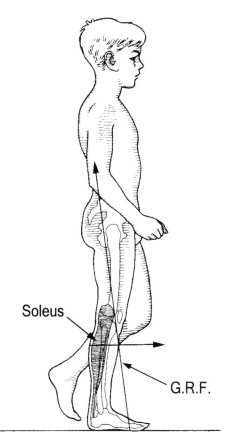

Soleus

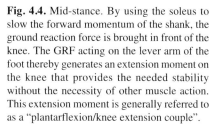

G.R.F.

Fig. 4.4. Mid-stance. By using the soleus to slow the forward momentum of the shank, the ground reaction force is brought in front of the knee. The GRF acting on the lever arm of the foot thereby generates an extension moment on the knee that provides the needed stability without the necessity of other muscle action. This extension moment is generally referred to as a "plantarflexion/knee extension couple".

Types of muscle fibers

Brooke and Kaiser (1970a, b) described three types of muscle fiber, each of which depends on different means of energy production. Type I (slow-twitch) fibers have a small diameter and a high oxidative potential. Type II (fast-twitch) fibers have two subtypes: IIa has a high oxidative potential, while IIb has a low oxidative potential.

Burke et al. (1973) classified muscle fibers on the basis of contraction time, sag (defined as decrease in force in a 500 millisecond period), and degree of fatigability. On the basis of this he arrived at three fiber types that were essentially analogous to those of Brooke and Kaiser. They are S (slow) which are equivalent to type I, FR (fast, fatigue-resistant) equivalent to type IIa, and FF (fast, fatigable) equivalent to type IIb. FF and FR motor units contain more muscles fibers than S units. The fast (type II) units are ideal for producing large forces quickly, but cannot sustain contraction over a long period of time. Type I units generate forces more slowly but have high resistance to fatigue. Thus they are ideally suited to produce submaximal forces over long periods of time, and as such are found in abundance in the postural antigravity muscles. It is now known that the muscle fiber type is determined by its motor neuron and may change in response to conditioning, denervation/reinnervation

45

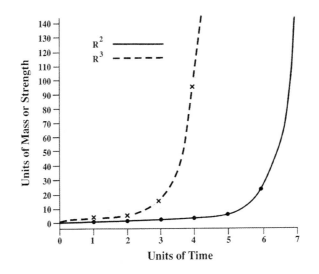

Fig. 4.5. The "law of magnitude". A graph of muscle power which is proportional to its cross-sectional area (πr^2), versus mass which is cubic (r^3). It can be readily seen that with time and growth, mass increases at a much faster rate than strength.

or in certain neuromuscular conditions (Alway et al. 1988). Muscles fibers and fiber types are discussed more fully in Chapter 9.

Muscle power

Muscle power relates primarily to its cross-sectional area and secondarily to factors such as pennate structure, fiber type and degree of fatigue. It is equal to roughly 2 kilograms per cubic centimeter of cross-sectional area. In muscle, power is defined as force times velocity. It is optimal when the muscle is contracting at about one-third of its maximal velocity (Lieber 1986).

A muscle's pennate structure also determines its power and range since the pennates function as internal levers within the muscle. Isometric stabilizers such as the gluteus medius have relatively horizontal pennates within their structure that acts to greatly amplify the muscles force production at the expense of speed and range of motion (Rab 1994).

As a child grows, muscle strength and overall body mass both increase. Since muscle power is related to cross-sectional area, it can be estimated by multiplying π times the square of the muscle's radius. However, weight or mass is a function of volume, which is cubic. For example, the mass of a cubic volume of water which measures 2cm on a side would be $2 \times 2 \times 2 = 8cc \times$ density of water. The implication is that as a child grows, her/his mass increases as a function of the cube, but strength increases only as a function of the square. In other words, young children are relatively Herculean for their weight, i.e. they have a much greater power to mass ratio than adults. Simply stated, as children grow their strength does not keep pace with their mass. J.M. Cary (in a personal communication) referred to this as the "Law of Magnitude" (Fig. 4.5). This is an important treatment principle to remember when treating children with cerebral palsy, because if a young child is ambulating marginally, s/he may cease walking in the midst of the adolescent growth spurt because of the falling power/mass ratio. If surgery is performed with the goal of improving ambulation at that time, it will not be successful unless it significantly lowers the child's energy requirements, i.e. makes the child's gait more efficient. In the light of this, there is now a great deal of interest in measuring energy consumption in children with neuromuscular disabilities, because the expectation is that such data may be useful both in assessing outcomes of treatment and in determining their future ambulation potential.

A muscle's tension also affects its power. Cavagna et al. (1968) showed that if a muscle is stretched just prior to contraction it will contract with greater power. It is interesting to note that during normal gait, inertial and/or ground reaction forces stretch most of the major muscle groups of the lower-extremity muscles just before the onset of their contraction. The hamstrings in terminal swing are just one example of this.

Types of muscle contraction
Muscles work in one of three modes. (1) In concentric contraction (shortening contraction), the muscle does positive work. All accelerators work in this mode. The iliopsoas acting in pre-swing and initial swing is an example of this type of contraction. (2) In eccentric or lengthening contraction the muscle does negative work. All decelerators and/or shock absorbers work in this mode. Alexander (1992) cites studies that indicate that the efficiency of negative work by a muscle is greater than that of positive work. The energy conservation potential of negative work may be part of the explanation as to why it is the most frequent type of contraction in normal gait. The soleus contracting in midstance is an example of this type of contraction. (3) In isometric contraction the muscle length is static. Stabilizers work in this mode. Most of these are postural, antigravity muscles. The gluteus medius during the period of single limb support is an example of this type of contraction.

Muscle forces can be much more easily understood if we picture them as part of a force couple or moment. As stated previously, muscles produce internal moments that resist the external ground reaction and/or inertial forces. In every case, the lever arm upon which the muscle is acting is the bone and the axis about which it is acting is the joint center. If the muscle is acting perpendicular to the axis of rotation, the moment of force which is produced is always equal to the muscle force times its distance from the axis of joint rotation (Fig. 4.6).

A simple way of illustrating force moments is to think of two children on a teeter-totter (see-saw). Each child is creating a moment around the axle to which the teeter-totter is attached, and since the moments are in opposite directions, they are tending to balance each other (Fig. 4.7). A lighter child can balance a heavier one so long as he sits further from the center of the teeter-totter because he has a "mechanical advantage". In the same way, the length of the lever arm on which a muscle is acting is frequently spoken of as its "mechanical advantage". Inman et al. (1981) pointed out that particular joint positions are assumed in daily activities because they allow the maximum moment for the muscles acting on that joint. Because muscles can exert maximum power at only one fiber length, the skeleton has provided certain compensatory mechanisms. First, as the muscle shortens and becomes

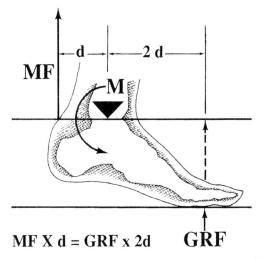

$$MF \times d = GRF \times 2d \qquad GRF$$

Fig. 4.6. The relationship between the external moment produced by the GRF, and the internal moment produced by the muscles. In each case they act on a skeletal lever and their fulcrum is the joint center. Since in this illustration the lever arm of the ground reaction force is twice as long as that of the muscles, its magnitude would be only half as much: d (MF) = 2d (GRF). Dividing through by d, MF = 2 (GRF).

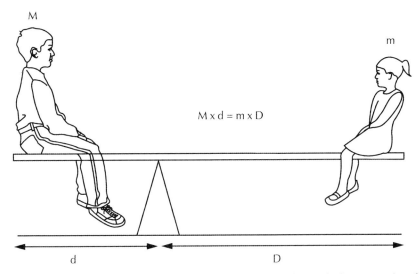

Fig. 4.7. The relationship between a man and a child on a teeter-totter is exactly the same as that of the muscle and the ground reaction forces at each of the lower-extremity joints, and the pivot point or fulcrum is always the joint center.

weaker, the effective lever arm of the muscle lengthens. Since the magnitude of a moment is given as force times distance, the effect of this phenomenon is to produce a force couple with a relatively constant magnitude. Quadriceps action at the knee is an example of this,

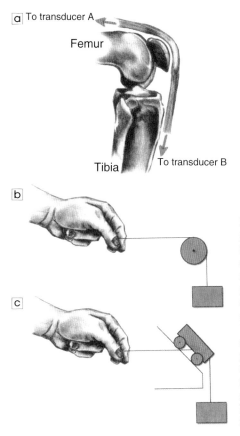

Femur

Tibia To transducer B

b

c

Fig. 4.8. Diagram showing how the motion of the patella affects the excursion of the knee. (a) Schematic drawing of the knee joint; (b) rope running over a fixed pulley; (c) model that magnifies movement by the same principle as the patellar–femoral joint. In (b), for every 1 cm movement of the hand there will be 1 cm of movement of the weight, whereas in (c) for every 1 cm of movement of the hand there will be 2 cm of movement of the weight because as the rope is pulled, the cart will move up the incline. Consequently the force exerted by the hand must be twice that of the weight, because the work (force multiplied by distance) done on the weight cannot be more than the work done by the hand (Adapted from Alexander 1992, by permission.)

since the patella acts to amplify knee motion in mid-range where the muscle has a strong mechanical advantage, but not in terminal extension where the muscle is working near end-range (Fig. 4.8). Secondly, a muscle that passes over two joints can be maintained at a favorable resting length by simultaneous and related movements of the other joint over which the muscle passes. For example, the hamstrings in sitting undergo little change in length since the hip and knee are flexing simultaneously with elongation at the former joint and shortening at the latter.

The prerequisites of normal gait

Normal gait has four attributes or prerequisites that are frequently lost in pathological gait (Perry 1985). These are, in order of importance: (1) stability in stance, (2) sufficient foot clearance during swing, (3) appropriate swing phase pre-positioning of the foot, and (4) an adequate step length. To these we need to add a more global fifth prerequisite: energy conservation (Gage 1991).

Stability in stance is challenged by two major factors. (1) The body is top-heavy, so that the center of mass (CoM) lies above the base of support, just in front of the S2 vertebra.

(2) Walking continually alters segment alignment. As an individual walks, the CoM—which remains within the base of support while standing—moves forward with each step from one base of support to another. This means that the body must constantly alter the position of the trunk in space in order to maintain balance over the base of support and/or to maintain balance when moving.

Therefore stability in stance involves much more than a stable foot. In addition to having the stance foot stable on the floor, the major lower-extremity joints must function to: (1) allow advancement of the limb in swing, (2) maintain balance, (3) provide propulsion, and (4) ensure appropriate position of the structures above.

Clearance in swing requires: (1) appropriate position and power of the ankle, knee and hip on the stance side; (2) adequate ankle dorsiflexion, knee flexion and hip flexion on the swing side; (3) stability of the stance foot; and (4) adequate body balance.

Pre-position of the foot in terminal swing necessitates: (1) appropriate body balance, (2) stability, power and proper position on the stance side, and (3) adequate ankle dorsiflexion, balance between inverters and everters of the foot, appropriate knee position, and proper foot position.

An *adequate step-length demands* that there is (1) adequate body balance, (2) a stable and properly positioned stance side, (3) adequate hip flexion and knee extension on the swing side, and (4) neutral dorsiflexion, inversion and eversion of the foot on the swing side.

Finally, *energy conservation* requires that, when possible: (1) joint stability is provided by the ground reaction force (GRF) in conjunction with ligaments instead of muscles; (2) the center of mass excursion is minimized in all planes; and (3) muscle forces are optimized. Optimizing muscle forces may involve a number of factors: eccentric muscle forces (as opposed to concentric) are used to the greatest extent possible during gait; "stretch energy" in tendons and muscles is returned as kinetic energy, since in normal gait muscles tend to be "pre-stretched" before they fire concentrically; biarticular muscles serve to transfer energy from one segment to another; and walking is accomplished in a manner that minimizes the forces in our muscles (Alexander 1992).

In a toddler, ambulation begins without these prerequisites. Initially the knees are relatively stiff and the child walks with a wide base of support. Gradually, as the toddler develops balance and equilibrium, gait evolves toward the adult pattern. Sutherland and colleagues (1980) pointed out that although walking usually starts at about one year of age, children do not develop an adult, heel–toe gait until at least 42 months. What is remarkable, however, is that despite the fact that we all learn to walk without instruction; there is very little deviation from the norm. Sutherland and colleagues (1988) suggested that walking is "instinctive rather than cognitive" and is dependent upon progressive maturation of the central nervous system. Contrast this with other activities such as swinging a golf club or throwing a ball in which individuals have their own unique style and no built-in system of optimization exists.

A number of authors have studied energy expenditure as a function of walking-speed and found that if the curve of energy cost is plotted on the ordinate versus speed on the abscissa, the curve is parabolic. As such it exhibits a minimum value at a particular speed (Fig. 4.9) (Rose et al. 1994). Dr H.J. Ralston is credited with the hypothesis that if a person

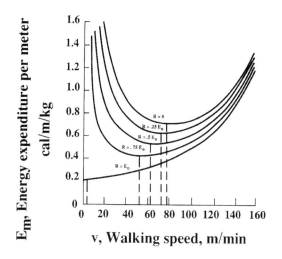

Fig. 4.9. Gross energy expenditure per meter as a function of walking-speed (V) for a typical subject walking naturally at different speeds. The lower curves show that as increasing amounts of energy (R) are subtracted from the gross energy expenditure per minute, the optimal speed corresponding to minimal Em becomes smaller and smaller. (Reproduced from Rose J, Ralston HJ, Gamble JG, 1994, Energetics of walking. In: Rose J, Gamble JG, editors, *Human Walking*, 2nd edn. Baltimore: Williams and Wilkins. p. 45–72, by permission.)

is allowed to walk at her/his natural rate, s/he will select a speed that allows minimum energy expenditure (see Inman et al. 1981). The hypothesis was confirmed by Corcoran and Brengelmann (1970). To my mind this also explains why gait is so uniform, i.e. during walking the body integrates the motion of the various segments such that energy expenditure is minimized. Winter (1991) noted that with increasing linear velocity, the angular velocities of the hip, knee, and ankle increase in nearly identical proportions. He also noted that the timing of the power patterns during the gait cycle is identical at all walking-speeds and only the gain increases with cadence. Both of these observations give evidence to a finely tuned proprioceptive feedback system. The other inference, which can be drawn from Ralston's hypothesis, is that any deviation of gait from the norm will interfere with this mechanism and therefore increase energy cost.

The gait cycle
When dealing with human gait it is conventional to do so in terms of the "gait cycle". A complete gait cycle or stride begins when one foot strikes the ground and ends when the same foot strikes the ground again. Perry (1992) subdivided the gait cycle according to phases, tasks, and periods. These periods include initial contact (IC), loading response (LR), mid-stance (MSt), terminal stance (TSt), pre-swing (PSw), mid-swing (MSw), and terminal swing (TSw) (Fig. 4.10). The cycle is divided into two major phases, stance and swing. Using Dr Perry's scheme, the three tasks that must be accomplished during the cycle are weight acceptance, single limb support, and limb advancement (Fig. 4.11). Weight acceptance occurs during the first two periods (IC and LR), single limb support during the second two

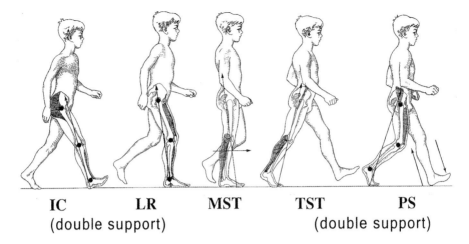

IC　　　　LR　　　　MST　　　TST　　　　PS
(double support)　　　　　　　　　(double support)

Fig. 4.10. The stance phase of gait. Stance phase constitutes roughly 60% of the cycle and is divided into five subphases: initial contact (IC), loading response (LR), mid-stance (MST), terminal stance (TST) and pre-swing (PS).

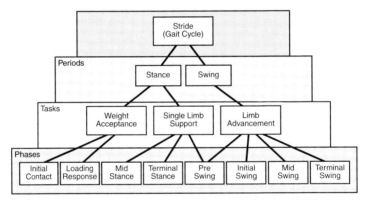

Fig. 4.11. The gait cycle consists of one stride, which is subdivided into two periods, stance and swing. The tasks that must be accomplished during a single cycle include weight acceptance, single-limb support and limb advancement. These occur during the phases shown in the bottom row (Adapted from Perry 1992, by permission.)

(MSt and TSt), and limb advancement during the final four (IS, PS, MSw, and TSw). Stance phase begins with initial contact, which in normal gait is with the heel, and ends at toe-off when swing phase begins. Events in the gait cycle are defined sequentially as occurring at specific percentages of the cycle. Initial contact is defined as occurring at 0% and 100% of the gait cycle. During normal walking, toe-off occurs at approximately 60% of the cycle. Therefore stance represents approximately 60% of the gait cycle and swing 40%. Opposite toe-off and opposite heel strike occur at 10% and 50% of the cycle respectively. This means that during walking there must be two periods of "double support" when both feet are on the ground and that each of these periods constitutes about 10% of the cycle. The first

52

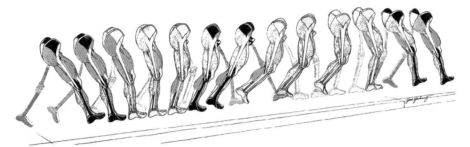

Fig. 4.12. A schematic of the complete gait cycle. Muscle activity is denoted by the intensity of color. Note that most of the muscles are active at the beginning and end of swing and stance phases from (Reproduced from Inman VT, Ralston HJ, Todd F, 1981, Human walking. In Lieberman JC, editor. *Human Walking*. Baltimore: Williams, p85–117, by permission.)

period occurs immediately after initial contact and the second just prior to toe-off. Loading response is a period of deceleration when the shock of impact is absorbed. This is followed by a period of single stance occupying about 40% of the cycle during which the opposite limb is going through its swing phase. Thus, in walking, single support on the stance side must be equal to the period of swing of the opposite limb. In late stance there is a second period of double support called pre-swing which begins at approximately 50% of the gait cycle and lasts until toe-off on the stance side. Therefore loading response is equivalent in time and is, in fact, the same event as pre-swing on the opposite side. Since normal gait is symmetrical, it is important to remember these relationships in order to form a mental picture of where the opposite limb is in the cycle. The period of single stance can be subdivided into mid-stance and terminal stance. During mid-stance, the body's center of mass is decelerating as it climbs to its zenith and passes over the base of support. In terminal stance the center of mass has passed in front of the base of support and is accelerating as it falls forward and toward the unsupported side. During this period of acceleration an amount of energy equivalent to that lost earlier in the gait cycle must be added back into the cycle if steady-state walking is to be maintained. Walking has been likened to the action of a pendulum, whereas running has been compared to the action of a pogo-stick. Notice that in walking the activity of muscles tend to be concentrated at the beginning and end of swing and stance phases, since their principal actions seem to be to accelerate and decelerate the pendulum movements of the legs (Fig. 4.12).

In swing phase, the swinging limb behaves as a compound pendulum and as such the period of swing is determined by the mass moment of inertia of its segments (Hicks et al. 1985, Tashman et al. 1985). If the swing period of the pendulum could not be altered, variation of cadence during gait would be impossible. In order to accelerate cadence, the swinging compound pendulum must be accelerated early in swing and then decelerated in the latter part of swing. As such, swing must consist of three periods: a period in which the rate of swing can be altered (accelerated or decelerated), a transition period, and a final period in which the alteration is reversed. These three periods are known as initial swing, mid-swing, and terminal swing (Fig. 4.13).

Running is differentiated from walking by the fact that the two periods of "double support"

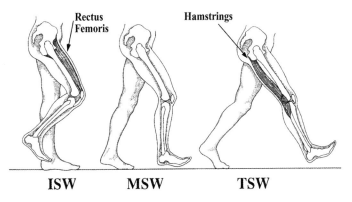

Fig. 4.13. Swing phase consists of three periods known as initial swing, mid-swing and terminal swing. Mid-swing is a switching period when no muscles are active. During running or fast walking, the rectus femoris accelerates the shank in initial swing, while the hamstrings decelerate it in terminal swing.

are replaced by periods of "double float" when neither foot is on the ground. To accommodate the periods of "double float" during running, therefore, the period of time spent in stance must always be shorter than the time spent in swing. (Fig. 4.14).

Temporal gait measurements

Further characterization of the gait cycle can be done with temporal measurements such as walking velocity, cadence, step length and stride length. Step length is defined as the longitudinal distance between the two feet. Thus the right step length is measured from the point of contact of the trailing left foot to the point of contact of the right foot. One stride length is the distance covered during a complete gait cycle and represents the sum of the right and left step lengths, or stated another way; it extends from the initial contact of one foot to the following initial contact of the same foot. Walking velocity is usually expressed in centimeters/second or meters/minute and is equal to step length times cadence.

Components of the gait cycle during stance phase

As mentioned earlier, the stance phase of walking can be broken down into five separate parts, while swing phase can be broken down into three. Each of these subphases has a specific purpose and is marked by particular events in the gait cycle. Consequently, we now need to spend a bit of time looking at the purpose and mechanism of each of these gait segments.

The foot rockers

Perry has described the action of the ankle and foot during *loading-response*, *mid-stance*, and *terminal stance* in stance in terms of three rockers (Fig. 4.15) (Perry 1992). The *first rocker* (heel rocker) begins at initial contact and extends through loading response. In normal gait the fulcrum of this rocker is the heel. Posterior protrusion of the heel creates a lever equal to 25% of the foot's total length. Because the GRF acting on this lever is passing through the heel at initial contact, its immediate effect is to thrust the entire foot towards

WALKING

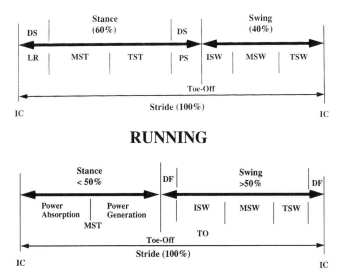

RUNNING

Fig. 4.14. Walking (above) versus running (below). Walking features two periods of double support (DS) when both feet are on the ground. In running these are replaced by two periods of "double float" (DF) when neither foot is on the ground. Thus, in walking, stance always occupies more than 50% of the gait cycle, whereas stance is always less than 50% in running. LR, loading response; MST, mid-stance; TST, terminal stance; PS, pre-swing; ISW, initial swing; MSW, mid-swing; TSW, terminal swing; IC, initial contact; TO, toe-off.

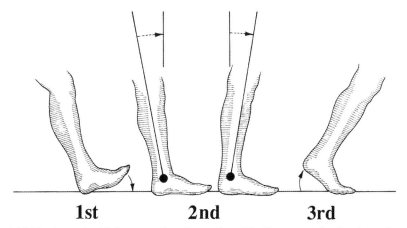

1st   2nd   3rd

Fig. 4.15. The foot and ankle in stance: three foot-rockers. The first two are deceleration rockers and so their respective muscles are acting eccentrically, i.e. undergoing a lengthening contraction with energy absorption (negative work). Third rocker is an acceleration rocker and so the plantarflexors must act concentrically, i.e. produce positive work. Notice that the point of application of the ground reaction force is forced to move forward with each successive rocker, thus allowing the center of mass to move forward with it.

the floor. This external moment is resisted by the internal moment of the pre-tibial muscles (tibialis anterior, extensor digitorum longus, and peroneus tertius) as they undergo controlled, eccentric contraction. Eccentric (lengthening) contraction is always associated with deceleration. Remember that the body has been accelerated by gravity as it fell from its zenith at mid-stance to its nadir at loading response so that the total force on the limb as it impacts the floor is about 120% of body weight. Thus the purpose of first rocker is shock absorption, i.e. to decelerate the body's inertia at initial contact.

Mid-stance begins with the entire plantar surface of the foot is in contact with the floor. The ground reaction force has passed anterior to the center of the ankle joint and is now producing a dorsiflexor moment that must be resisted by the ankle plantarflexors. This restraint comes chiefly from eccentric contraction of the slow-twitch soleus muscle with later assistance by the gastrocnemius and long toe-flexors. This is the period of *second rocker* (ankle rocker), during which the fulcrum has moved from the heel to the center of the ankle joint as the tibia hinges forward on the stationary foot. The purpose of second rocker is to control the position of the ground reaction force referable to the joints above. Since the ground reaction force is now anterior to the knee, it acts to extend the knee against the posterior capsule. Since the knee is stable in full extension, joint extension can now be maintained without quadriceps action. In a similar manner, if the ground reaction force is posterior to the hip, the hip is also stable in extension against the iliofemoral ligament. In normal gait, this situation occurs in the latter half of mid-stance.

Towards the end of mid-stance, the combined action of the plantarflexors act to arrest the forward progression of the tibia. This forces the fulcrum of the pivot forward to the metatarsal heads as the heel rises off the ground. Thus, in *third rocker* (forefoot rocker), the fulcrum has moved forward from the ankle to the metatarsal heads. The action of the plantarflexors has now switched from eccentric to concentric. By definition, concentric contraction of muscle produces acceleration. The necessity for this acceleration is apparent if one remembers that in steady-state walking the sum of the forces and the moments is equal to zero. Thus the deceleration of the first two rockers must be balanced by the acceleration produced by the third. Pre-swing begins with the onset of double support at the conclusion of opposite swing. The accelerative force of third rocker peaks at the end of terminal stance and then falls rapidly to zero by the end of pre-swing (Õunpuu et al. 1991) (Fig. 4.16).

Components of the gait cycle during swing phase
Swing phase constitutes 38% of the gait cycle. It is divided into initial swing, mid-swing, and terminal swing. The purpose of swing is: (1) to advance the limb, (2) to provide foot clearance, (3) to allow variation in cadence, and (4) to conserve energy.

Consequently in order for swing to occur in a normal fashion, several prerequisites must be met. (1) The hip, knee, and ankle must flex sufficiently to allow adequate clearance (at least 60° of knee flexion needed in initial swing to clear the toe). (2) Since the duration of swing varies in proportion to cadence, a mechanism is needed to allow this. (3) Muscles need to provide adequate power to carry the limb through swing and to alter the period of swing. (4) Energy transfers between body segments are necessary in order to conserve

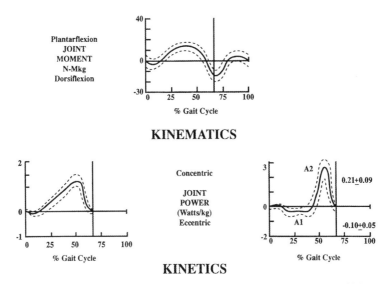

KINEMATICS

KINETICS

Fig. 4.16. An illustration of the kinematics and kinetics of the normal ankle. The units of joint moments and powers are Newton meters and watts respectively. A plantarflexor moment begins at the end of loading response, reaches its peak at terminal stance, and then rapidly falls to zero during pre-swing (double support). Power is obtained by multiplying the moment times the joint angular velocity. The sign convention is such that a negative power indicates negative work, i.e. the muscle is contracting eccentrically and absorbing energy. Positive power indicates that the muscle is contracting and performing positive work, i.e. producing acceleration. The numbers on the right of the power graph are an integration of all positive and negative powers ±1 S.D. and represent the total work done in joules. Hence the total positive work done during one gait cycle is 0.21 ± 0.09 joules/kg. Kinematics and kinetics will be discussed in detail in Chapters 7 and 8.

energy and minimize the work of walking.

During swing phase, the lower-extremity functions as a compound pendulum. That is, the period of time that it takes the swinging limb to go through to through its arch of motion is constant unless internal or external forces act upon it. In physics, the period (the time it takes a pendulum to go through one full swing arc) is given by the formula:

$$T = 2\pi \sqrt{I_a/mgh}$$

where T = the period of the pendulum (leg), Ia = the mass moment of inertia of the leg, m = mass, g = acceleration due to gravity, and h = distance from point of suspension to the center of mass.

At our "normal" or "usual" speed and cadence of walking, the period of passive swing depends upon the mass moment of inertia of the shank (Fig. 4.17). That is, we all select a walking-speed at which our limb swings freely (without extraneous muscle action) so that the amount of energy expended is minimal. This concept was discussed earlier in this chapter when we discussed energy conservation as one of the five prerequisites of normal gait. When we accelerate or decelerate the normal pendulum swing of our lower limb, muscle action is required. If walking-speed is to be increased, kinetic energy must be increased. Therefore the muscles that accelerate the limb (the ankle-plantarflexors and hip-

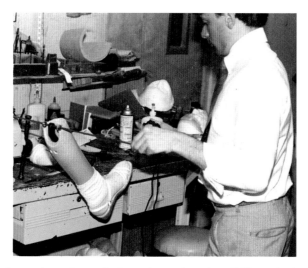

Fig. 4.17. A simple experiment that can be done using an above-knee (AK) prosthesis with a single-axis knee. The leg acts like a pendulum and its period is dictated by its mass moment of inertia. Since the lower-extremity functions as a compound pendulum in gait, the period of the pendulum (in this case the shank) will be equal to the cadence of the individual to whom it belongs. Given that the cadence of swing is usually found to be much lower than normal in these experiments, a strong argument could be made to bring the mass moment of inertia closer to the fulcrum by minimizing the weight distally and/or adding weight proximally.

flexors) must provide more energy. Because the knee is caught between these two forces, it will flex excessively in a manner similar to an above-knee amputee's prosthetic knee joint that lacks sufficient friction. However, the period of flexion will not change. During rapid gait, therefore, the amount of knee flexion must be limited and the period of knee flexion must be shortened. This is accomplished by active muscle action of the biarticular muscles that cross the knee (the rectus femoris and the hamstrings). Because the rectus femoris originates from the anterior–inferior spine of the ileum and inserts into the patella, when it contracts isometrically, it acts to limit flexion of the knee and augment flexion of the hip. Essentially it acts like a spring or a semi-elastic strap to carry the inertial energy of the shank up to the hip where is can be used to flex the hip. Its major period of activity is during pre-swing and initial swing.

Swing phase has been subdivided into three periods: (1) initial swing, (2) mid-swing, and (3) terminal swing.

Summary of muscle action in the sagittal plane during gait

Perry has pointed out that there is a coordinated flow of muscle activity in normal walking during stance and swing, which in general, starts proximally and flows distally (Fig. 4.18). During walking these muscles are sequentially activated in response to the stance and swing demands that are imposed on the limb. She feels that the simple classifications of the past in which muscles are classified as acting at the hip, knee, ankle or foot are inadequate since, in walking, the total limb requirements require a subtle overlap of muscle functions. She

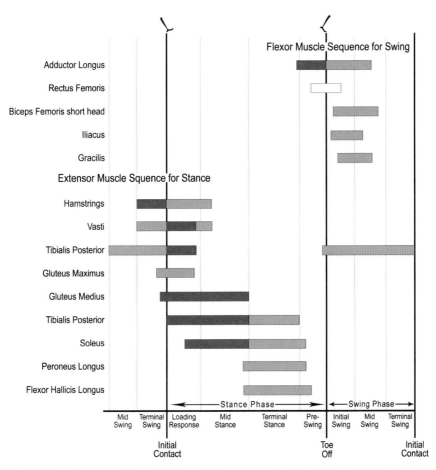

Fig. 4.18. Perry's concept of muscle flow, which starts proximally and flows distally. According to Perry, there are two periods of transition when this sequential activation is initiated, which are terminal swing and pre-swing. The former is the transition from swing-to-stance and the latter from stance-to-swing.

further points out that two phases of gait are devoted to the transition from swing-to-stance and stance-to-swing: these are terminal swing and pre-swing, respectively. Because of this, when Perry (1988) discusses muscle function, she begins the gait cycle with terminal swing rather than initial contact. The following is a list of the muscle activities during each of the subphases of gait. The period of activity is taken from Perry's data, although I have modified the muscle actions in some cases based on our work and the work of others with joint kinetics (Anderson and Pandy 2003)

Stance-phase limb control
1. TERMINAL SWING (Fig. 4.19)
Muscle function
Muscle control ends swing and prepares limb for stance.

59

Fig. 4.19. Terminal swing. The color of the muscle denotes the type of its activity (green, concentric contraction; red, eccentric contraction; yellow, isometric contraction). The illustration illustrates rapid gait. Note that the hamstrings are yellow (isometric) because they are acting like elastic straps to slow the rate of extension of the knee and accelerate the rate of extension of the hip. That is, they are absorbing or harnessing the kinetic energy of the shank and transferring it up to the hip. This is one of the body's methods of conserving energy.

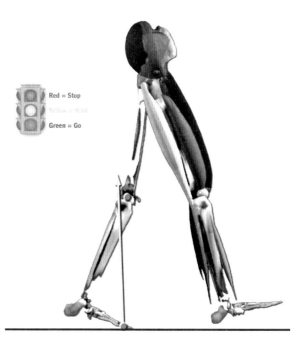

Red = Stop
Yellow = Hold
Green = Go

Specific muscle actions

Hip-flexors: these muscles are usually not active at this time.

Hamstrings: action on hip and knee decelerates the forward swing of the thigh and leg during rapid gait.

Quadriceps: knee extension in slow gait extends the limb for stance.

Tibialis anterior: ankle dorsiflexion supports ankle at neutral to prevent foot drop and maintains heel in proper position for contact.

Synopsis of activity

With the onset of terminal swing, eccentric hamstring activity begins to decelerate both the hip and knee. Terminal swing is the analog of initial swing and so again, three muscle states are possible.

(1) Normal walking-speed: the limb swings passively with no muscles activity except the tibialis anterior, which is working as an accelerator to lift the foot out of equinus.

(2) Slow walking-speed: hip and knee extension must be augmented. This is accomplished by action of the vasti and/or the rectus femoris.

(3) Rapid walking-speed: hip and knee extension must be restrained. As the rectus femoris acted to restrain knee flexion in initial swing, the foot and shank was negatively accelerated. In the same way, without the action of the hamstrings, there would be excessive stress on the posterior cruciate ligament and knee capsule during rapid gait. The hamstrings are also biarticular muscles that insert proximal to the hip joint, so the inertial energy of the shank is again carried up to the hip, which has the beneficial effect of augmenting hip

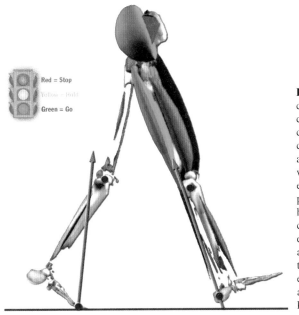

Red = Stop
Yellow = Hold
Green = Go

Fig. 4.20. Initial contact. The same color convention is used (green, concentric contraction; red, eccentric contraction; yellow, isometric contraction). The quadriceps and anterior tibial musculature are working eccentrically to limit (decelerate) knee flexion and ankle plantarflexion respectively. The hamstrings and gluteus maximus are contracting concentrically as hip-extensors. Although the hamstrings are biarticular muscles, they are able to work as accelerators of the lower extremity at the hip because the vasti are preventing their action at the knee.

extension while still conserving energy. This phenomenon can easily be observed in an above-knee amputee if the friction at the knee joint is excessively reduced. In initial swing there is excessive knee flexion and in terminal swing the knee is driven into extension with a loud snap or bang. I have always considered this beautiful mechanism as a small testament to the cleverness of our Creator. The whole thing could have been accomplished with monoarticular muscles, but then the muscles would have had to transfer their absorbed energy to the bone in the form of heat. The unfortunate result would not only be excessive energy consumption during running, but also "hot thighs".

2. INITIAL CONTACT (Fig. 4.20)
Muscle function
Muscles act to allow smooth progression and stabilize joints while simultaneously decelerating body's inertia.

Specific muscle actions
Gluteus maximus: controls flexor moment produced by ground reaction forces.
Hamstrings: inhibit knee hyperextension and assists in controlling flexion moment at hip.
Tibialis anterior: initiates the heel rocker.

Synopsis of activity
Initial contact begins the gait cycle when the lead foot contacts the floor. As such it is an

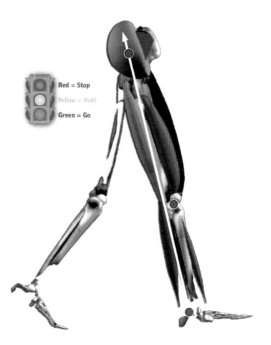

Red = Stop

Yellow = Hold

Green = Go

Fig. 4.21. Loading response. The purpose of loading response is shock absorption. The vasti and tibialis anterior muscles are acting eccentrically during the period of first rocker as shock absorbers at the knee and ankle respectively. The gluteus maximus and hamstrings continue to work as accelerators at the hip (green, concentric contraction; red, eccentric contraction; yellow, isometric contraction).

instantaneous event that occurs when the lead foot contacts the ground or floor. Since the trailing foot is still on the ground, this initiates the beginning of double support. In normal walking initial contact is made with the heel and as such the ground reaction force is posterior to the ankle and knee joints, and at or slightly anterior to the hip joint. Because the control system anticipates the forces that the ground reaction will deliver, the hip-extensors, vasti, ankle-dorsiflexors, and toe extensors are all active and ready to absorb the force of impact.

3. LOADING RESPONSE (Fig. 4.21)

MUSCLE FUNCTION

Muscles act to allow smooth progression and stabilize joints while simultaneously decelerating body's inertia.

Specific muscle actions

Hamstrings: concentric action unlocks the knee; the magnitude of their action is low and their intensity brief.

Tibialis anterior: decelerates foot fall and pulls the tibia anterior to the body's weight line which results in knee flexion.

Quadriceps: act as eccentric knee-extensors to decelerate flexion and absorb the shock of floor contact.

Gluteus maximus: acts concentrically as a hip-extensor to accelerate the trunk over the femur. Its action through the iliotibial band contributes to knee extension.

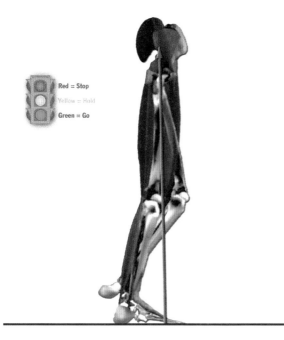

Red = Stop

Yellow = Hold

Green = Go

Fig. 4.22. Mid-stance. The purpose of mid-stance is energy conservation. Since the GRF is now anterior to the knee-joint center, the forefoot acts like a lever to push the knee back into extension so that the knee is stabilized by the posterior capsule thereby obviating the need for muscle action of the vasti. The only muscle action that is required to accomplish this is eccentric action of the soleus.

Adductor magnus: acts to advance and internally rotate the pelvis on the stance limb.

Gluteus medius: eccentric action as hip abductor stabilizes pelvis to minimize contralateral pelvic drop.

Synopsis of activity

The purpose of loading response is shock absorption or weight acceptance. It begins when the foot touches the floor and lasts until opposite toe-off. In the motion analysis laboratory, the force plate registers about 120% of body weight at this phase of the gait cycle. The extra 20% represents the inertial force of the falling body that must be decelerated. This is accomplished via eccentric contraction of the ankle dorsiflexors and long toe-extensors at the ankle and the vastus medialis, lateralis, and intermedius at the knee (the rectus femoris is not active at this time). The hip does not participate in this deceleration. On the contrary, since double support is the nadir or lowest point of the body during the gait cycle, the gluteus maximus and hamstrings act concentrically at the hip to provide the energy needed to provide forward propulsion and to lift the body up to its high point in mid-stance. Loading response is also known as the period of "*first rocker*" or "*heel rocker*". During loading response, the opposite limb is in pre-swing.

4. MID-STANCE (Fig. 4.22)

Muscle function

Muscles act to allow smooth progression over a stationary foot while simultaneously controlling the position of the GRF referable to the hip and knee.

Fig. 4.23. Terminal stance. The color of the calf has now changed from red to green (green, concentric contraction; red, eccentric contraction; yellow, isometric contraction). Since the gastrocnemius has now joined the soleus, their resultant force is sufficient to drive the ankle into plantarflexion. The force generated by the triceps surae in terminal stance accounts for about 50% of the total propulsive power needed in walking. Note too that the ground reaction force has now moved behind the hip joint thereby generating a hip-extension moment that renders the joint stable against the iliofemoral (Bigalow's) ligament. Consequently gluteus maximus activity is no longer required for stability.

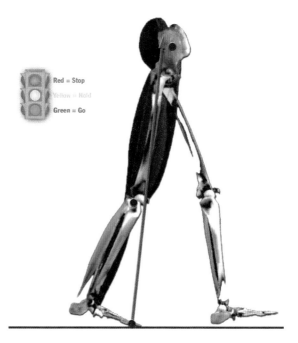

Red = Stop
Yellow = Hold
Green = Go

Specific muscle actions

Soleus: this muscle, which is made up primarily of slow-twitch fibers, acts eccentrically to decelerate ankle dorsiflexion thereby stabilizing the tibia during the period of second rocker.

Quadriceps: stabilize the flexed knee. Their action ceases as soon as the GRF vector passes in front of the knee.

Gluteus maximus: muscle ceases to act at the point at which the GRF passes posterior to the hip.

Synopsis of activity

Mid-stance constitutes the first half of single limb support. It begins with toe-off of the contralateral limb and ends with heel-rise on the ipsilateral side. The purpose of mid-stance is energy conservation. The muscles act to allow smooth progression over the stationary foot while simultaneously controlling the position of the GRF referable to the hip and knee. This is accomplished via eccentric contraction of the ankle plantarflexors (principally the soleus), which act to retard forward motion of the tibia. This in turn allows the GRF to pass in front of the knee so that it acts to produce an extension moment at that joint. Once the knee joint has been stabilized by the GRF, the action of the quadriceps is no longer needed. Consequently the vastus muscles are quiescent during mid-stance. As the body moves forward over the planted foot, the GRF moves posterior to the hip. When this occurs, the hip becomes stable, because the anterior capsule (Bigalow's ligament) limits further hip extension. Consequently, hip extensor activity ceases during mid-stance as well. Mid-stance is also known as the period of "*second rocker*" or "*ankle rocker*". During mid-stance, the opposite limb is in mid-swing.

5. TERMINAL STANCE (Fig. 4.23)
Muscle function
Muscles act to provide acceleration and adequate step length.

Specific muscle actions
Soleus: intensity of action increases to limit ankle dorsiflexion. It also acts as an inverter of the subtalar joint to provide stability against eversion forces.

Gastrocnemius: this muscle, which is made up primarily of fast-twitch fibers, acts as an accelerator to stop forward motion of the tibia and begin active plantarflexion of the ankle. This provides the necessary power to advance the limb and flex the knee. The gastrocsoleus complex provides about 50% of the acceleration force necessary to maintain steady state walking.

Tibialis posterior: acts as a strong inverter to stabilize the foot against eversion forces.

Peroneals: act as an everter to stabilize the foot against inversion forces.

Long toe-flexors: stabilize the MP joints thereby adding toe support to augment forefoot support.

Synopsis of activity
Terminal stance constitutes the second half of single-limb support. It begins with heel-rise of the ipsilateral limb and ends with initial contact on the contralateral side. The purpose of mid-stance is propulsion. The muscles act to provide forward and upward acceleration of the limb and trunk. At the ankle the gastrocnemius and long toe-flexors have joined the soleus to produce enough force to arrest dorsiflexion and initiate active ankle plantarflexion. This provides the necessary power to advance the limb and flex the knee. The tibialis posterior and peroneals are also active to stabilize the foot against eversion and inversion forces respectively. Since weightbearing is now occurring mainly on the forefoot, the long toe-flexors act to stabilize the metatarsal–phalangeal joints thereby adding toe support to augment forefoot support. The combined actions of the muscles of the posterior calf generate nearly half of the total propulsive force needed for walking. Terminal-stance is also known as the period of "third rocker" or "forefoot rocker". During terminal-stance, the opposite limb is in terminal swing.

Swing-phase limb control
6. PRE-SWING (Fig. 4.24)
Muscle function
Muscle control ends stance and prepares limb for swing.

Specific muscle actions
Gastrocnemius: during its brief period of activity it unlocks the knee so knee flexion can begin.

Psoas: acts to advance thigh and works in conjunction with shank inertia to create knee flexion.

Adductor longus: since the pelvis is oblique to the line of progression, concentric action of this muscle acts to advance the thigh. Knee flexion follows by tibial inertia.

Fig. 4.24. Pre-swing. Muscle activity here depends upon the rate of cadence. In slow gait, knee flexion has to be augmented; in rapid gait it has to be restrained. Augmentation is brought about by concentric action of the sartorius, gracilis, and/or short head of biceps femoris. Restraint is accomplished by isometric action of the rectus femoris, which acts like an isometric strap to decelerate the knee and transfer the kinetic energy of the shank proximally to augment hip flexion. Rapid gait is pictured here (green, concentric contraction; red, eccentric contraction; yellow, isometric contraction).

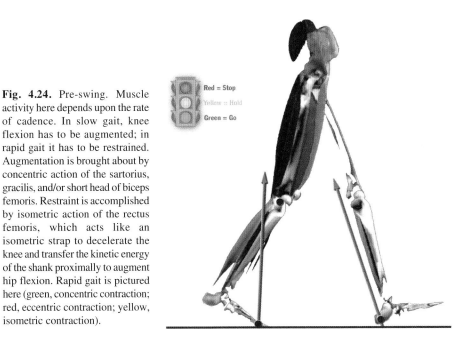

Red = Stop
Yellow = Hold
Green = Go

Rectus femoris: this biarticular muscle acts eccentrically during rapid gait. Via isometric action, its distal end decelerates the inertia of the shank. At the muscles proximal end, it acts to augment hip flexion. In essence then it is acting to transfer energy, which would otherwise be wasted, from the shank to the hip.

Synopsis of activity

Pre-swing begins when the swinging foot strikes the ground and two limbs once again support the individual. The purpose of pre-swing is to prepare the stance limb for swing by transferring weight from the trailing limb to the front limb. Body weight and inertia move rapidly forward on to the front limb. Residual body weight on the trailing limb has moved forward to the forefoot; so that the GRF is now well behind the knee, thus creating a strong flexion moment. The gastrocsoleus complex is just completing its activity and the force it has imparted to the trailing limb is driving it forward and upward. Furthermore, at the instant the knee started to flex, the action of the gastrocnemius switched from ankle plantarflexion to knee flexion, since it spans both joints. At the upper end of the femur, the hip-flexors and the superficial adductors (adductor longus, brevis and gracilis) are pulling the hip into flexion, which also has the effect of producing knee flexion. Thus the knee, driven from the inertial forces of ankle plantarflexion and hip flexion, begins to flex rapidly. It addition a knee flexion moment is produced by the gastrocnemius. At normal speed and cadence, the knee flexion produced by these forces drives the knee into about 60° of flexion, which is just enough to just enough to clear the swinging foot. During rapid gait, these forces are excessive, and so knee flexion must be restrained. With slow cadence the forces are inadequate and so knee flexion must

66

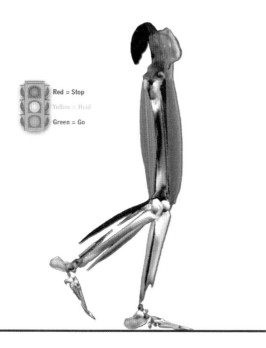

Red = Stop
Yellow = Hold
Green = Go

Fig. 4.25. Initial swing (slow gait). Knee and hip flexion are augmented by concentric action of the sartorius and gracilis. The short head of the biceps can also work concentrically to augment knee flexion during slow gait (green, concentric contraction; red, eccentric contraction; yellow, isometric contraction).

be augmented. Knee-flexion restraint is provided by isometric action of the rectus femoris in pre-swing and initial swing and by the hamstrings in terminal swing (Piazza and Delp 1996). With slow cadence, the sartorius, gracilis, and/or short head of the biceps femoris augment knee flexion in pre-swing and initial swing. Since they span both the hip and the knee, the first two muscles also act simultaneously to augment hip flexion. However augmentation of knee flexion in initial swing means that extension of the knee must also be augmented in terminal swing. During slow walking, this can be accomplished by concentric action of the rectus femoris and/or the vasti. Since the rectus femoris spans both the knee and the ankle, it will assist in hip flexion. During pre-swing, the opposite limb is in loading-response.

7. INITIAL SWING (Figs 4.25, 4.26)
Muscle function
Muscle control provides the ability to vary cadence and maintain foot clearance. Foot clearance is accomplished by muscle action that acts to increase the range of knee flexion in slow gait and limit knee flexion in rapid gait.

Specific muscle actions
Hip-flexor group: the iliacus, adductor longus, sartorius and gracilis act to advance the thigh and work in conjunction with shank inertia to create knee flexion.

    Rectus femoris: isometric action restrains knee flexion and augments hip flexion during rapid gait.

    Biceps femoris: short head of biceps along with sartorius and gracilis augments knee

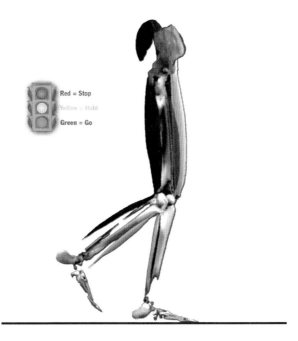

Red = Stop
Yellow = Hold
Green = Go

Fig. 4.26. Initial swing (fast gait). The rectus femoris is working as an isometric strap to restrain knee flexion and augment hip flexion. In a sprinter the periods of gastrocnemius and rectus femoris activity are probably less than 0.1 second, which demands a great deal of precision from the control system; therefore it is not surprising that these muscles almost always function abnormally in spastic diplegia.

flexion during slow gait, when inertial forces are inadequate.

Tibialis anterior and long toe-flexors: work concentrically as dorsiflexors to lift the foot out of plantarflexion.

Synopsis of activity

Initial swing begins at toe-off and ends as the swinging limb passes the stance limb. Depending on the speed of walking, one of three muscle states will occur during initial swing.

(1) Normal walking-speed: the limb swings passively with no muscles activity except the tibialis anterior, which works as an accelerator to lift the foot out of equinus.

(2) Slow walking-speed: hip and knee flexion must be augmented. This is accomplished by action of the hip-flexors and the knee-flexors (the specific muscles that act at the knee are the sartorius, gracilis, and/or short head of the biceps) (Fig. 4.25)

(3) Rapid walking-speed: hip and knee flexion must be restrained. From terminal stance through pre-swing, increased power to supply the kinetic energy necessary to increase the limb's velocity was provided by the triceps surae and the hip-flexors. However, now the rectus femoris acts isometrically for a brief period to restrain the unwanted knee flexion that would otherwise result. That kinetic energy is transported up to the hip where it can be used to augment hip flexion. The period of required rectus femoris activity is about 20% of the gait cycle; so at a cadence of 120 steps per minute, the rectus femoris would be active for only 0.10 second. In terminal swing, the corresponding period of hamstring activity would be only slightly longer. Thus, to achieve normal gait, the control and timing of the biarticular muscles must be precise (Fig. 4.26).

68

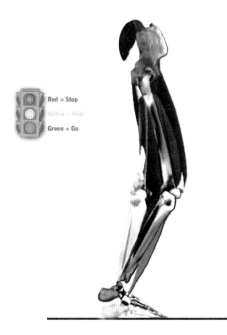

Red = Stop
Yellow = Hold
Green = Go

Fig. 4.27. Mid-swing is the switching period between acceleration and deceleration or vice versa. Inertial forces are propelling the limb, so very little muscle action is necessary.

8. MID-SWING (Fig. 4.27)

Muscle function

The switching period between acceleration and deceleration or vice versa. Inertial forces are propelling the limb, so very little muscle action is necessary.

Specific muscle actions

Tibialis anterior: supports ankle at neutral to prevent foot drop.

Synopsis of activity

Mid-swing is a switching period between the muscle activity that occurs in initial swing and the muscle activity in terminal swing, so there is no muscle activity across the knee-joint.

REFERENCES

Alexander RM. (1992) *The Human Machine*. London: Natural History Museum Publications.

Alway SE, MacDougall JD, Sale DG, Sutton JR, McComas AJ. (1988) Functional and structural adaptations in skeletal muscle of trained athletes. *J Appl Physiol* **64:** 1114–1120.

Anderson FC, Pandy MG. (2003) Individual muscle contributions to support in normal walking. *Gait Posture* **17:** 159–169.

Brooke MH, Kaiser KK. (1970a) Three "myosin adenosine triphosphatase" systems: the nature of their pH lability and sulfhydryl dependence. *J Histochem Cytochem* **18:** 670–672.

Brooke MH, Kaiser KK. (1970b) Three human myosin ATPase systems and their importance in muscle pathology. *Neurology* **20:** 404–405.

Burke RE, Levine DN, Tsairis P, Zajac FE 3rd. (1973) Physiological types and histochemical profiles in motor units of the cat gastrocnemius. *J Physiol* **234:** 723–748.

Cavagna GA, Dusman B, Margaria R. (1968) Positive work done by a previously stretched muscle. *J Appl Physiol* **24:** 21–32.

Corcoran PJ, Brengelmann GL. (1970) Oxygen uptake in normal and handicapped subjects, in relation to speed of walking beside velocity-controlled cart. *Arch Phys Med Rehabil* **51:** 78–87.

Gage GT. (1991) *Gait Analysis in Cerebral Palsy,* London: Mac Keith Press. p 61–95.

Hicks R, Tashman S, Cary JM, Altman RF, Gage JR. (1985) Swing phase control with knee friction in juvenile amputees. *J Orthop Res* **3:** 198–201.

Inman VT, Ralston HJ, Todd F. (1981) Human walking. In: Lieberman JC, editor. *Human Walking.* Baltimore: Williams and Wilkins. p 85–117.

Lieber RL. (1986) Skeletal muscle adaptability. I: Review of basic properties. *Dev Med Child Neurol* **28:** 390–397.

Õunpuu S, Gage JR, Davis RB. (1991) Three-dimensional lower extremity joint kinetics in normal pediatric gait. *J Pediatr Orthop* **11:** 341–349.

Perry J. (1985) Normal and pathologic gait. In: Bunch WH, editor. *Atlas of Orthotics,* 2nd edn. St Louis: C.V. Mosby. p 76–111.

Perry J. (1988) *Gait Analysis Instructional Course: normal muscle control sequence during walking.* Paper presented at the Annual Meeting of the American Academy of Cerebral Palsy and Developmental Medicine, Toronto, Canada.

Perry J. (1992) *Gait Analysis: Normal and Pathological Function.* Thorofare, NJ: Slack. p 1–19.

Piazza SJ, Delp SL. (1996) The influence of muscles on knee flexion during the swing phase of gait. *J Biomech* **29:** 723–733.

Rab GT. (1994) Muscle. In: Rose J, Gamble JG, editors. *Human Walking,* 2nd edn. Baltimore: Williams and Wilkins. p 101–122.

Rose J, Ralston HJ, Gamble JG. (1994) Energetics of walking. In: Rose J, Gamble JG, editors. *Human Walking,* 2nd edn. Baltimore: Williams and Wilkins. p 45–72.

Sutherland DH, Olshen R, Cooper L, Woo SL. (1980) The development of mature gait. *J Bone Joint Surg Am* **62:** 336-353.

Sutherland DH, Olshen RA, Biden EN, Wyatt M.P (1988) *The Development of Mature Walking.* London: Mac Keith Press.

Tashman S, Hicks R, Jendrejczyk D. (1985) Evaluation of a prosthetic shank with variable inertial properties. *Clin Prosthet Orthot* **9:** 23–25.

Winter DA. (1991) *The Biomechanics and Motor Control of Human Gait: Normal, Elderly, and Pathological,* 2nd edn. Waterloo: Ontario: University of Waterloo Press. p 31.

5
PHYSICAL ASSESSMENT AND OBSERVATIONAL GAIT ANALYSIS

Joyce Trost

Clinical evaluation

In the assessment of children with cerebral palsy, many pieces are needed to complete the puzzle. The best way to start is with a complete history and physical exam (Bleck 1987). Gait analysis is also a critical part of the assessment (Gage 1994). In order to prepare treatment plans and accurately assess outcomes of treatment, a balanced combination of history, detailed physical examination, observational gait analysis and computerized gait analysis must be interpreted together.

HISTORY TAKING

The history should include a collection of information regarding birth, developmental milestones, medical problems, surgical history, current physical therapy treatment, and patient and family expectations or goals. Current functional walking level at home, school and in the community, as well as other functional skills such as stair climbing, jumping and running may also have an effect on treatment plans and outcome analysis. An outcome evaluation tool entitled Functional Assessment Questionnaire (FAQ) has been developed at Gillette Children's to evaluate these skills (Novacheck et al. 2000). Please see the final chapter of this book for a complete discussion of this document.

Birth history and other medical problems are important pieces of information for accurate diagnosis. For example, treatment of spasticity using a rhizotomy is most effective when done on children with pure spasticity caused by damage to the pyramidal system (see Chapter 18). This is most often true in children born preterm, as discussed in Chapter 2. Developmental milestones give information regarding the maturity of a skill such as walking. When considering surgical treatment, it is important to obtain the actual operative reports of previous surgeries to accurately assess current deformities, iatrogenic deviations and necessary compensations. For example, if iatrogenic weakness of the soleus muscle was caused by heelcord lengthening, the treatment plan may be different from that recommended for primary soleus weakness.

PHYSICAL EXAMINATION

In the Center for Gait and Motion Analysis at Gillette Children's, we use a standard physical assessment form as part of the evaluation (Fig. 5.1). The physical examination has six main goals: (1) to determine strength and selective motor control of isolated muscle groups; (2)

Gillette Children's Specialty Healthcare
Physical Assessment

Name:
MR#:
DOB:

MOTION   SELECTIVITY, STRENGTH   FOOT POSITION

            R   L   R   L   R   L

HIPS   FOOT NON-WEIGHTBEARING
 Flexon   ___   ___   ___   ___   Subtalar neutral ___   ___
 Extension   ___   ___   Hindfoot pos.   ___   ___
 Thomas test ___   ___   Hindfoot motion
  knee 0   ___   ___   eversion   ___   ___
  knee 90   ___   ___   inversion   ___   ___
 Abduction   Midfoot motion   ___   ___
  hips ext   ___   ___   Forefoot pos.   ___   ___
  hips flx   ___   ___
 Adduction   ___   ___   Bunion def.   ___   ___
 Ober test   ___   ___   1st MTP DF   ___   ___
 Int rotation ___   ___
 Ext rotation ___   ___
 Anteversion ___   ___
                                                        FOOT WEIGHTBEARING
KNEE   Hindfoot pos.   ___   ___
 Extension   ___   ___   ___   ___   Midfoot pos.   ___   ___
 Flexion   Forefoot pos.   ___   ___
  prone   ___   ___   ___   ___
  supine   ___   ___   SPASTICITY (Ashworth scale)
 Popliteal angle
  unilateral ___   ___   Hip flexors   ___   ___
  bilateral ___   ___ | Selectivity grade key | Adductors   ___   ___
 HS Shift   ___   ___ | | Hamstrings   ___   ___
                            | 0 - Only patterned | Rectus femoris   ___   ___
 Extensor lag ___   ___ | movement observed | Plantarflexors   ___   ___
 Patella alta ___   ___ | | Posterior tibialis ___   ___
TIBIA | 1 - Partially isolated| Ankle clonus   ___   ___
 TF angle   ___   ___ | movement observed | _____
 BM axis   ___   ___ | | | ASHWORTH SCALE |
 2nd toe test ___   ___ | 2 - Completely isolated| | 1. No increase in tone |
                            | movement observed | | 2. Slight increase in tone|
ANKLE SUBTALAR: | | | 3. More marked increase in tone |
 Dorsiflexion | Range of Motion | | 4. Considerable increase in tone |
  Knee 90   ___   ___ | Neu = Neutral w/ Stretch| | 5. Affected part rigid |
  Knee 0   ___   ___   _____
 Confusion test ___ ___
 Plantarflexion ___ ___   ___   ___   POSTURE/TRUNK
 Ant tibialis   ___   ___
 Post tibiallis   ___   ___   Abdominal Strength   ___
 Peroneus longus   ___   ___   Back Extensor Strength ___
 Peroneus brevis   ___   ___
 Extensor hallucis longus   ___   ___   LEG LAXITY: ___   ___
 Flexor hallucis longus   ___   ___   LEG LENGTH: ___   ___

STANDING POSTURE:

COMMENTS:

Fig. 5.1. Physical examination is an important part of the problem-solving process. It is most helpful in measurements of torsional deformities, foot deformities and muscle tone.

to evaluate muscle tone and the influence of positional changes on tone; (3) to estimate the degree of static deformity and/or muscle contracture at each joint; (4) to assess torsional and other deformities of the bone; (5) to describe fixed and mobile foot deformities; and (6) to assess balance, equilibrium responses and standing posture.

Clinical examination has limitations and benefits. The information collected during a clinical examination is based on static examination where as functional activities such as walking are dynamic. Tone patterns often change significantly with the position of the child, whether s/he is moving or at rest, the level of excitement or irritability, or the time and/or day of the assessment. Objective evaluation of muscle strength is difficult to measure in small children and children with neurological impairments (Bohannon 1989). In addition, motor control is a subjective measurement that relies heavily on the experience and expertise of the examiner.

Clinicians who treat gait abnormalities are interested in the dynamic aspects of walking. However, physical examination can lead the interpretation of the gait data and is helpful in separating structural or functional problems from gait compensations or "coping responses" which children develop to circumvent their primary gait problems.

MUSCLE STRENGTH AND CONTROL

Strength evaluation is necessary and is extremely important to ensure optimal clinical outcomes. Muscle strength evaluation is done using the Kendall scale (Kendall et al. 1971). Children with cerebral palsy have an impaired ability to isolate and control movements. Therefore the muscle grading scale has been adapted by adding a selectivity scale that includes three levels of control: no ability to isolate movement (0), partially isolated movement (1), and complete isolation of movement (2).

During a static examination, a child with hemiplegia may not be able to actively dorsiflex his foot on the involved side without a mass flexion pattern including hip and knee flexion. On examination muscle strength may measure 3/5, but with a selectivity grade of 0/2. During gait analysis this child may have difficulty with clearance of his foot in early swing phase. In mid-swing, however, dorsiflexion with inversion occurs (Perry et al. 1978, Gage 1991). In this example, adequate knee flexion and dorsiflexion occur, but the timing is late when compared to a walk of a child with good motor control.

The inability to move the foot actively into plantarflexion or perform a heelrise with knees flexed would suggest weakness of the soleus. The most frequent iatrogenic cause of crouch gait is soleus weakness as a result of tendo-Achilles lengthening (TAL) (Gage 1991). A TAL will lengthen both the gastrocnemius and soleus muscles equally and allow excessive knee flexion in midstance phase. This occurs because the gastrocnemius, which is trying to assist the weakened soleus, also acts as a knee flexor.

Hamstring weakness can also contribute to crouch gait since these muscles are biarticular and act as extensors of the hip (Delp et al. 1990, Delp and Loan 1995). Strength and selectivity testing of the hip extensors, hip abductors and abdominal muscles can provide information on whether the deviations observed at the trunk and pelvis are primary (due to weakness and impaired control) or secondary (due to pathology occurring more distally in the limbs). Increased pelvic tilt and decreased hip extension in stance have many etiologies, which include hip extensor and abdominal weakness. This loss of proximal control allows the pelvis to rotate anteriorly during static standing and periods of the gait cycle when these muscle groups are unable to provide the needed control and power.

Muscle groups such as the quadriceps may become functionally long, due to biomechanical malalignments causing a stretch weakness at the end range of motion. Assessment of the active versus passive range of motion of a joint can give insight into true strength and control deficits.

Knee extensor lag as a measure of inadequate full range quadriceps strength is done with the hips in extension to eliminate the influence of hamstring tightness or shift.

Assessment is most easily done supine with legs hanging over the edge of the table. Ask the child to extend his knee fully without manual resistance and measure the angle of the missing range of motion. Children who walk with a crouch gait pattern may not have the ability to fully extend the knee at the end range of motion, but may have good isolation and strength through the rest of the range.

MUSCLE TONE

Tone is influenced by the degree of apprehension or excitement present in the patient as well as the position of the assessment. This will then affect the degree of both dynamic and sometimes false static contracture. To get the best overall assessment of variations in muscle tone and the interference on movement, several different practitioners should do an assessment on several different occasions. Time spent playing or talking with a child before and during the examination will often help with the accuracy of the examination.

When examining a child with cerebral palsy, it is important to determine the nature and extent of abnormal tone. As discussed in Chapter 3, spastic tone results from damage to the corticobulbar, reticulospinal and vestibulospinal tracts, and has certain characteristics that can be easily identified by history and clinical examination. Spasticity is velocity dependent, increasing with increased speed of movement. The modified Ashworth scale is used to quantify the severity of this type of movement disorder (Bohannon and Smith 1987).

Dyskinesias are defined as abnormal motor movements that are seen when the patient initiates a movement. The motor patterns and posture of patients with dyskinesias are secondary to inadequate regulation of muscle tone and coordination caused by damage to the extrapyramidal system (Kyllerman et al. 1982). When the patient is totally relaxed, usually in the supine position, a full range of motion and decreased muscle tone is evident. Increased deep tendon reflexes are invariably increased in spasticity, but are normal or diminished in disorders of the extrapyramidal system. Patients with dyskinesia are subdivided into two subgroups.

The children with *hyperkinetic or choreoathetoid motor impairment* have massive involuntary movements with motor overflow. That is, the initiation of a movement of one extremity leads to movement of other muscle groups. Posturing of the fingers or limbs is frequently present, particularly when attempting to carry out a voluntary activity.

Patients with *dystonia* have abnormal shifts of general muscle tone induced by movement. Typically, abnormal and distorted postures are assumed and retained in the same stereotyped patterns. Dystonia may be confused with spasticity, because passive range of motion in both situations may be difficult and limited. Examining the patient in the supine position commonly will not alter the muscle tone in the spastic patient, but usually will reveal low tone in the patient with dystonia. Moving a joint with dystonic rigidity produces a plastic or "cogwheel" type of resistance to passive manipulation, where spasticity reveals a "clasped knife" feel. Dystonic tone will often "shake loose". That is, if the limb is shaken, the tone will normalize for a few moments. This is not true in spasticity, and can be used to differentiate between the two. Spasticity will cause an increase in the deep tendon reflexes where dystonia will not.

Dystonia tends to affect central, postural musculature whereas choreoathetosis is more prominent in the limbs. However, both types of dyskinesia may occur either together or independently in the same patient.

Mixed tone is more difficult to diagnosis and quantify than pure spasticity. In children with cerebral palsy, however, it is important to assess the degree of extrapyramidal tone present, since the outcome of surgery is inconsistent for all but the patient with pure spasticity. Fortunately, dynamic EMG and motion analysis is also useful in determining when athetosis and mixed tone are present.

RANGE OF MOTION/CONTRACTURE

Differentiation between static and dynamic deformity may be difficult in the non-anesthetized patient (Perry et al. 1974). However, static examination of muscle length will provide some insight into whether contractures are static or dynamic. Spasticity is velocity dependent. Therefore it is important that assessment of range of motion is carried out slowly. Comparison of joint range of motion with slow and rapid stretch, however, is useful in the differentiation between spasticity and contracture (Boyd and Graham 1999). Static examination can also help distinguish deviations caused by weakness rather than shortness of the antagonistic muscle group. Dynamic contracture will disappear under general anesthesia. Every surgeon should repeat the range of motion examination under general anesthesia prior to beginning the surgery. The degree of muscle lengthening and/or the use of botulinum toxin injection can then be decided.

When assessing muscle contracture and muscle length either statically or dynamically by gait analysis, awareness of the interaction of multiple muscle groups at a variety of levels is important. There are three common lower extremity tests that are designed to differentiate between contracted biarticular and monoarticular muscles. These are the Silfverskiöld test for the gastrocsoleus complex (triceps surae) (Fig. 5.2a, b), the Duncan–Ely test for the monoarticular vasti and the rectus femoris (Fig. 5.3), and Phelps test for the biarticular adductor gracilis and the other monoarticular hip adductors. The gracilis arises from the adductor region of the ischium and inserts on the pes anserine of the tibia. The gracilis functions as a hip adductor and knee flexor. For assessment, the patient should be prone, with knee flexed and hip abducted. If the ipsilateral hip adducts as the knee is extended, tightness of the gracilis is confirmed. Perry et al. (1976) showed that when these tests are performed in conjunction with fine wire electromyography, both the monoarticulator and the biarticular muscles crossing the joint will contract. For example, the Duncan–Ely test will induce EMG activity of not only the rectus femoris but also the iliopsoas, and the Silfverskiöld test will induce EMG activity of both the gastrocnemius and the soleus. Under general anesthesia, however, these biarticular muscle tests will reliably demonstrate contracture of the biarticular muscle involved. Consequently, they should be included as part of the presurgical examination under anesthesia.

HIP

The Thomas test is used to measure the degree of hip flexor tightness supine with the pelvis held in a position where the anterior and posterior superior iliac spines (ASIS and PSIS,

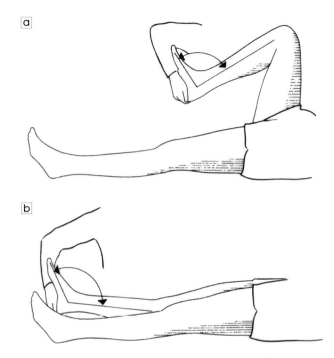

Fig. 5.2. The Silfverskiöld test differentiates tightness of the gastrocnemius and the soleus. In this test the knee is flexed to 90°, the hindfoot is positioned in varus, and maximal dorsiflexion is obtained (a). As the knee is extended, if dorsiflexion is lost, tightness/contracture of the gastrocnemius is present (b).

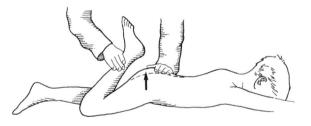

Fig. 5.3. The Duncan–Ely test, sometimes referred to as the "prone rectus test" since it is based upon the fact that the rectus femoris spans both the knee and the hip. With the patient lying prone, the knee is flexed quickly. The examiner looks for a rise of the buttocks and feels for increased tone within the limb.

respectively) are aligned vertically. Defining the pelvic position consistently rather than using the "flatten the lordosis" method will improve reliability. Hip adductor tightness can be distinguished from medial hamstring tightness by measuring hip abduction with the hips both flexed and extended.

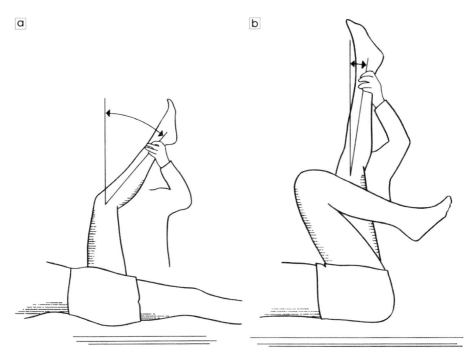

Fig. 5.4. The hamstring shift is measured by comparing the unilateral and bilateral popliteal angles. The unilateral popliteal angle is measured with the ipsilateral hip flexed to 90° and the contralateral hip extended so that the child's typical lordosis is unaffected (a). The bilateral popliteal angle is measured with the contralateral hip flexed until the ASIS and PSIS are vertical (b). The difference between the two measured popliteal angles is the "hamstring shift".

KNEE

A knee flexion contracture can be caused by (1) shortened hamstrings, (2) shifted hamstrings due to excessive anterior tilt, (3) shortened proximal gastrocnemius, and (4) capsular contracture. Measurements that reflect positional changes of the biarticular muscle groups are especially important at the knee since many biarticular muscles cross this joint including the gastrocnemius, rectus femoris, medial and lateral hamstrings, and the adductor-gracilis. In addition to the Silfverskiöld, Duncan–Ely and Phelps tests for the gastrocnemius, rectus femoris and gracilis respectively, we routinely evaluate the degree of "hamstring shift". Hamstring shift is calculated by first measuring the unilateral popliteal angle, then the bilateral popliteal angle, and finding the difference between the two (Fig. 5.4). "Unilateral popliteal angle" is measured with a normal resting lordosis. The contralateral hip is fully extended, while the ipsilateral hip is flexed to 90°. The knee is then extended until the first endpoint of resistance is felt (Fig. 5.4a). The measurement of the degrees of motion lacking from full extension will give the connective tissue and resting muscle extensibility. Cusick (1990) stated that the findings pertaining to the initial endpoint are more significant to functional ability than the stretched endpoint findings. The "bilateral popliteal angle" measurement is done with the ipsilateral hip flexed to 90° and the contralateral hip flexed until the ASIS and PSIS are aligned vertically (Fig. 5.4b). If there is a significant "hamstring shift", the popliteal angle, which is a measure of hamstring contracture, will significantly decrease as the pelvis is tipped posterior. The value of the popliteal angle with a neutral pelvis is a measure of the "true hamstring contracture" and the value with the lordosis present is the "functional hamstring contracture". The difference between the two represents the degree of hamstring shift. Measurement of capsular tightness by fully extending the knees should also be done to complete the assessment at the knee.

Various papers have pointed out that excessive anterior pelvic tilt, which is common in diplegic and quadriplegic cerebral palsy, will produce a "hamstring shift" in conjunction with an apparent knee flexion contracture (Hoffinger et al. 1993, Delp et al. 1996, Schutte et al. 1997). Suprisingly, hamstring length is frequently normal or even long in children with crouch gait. Consequently, surgical lengthening of the hamstrings often serves to produce further weakening of the hip extensors with resultant additional hip flexion, anterior pelvic tilt and lumbar lordosis. Based on the relative length of the hamstring moment arm at the hip and knee, Delp and colleagues (1996) have estimated that for every 1° of excessive pelvic lordosis, there is 2° of hamstring shift. A hamstring shift > 20° is usually indicative of excessive anterior tilt, from tight hip flexor musculature, weak abdominals, and/or weak hip extensors. Normal popliteal angle measurements should be no greater than 20° for optimal function (Gage 1991). Because of the difficulty in establishing dynamic hamstring length on physical exam and the danger of iatrogenic problems with excessive lengthening, dynamic hamstring length should be evaluated using gait analysis prior to consideration of any hamstring lengthening surgery.

ANKLE/FOOT

In children with spastic diplegia and quadriplegia, Rose et al. (1993) and Delp et al. (1995) have reported that generally the gastrocnemius is contracted and the soleus is of normal length. In the few cases in which both muscles are contracted the gastrocnemius contracture is greater than that of the soleus. This can frequently be determined during the clinical examination and always under anesthesia by simply employing the Silfverskiöld test. For normal mature walking, 10° of ankle dorsiflexion with knee extension is needed. The task of the soleus (as was discussed in the previous chapter) is to restrain ankle dorsiflexion during mid-stance. Excessive length or loss of soleus strength allows the ankle to move into excessive dorsiflexion, which promotes crouch gait. In order to assess the true length of the triceps surae and not be misled by motion in the midfoot, the measurement of ankle dorsiflexion should be taken with the foot structures in slight subtalar varus position and then measured first with the knee flexed and then with the knee extended (Fig. 5.2).

The length of other soft tissues around the foot and ankle that should be assessed include posterior tibialis, anterior tibialis, and in the case of severe planovalgus foot deformities, adequate length of the peroneals. Great toe metatarsophalangeal joint (MTP) dorsiflexion range of motion should measure 65°–75° to allow adequate roll over in mid-stance and terminal stance (Mann and Hagy 1979).

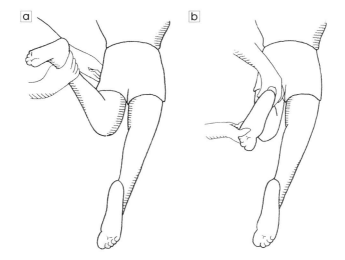

Fig. 5.5. Femoral anteversion can be estimated by flexing the knee to 90°, rotating the limb to the point of maximum trochanteric prominence, and then measuring the angle of the shank from the vertical (a). In a similar manner, the foot-progression angle, which is the angle between the long axis of the thigh and the line of progression of the foot, yields a fairly good estimate of tibial torsion so long as care is taken to be sure that the heel is in a neutral position. In order to eliminate varus or valgus bias from the foot, it is best to start with the foot into full equinus, neutralize the heel with respect to varus/valgus and then carefully bring the ankle to the neutral position to measure the ankle. One must also focus on the alignment of the hindfoot to the thigh rather than the foot as a whole as a persistent forefoot adduction will often mask an external tibial torsion (b).

Bone deformity

ANTEVERSION

Anteversion refers to the relationship between the axes of the femoral neck and the femoral condyles. These deformities are most easily and reliably assessed as part of the static examination in the prone position. Anteversion is best evaluated by comparing internal and external hip rotation, as well as palpation of the point of maximal trochanteric prominence (Ruwe et al. 1992, Davids et al. 2002) (Fig. 5.5a).

Children with spastic diplegic, quadriplegic, and/or severe hemiplegic cerebral palsy commonly have femoral anteversion, as do children with hypotonia and/or ligamentous laxity. In children with excessive joint laxity, however, the failure of remodeling comes from a different mechanism. In utero, femoral anteversion is about 55°. With the onset of walking, anteversion remodels so that by adulthood it measures on average 10°–15° (Ryder and Crane 1953). Hip extension against the anterior iliofemoral (Bigalow's) ligament is the mechanism by which this remodeling occurs. When a child starts to pull to stand and pulls his/her hips into full extension, the soft and cartilaginous femoral head and neck are pushed back towards normal adult alignment by Bigalow's ligament. In a child with excessive ligamentous laxity, Bigalow's ligament stretches over the femoral head and neck with insufficient tension to bring about normal remodeling. In discussing anteversion in the child with ligamentous laxity, Sommerville (1957) coined the term "persistent fetal alignment" to denote the failure of remodeling that may occur. In a child with cerebral palsy, the onset of walking is significantly delayed. By the time the child starts to stand, the femoral neck and head are largely ossified and less able to remodel. Furthermore, when the child does start to walk, s/he usually does so with the hips in flexion so that Bigalow's ligament does not come into play. Finally, the muscles that internally rotate the femur (anterior gluteals and medial hamstrings) tend to be more dominant and spastic than their antagonists so that as the child grows these abnormal muscle forces promote the development of more anteversion.

When coping with femoral anteversion, in order to seat the femoral heads congruously into the acetabulum the child is forced to do two things: (1) internally rotate the femur, which results in excessive internal rotation of the entire lower limb, and (2) increase pelvic tilt. This, in turn, promotes the posture of internal limb rotation and excessive lumbar lordosis during gait that is common in children with spastic diplegia.

PATELLA ALTA
Patella alta is common in children who walk with excessive knee flexion. To screen for patella alta, position the patient supine with knees extended. Palpate the top of the patella. The superior edge of the patella is typically one finger width proximal to the adductor tubercle. When the patient is examined lying supine with the lower leg over the edge of the table, an extensor lag in the absence of a knee flexion contracture is suggestive of patella alta and/or quadriceps insufficiency. To confirm patella alta, a lateral X-ray must be obtained with the knee in full extension. The top of the patella should be at the level of the distal femoral growth plate.

TIBIAL TORSION
Tibial alignment can be measured in three ways: (1) by measurement of a thigh–foot angle (Fig. 5.5b), (2) by measurement of a bimalleolar axis, or (3) using the second toe test (Fig. 5.6). Often in a child with foot deformities, the bimalleolar axis is more accurate than the thigh–foot angle. The second toe test allows one to visualize the foot progression angle with the knee extended. As such, it eliminates the rotational component of knee movement, but requires aligning the foot at a right angle to the axis of the ankle mortise. Therefore, in children with equinus contracture and/or severe varus or valgus foot deformities, it is difficult to perform this test accurately. Despite the absence of tibia torsion, the presence of a true knee valgus will increase the measurement of the second toe test by the amount of true valgus that is present. However, assuming that the foot can be brought into a plantargrade position so that the test can be preformed accurately, the second toe test is reliable, particularly if the patient is under anesthesia.

SUBTALAR POSITION AND MOBILITY
Complete examination of the foot includes both physical examination in open and closed kinetic chain positions and the use of X-rays. Establishing a subtalar neutral (STN) position prior to examination of the hindfoot and forefoot in non-weightbearing provides consistency

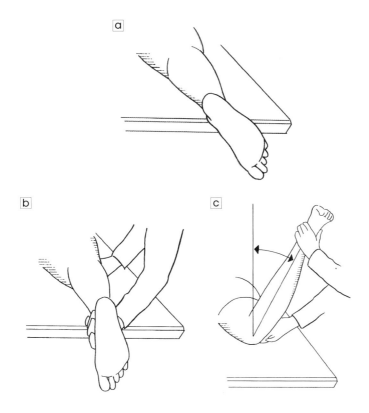

Fig. 5.6. The second toe test is a third method of measurement of tibial torsion. To perform this test, the foot must either be well aligned or flexible enough to hold in normal alignment (a). The test begins with the patient's knee fully extended. The lower extremity is then rotated until the second toe is pointing directly towards the floor (b). Without changing the rotation of the thigh, the knee is flexed to 90°. The angle between the vertical line and the shank is equal to the amount of external tibial torsion present (c)

in positioning (Oatis 1988). The subtalar joint is aligned within all three planes and is therefore considered a triplanar joint. In the normally aligned foot, the motions of inversion and eversion occur at the subtalar joint. The pitch or alignment of the subtalar joint determines the axis about which inversion and eversion occurs. If the medial longitudinal arch is to be maintained, the ligaments and the muscles around the subtalar joint must be balanced. If the axis of the subtalar joint is abnormal, either cavus or planus will occur with weightbearing. Assessment of the subtalar joint and surrounding structures is most reliably done from a sagittal plane perspective with the patient either lying prone or sitting on the examining table with the knees flexed to 90° (Mann 1999). Goniometric measurements of the foot are highly unreliable therefore subjective descriptors of "normal, hyper-mobile, and restricted" give equal information as to the motions of the joint and should be defined for each laboratory testing situation (Cusick 1990).

To evaluate subtalar neutral, palpate the head of the talus while pronating and supinating

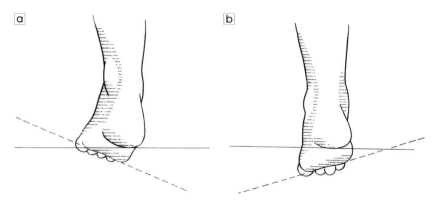

Fig. 5.7. In a normal forefoot, the plane of the metatarsals will be perpendicular to the axis of the calcaneus. Forefoot varus is present when the plane of the metatarsals is supinated to the plane of the calcaneus (a). Forefoot valgus is present when the plane of the metatarsals is pronated in relation to the axis of the calcaneus (b).

the plantarflexed foot. The midpoint, or point of neutrality, is the point at which the two sides of the talar head cannot be palpated, or the protrusion on both sides is equal. Once subtalar neutrality is found, "lock" the forefoot on the hindfoot by gently dorsiflexing the fourth and fifth metatarsal heads using a congruency grip. Relative positions of the hindfoot and forefoot can be consistently described from this position while in non-weightbearing. The hindfoot in relation to the leg will either be in neutral, varus, or valgus.

The forefoot will be in one of three positions in relation to the hindfoot: neutral, where the plane of the metatarsals and the calcaneus are perpendicular; forefoot varus (Fig. 5.7a), in which the plane of the metatarsals is supinated in relationship to the calcaneus; or forefoot valgus (Fig. 5.7b) where the metatarsal plane is pronated in relationship to the calcaneus (Mann 1999).

Forefoot varus (supination) is associated with pes planus in weightbearing. When the foot contacts the ground, the calcaneus must rotate into an everted position to bring the forefoot down to contact the floor (Root et al. 1977). Forefoot varus is usual when the hindfoot is in valgus and also is commonly associated with abduction of the forefoot on the hindfoot.

If a valgus (pronation) deformity of the forefoot on the hindfoot is rigid, in weightbearing the contact of the first metatarsal with the ground may force the hindfoot into varus. Confusion can then arise as to whether the hindfoot varus deformity is primary or secondary. Since appropriate surgical correction depends on this, the "Coleman block test" (Coleman and Chesnut 1977) is a very useful assessment tool (Fig. 5.8).

Evaluation of the position of the first ray to determine whether it is plantarflexed or dorsiflexed to the plane of the forefoot should not be confused with the overall position of the forefoot in relation to the hindfoot. If the first ray is plantarflexed, it may falsely suggest forefoot valgus (pronation). The position of the central metatarsal heads should be viewed as a separate group from the first or fifth rays. First ray mobility is also important for appropriate rollover and will therefore influence all other lower extremity biomechanics. Dorsiflexion of the first ray should be measured or at least noted if it is limited (Cusick 1990).

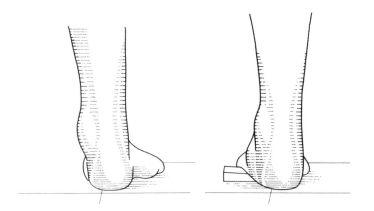

Fig. 5.8. The Coleman block test can be used to differentiate whether varus is emanating from the hindfoot or the forefoot. To perform this test, the heel and lateral border of the foot are placed on a 1-inch block, or a wedge is placed under the lateral portion of the forefoot which allows the first through fourth metatarsals to pronate. If a rigid forefoot valgus (pronation) is present in combination with a flexible hindfoot varus, the hindfoot varus will be eliminated or significantly reduced. If the hindfoot varus position is rigid, it will remain despite forefoot positioning. To document the results of the test, anteroposterior and lateral photographs as well as roentgenograms are taken.

The ratio of hindfoot motion is 2:1 inversion to eversion (Cusick 1990). This should be assessed with the foot gently dorsiflexed to eliminate frontal plane movements of the talus in the ankle mortise.

Metatarsus adductus occurs at the tarsal–metatarsal articulation. Forefoot adductus includes osseous abnormality of the tarsal bones and occurs at the midtarsal joints. These would be documented on video and recorded using a severity scale. A skew foot deformity includes both a metatarsus adductus, and hindfoot valgus in weightbearing. This may occur as children attempt to compensate for the in-toeing that the adductus has caused. Both of these deformities should be confirmed on X-ray.

In weightbearing, the closed kinetic chain connection between the foot and leg can be seen using a variety of wedges and close up video analysis. Small wedges are used under the foot to compensate for the deformities seen in the open kinetic chain evaluation. The mobility or rigidity of the observed deformities can then be appreciated and documented. Close-up video analysis in the current bracing system without shoes and socks may reveal whether the brace is able to support and correct the current deformities adequately.

Hindfoot valgus and forefoot pronation loosen the joints of the foot and allow it to function as a shock absorber, whereas hindfoot varus and forefoot supination tighten the foot so that it can function as a rigid lever during push-off (Inman et al. 1994). If a patient is unable to perform these motions during gait, biomechanics of the entire lower limb will be affected. Patterns of deformities and treatment consideration will be discussed in the following chapters.

LEG LENGTH

Good assessment of limb length inequality includes consideration of scoliosis, hip subluxation, pelvic obliquity, and unilateral contracture of the hip adductors, as well as other lower extremity biomechanical abnormalities that would contribute to a functional limb length inequality. Clinical assessment requires good precision for repeatability and accuracy. Clinical limb length is measured using the inferior border of the ASIS and the distal aspect of the medial malleolus.

POSTURE AND BALANCE

Assessment of posterior, anterior, and mediolateral equilibrium responses is important and often neglected when planning treatment. Many children with cerebral palsy will have delayed or deficient posterior equilibrium responses. According to Bleck (1987), the presence of mediolateral responses is a prerequisite for independent ambulation. Because of the poor base of support often found in children with cerebral palsy, posture and the ability to respond to a loss of balance are frequently impaired. Assessment of posture (including trunk, pelvis, and lower extremity posture in static standing and during walking in the sagittal and coronal planes) will often give insights into areas of weakness, poor motor control, and the compensation strategies that the child is using to circumvent them.

ROENTGENOGRAMS

Spine, hip and foot X-rays are taken regularly for all children with a diagnosis of cerebral palsy to follow the development of the skeletal system. Scoliosis and hip dysplasia are common in children with cerebral palsy, particularly those with quadriplegia. In young children, who are non-ambulatory, an anteroposterior (AP) X-ray of the pelvis should be taken for screening. The hips should be evaluated at each clinical visit and followed by X-ray at appropriate intervals until walking is well established and the hips are no longer at risk for subluxation. Lateral X-rays of the knees in full extension are useful to determine the presence of patella alta in children who walk with a persistent crouch gait pattern.

Pes planus with a relative subluxation of the talus on the calcaneous is very common in children with diplegia or quadriplegia. Pes cavus or cavovarus is more common in those with hemiplegia (Gage 1991). These deformities are best assessed with AP and lateral weightbearing X-rays of the foot and mortise X-rays of the ankle. Weightbearing X-rays can be used to measure the talar–first metatarsal angle, which should be close to zero on both the AP and lateral views (Fig. 5.9). Roentgenograms of the ankle mortise should also be obtained routinely, as a valgus ankle mortise often contributes significantly to valgus foot deformity in weightbearing.

VIDEOTAPE AND OBSERVATIONAL GAIT ANALYSIS

Observational gait analysis consists of observing a subject without the use of formal gait analysis equipment. To improve the ability to make appropriate determinations and address all deviations subtle and obvious, a systematic syllabus should be used. Various forms have been developed to assist the observer in organizing the analysis as well as for reporting the observations (Fig. 5.10) (Perry 1992). Krebs et al. (1985) reported that observational gait analysis is more consistent with a single observer and least consistent between multiple observers. He further observed that viewing a videotape of a patient walking is more

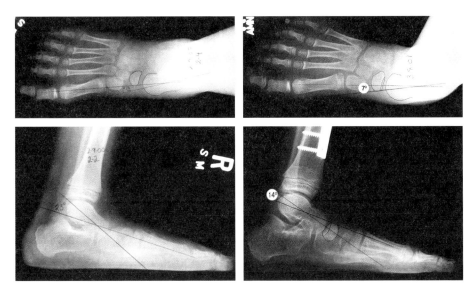

Fig. 5.9. *Left*: AP and lateral roentgenograms of a valgus foot taken before surgical correction. Note that prior to surgery the talar–first metatarsal angles, which should be zero on both views, were 23° and 10°, respectively. *Right*: AP and lateral roentgenograms of the same foot that were taken after lengthening of the os calcis and medial reefing of the talonavicular joint capsule. The valgus has been functionally corrected and the talar–first metatarsal angles are now improved to 7° and 14° (normal should be zero on both the AP and lateral views). Correction of the foot was done in conjunction with a distal tibial osteotomy, which was used to correct the associated external tibial torsion. Slight dorsal deviation of the distal end of the calcaneus such as is seen here frequently occurs following lengthening of the os calcis, but normally remodels rapidly and does not produce functional problems.

consistent both with single and multiple observers than viewing the subject live with repeated walks. Finally, if slow motion videotaping is employed, he found that the consistency of observation improved markedly. The speed at which we as observers are able to process what we see is much slower than the speed at which changes are taking place as someone walks. Many activities are occurring simultaneously at different joints and in different planes. Many gait abnormalities in the transverse plane cannot be seen without kinematic assistance. In addition, the compensations that the patient employs may mask the primary gait abnormalities.

Currently, computerized gait analysis cannot provide much information about foot deformities. Consequently, careful clinical examination, weightbearing X-rays and dynamic video in and out of current bracing or shoe wear is helpful. In addition, close up video of the feet from all sides as well as video documentation of a Root sign (Fig. 5.11) (Root 1970, Tachdjian 2002), and if necessary a Coleman block test should be done to assess the response of the foot to a variety of positions.

Finally, beginning with the feet during ambulation at initial contact, here are several questions, which should be asked to complete the gait by observation. (1) What is the position of the foot at the end of terminal swing? Is the foot neutral or is it in a varus or valgus position? (2) Is the ankle in a neutral position or equinus? (3) Which portion of the

85

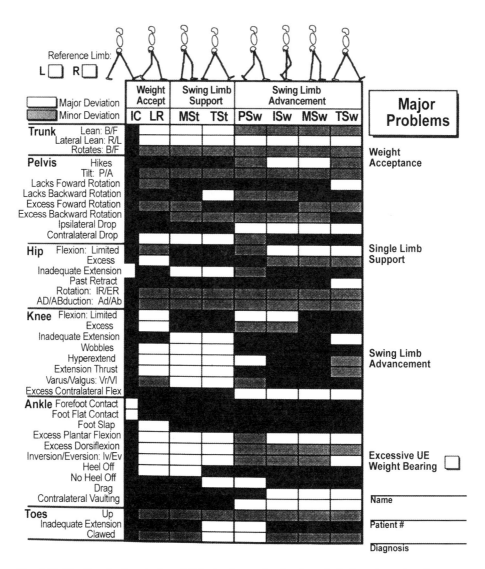

Fig. 5.10. The Rancho Los Amigos full body observational gait analysis form is used to document deviations during ambulation. Rows = gait deviations; columns = gait phases. Walking dysfunction is tabulated by checking the pertinent boxes. White boxes = major gait deviations; gray boxes = minor gait deviations; black boxes = not applicable. (Reproduced from Perry 1992, by permission.)

foot touches the floor first, and why? (4) What is the foot progression angle during stance and swing with respect to both the line of progression and the alignment of the knee? (5) Is the foot plantargrade in stance? Does the foot maintain its appropriate contour throughout stance? (6) At which point in the cycle does any deviation in the foot occur? (7) Does the foot go through the normal sequence of rockers, or is there premature plantarflexion, in

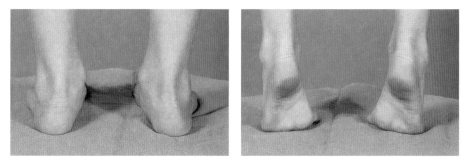

Fig. 5.11. Root test. This test is useful for differentiating between flexible and pathological pes planus. A positive Root test for flexible flat foot will demonstrate a reconstitution of the medial longitudinal arch with inversion of the hindfoot when the child is standing on tip-toe.

midstance or delayed dorsiflexion in terminal stance? (8) What are the positions of the toes in stance and swing? Is there toe clawing that is occurring in stance, or hyperextension of the first MTP joint in swing?

At the knee the following functions should be noted. (1) What are the positions of the knee at the end of terminal swing and at initial contact? (2) Is there a loading response present where the knee increases flexion right after initial contact? (3) Does the knee come to full extension at any point in stance? If so, when does this occur? (4) Does the knee hyperextend, or is the extension controlled? (5) What degree is the maximum knee flexion in swing? When does it occur? Is it adequate for clearance or is toe drag a problem? (6) What is the knee position during stance and swing? (7) Is the knee aligned with the foot? (8) Is the shank aligned with the thigh?

Observational gait analysis becomes more difficult as one moves proximally, since the mass of the trunk and the soft tissue around the hips and pelvis frequently obscures the motions that are occurring at these joints. Since selective motor control is best in the proximal and worse in the distal joints, compensatory motions for gait problems in the distal part of the limb often occur proximally via hip or trunk motion. However, without resorting to full, computerized gait analysis, it is difficult to determine whether the abnormal movements are compensations, or primary deviations. In looking at the trunk, pelvis, and hips it is necessary to note the following. (1) Are the thigh and knee aligned to the plane of progression at initial contact? If not is the malrotation internal or external? (2) Does the hip flex sufficiently at initial contact? (3) Is there full hip extension in terminal stance? (4) Is there excessive hip abduction in swing? (5) What is the pelvic position? Is it excessively anterior or posterior? (6) Is either asymmetric pelvic rotation and/or obliquity present? (7) What are the trunk movements in each plane? Are these appropriate? Are the abnormal motions likely to be primary or compensatory? (8) How are the arms moving during gait? Are they moving reciprocally or are they postured? Does the child elevate his/her arms to assist with balance?

And finally, some general questions. (1) Is the stride length adequate? (2) Are the step lengths symmetrical? (3) Does the walking pattern appear to be efficient or is there excessive body motion or other indications of excessive energy consumption? (4) What influence do assistive devices or orthotics have on the child's walking pattern?

This list will begin both the gait analysis and the problem solving processes. However, it is necessary to combine the clinical examination, roentgenograms, observational gait analysis and the motion analysis information together to get a complete problem list. Each piece of the examination process provides critical bits of information and it is necessary to gather all the pieces and fit them together to get a complete picture of the child's gait problems. Only when this has been done, can one devise a treatment plan that will ensure an optimal outcome.

REFERENCES

Bleck E. (1987) *Orthopaedic Management in Cerebral Palsy*. London: Mac Keith Press. p 17–64.

Bohannon RW. (1989) Is the measurement of muscle strength appropriate in patients with brain lesions? A special communication. *Phys Ther* **69:** 225–236.

Bohannon RW, Smith MB. (1987) Interrater reliability of a modified Ashworth scale of muscle spasticity. *Phys Ther* **67:** 206–207.

Boyd RN, Graham HK. (1999) Objective measurement of clinical findings in the use of botulinum toxin type A for the management of children with cerebral palsy. *Eur J Neurol* **6:** S23–S35.

Coleman SS, Chesnut WJ. (1977) A simple test for hindfoot flexibility in the cavovarus foot. *Clin Orthop* 60–62.

Cusick BD. (1990) *Progressive Casting and Splinting for Lower Extremity Deformities in Children with Neuromotor Dysfunction*. Tucson, Arizona: Therapy Skill Builders. p 129–168.

Davids JR, Benfanti P, Blackhurst DW, Allen BL. (2002) Assessment of femoral anteversion in children with cerebral palsy: accuracy of the Trochanteric Prominence Angle Test. *J Pediatr Orthop* **22:** 173–178.

Delp SL, Loan JP. (1995) A graphics-based software system to develop and analyze models of musculoskeletal structures. *Comput Biol Med* **25:** 21–34.

Delp SL, Loan JP, Hoy MG, Zajac FE, Topp EL, Rosen JM. (1990) An interactive graphics-based model of the lower extremity to study orthopaedic surgical procedures. *IEEE Transactions on Biomedical Engineering* **37:** 757–767.

Delp SL, Statler K, Carroll NC. (1995) Preserving plantar flexion strength after surgical treatment for contracture of the triceps surae: a computer simulation study. *J Orthop Res* **13:** 96–104.

Delp SL, Arnold AS, Speers RA, Moore CA. (1996) Hamstrings and psoas lengths during normal and crouch gait: implications for muscle-tendon surgery. *J Orthop Res* **14:** 144–151.

Gage JR. (1991) *Gait Analysis in Cerebral Palsy*. London: Mac Keith Press.

Gage JR. (1994) The role of gait analysis in the treatment of cerebral palsy (an Editorial). *J Pediatr Orthop* **14:** 701–702.

Hoffinger SA, Rab GT, Abou-Ghaida H. (1993) Hamstrings in cerebral palsy crouch gait. *J Pediatr Orthop* **13:** 722–726.

Inman VT, Ralston HJ, Todd F. (1994) Human locomotion. In: Rose J, Gamble JG, editors. *Human Walking*. Baltimore: Williams and Wilkins. p 1–22.

Kendall HO, Kendall FP, Wadsworth GE. (1971) *Muscle Testing and Function*. Baltimore: Williams and Wilkins. p 3–15.

Krebs DE, Edelstein JE, Fishman S. (1985) Reliability of observational kinematic gait analysis. *Phys Ther* **65:** 1027–1033.

Kyllerman M, Bager B, Bensch J, Bille B, Olow I, Voss H. (1982) Dyskinetic cerebral palsy. I. Clinical categories, associated neurological abnormalities and incidences. *Acta Paediatr Scand* **71:** 543–550.

Mann RA. (1999) Principles of examination of the foot and ankle. In: Coughlin MJ, Mann RA. *Surgery of the Foot and Ankle*. St Louis: Mosby-Year Book. p 31–49.

Mann RA, Hagy JL. (1979) The function of the toes in walking, jogging and running. *Clin Orthop* 24–29.

Novacheck T, Stout J, Tervo R. (2000) Reliability and validity of the Gillette Functional Assessment Questionnaire as an outcome measure in children with walking disabilities. *J Pediatr Orthop* **20:** 75–81.

Oatis CA. (1988) Biomechanics of the foot and ankle under static conditions. *Phys Ther* **68:** 1815–1821.

Perry J. (1992) *Gait Analysis: Normal and Pathological Function*. Thorofare, NJ: Slack.
Perry J, Hoffer MM, Giovan P, Antonelli D, Greenberg R. (1974) Gait analysis of the triceps surae in cerebral palsy. A preoperative and postoperative clinical and electromyographic study. *J Bone Joint Surg Am* **56:** 511–520.
Perry J, Hoffer MM, Antonelli D, Plut J, Lewis G, Greenberg R. (1976) Electromyography before and after surgery for hip deformity in children with cerebral palsy. A comparison of clinical and electromyographic findings. *J Bone Joint Surg Am* **58:** 201–208.
Perry J, Giovan P, Harris LJ, Montgomery J, Azaria M. (1978) The determinants of muscle action in the hemiparetic lower extremity (and their effect on the examination procedure). *Clin Orthop* 71–89.
Root L. (1970) Functional testing of the posterior tibial muscle in spastic paralysis. *Dev Med Child Neurol* **12:** 592–595.
Rose SA, DeLuca PA, Davis RB 3rd, Õunpuu S, Gage JR. (1993) Kinematic and kinetic evaluation of the ankle after lengthening of the gastrocnemius fascia in children with cerebral palsy. *J Pediatr Orthop* **13:** 727–732.
Ruwe PA, Gage JR, Ozonoff MB, DeLuca PA. (1992) Clinical determination of femoral anteversion. A comparison with established techniques. *J Bone Joint Surg Am* **74:** 820-830.
Ryder CT, Crane L. (1953) Measuring femoral anteversion; the problem and a method. *J Bone Joint Surg Am* **35:** 289.
Schutte LM, Hayden SW, Gage JR. (1997) Lengths of hamstrings and psoas muscles during crouch gait: effects of femoral anteversion. *J Orthop Res* **15:** 615–621.
Sommerville EW. (1957) Persistent foetal alignment of the hip. *J Bone Joint Surg Br* **39:** 106.
Tachdjian MO. (2002) Disorders of the foot. In: Herring JA, editor. *Pediatric Orthopaedics*. Philadelphia: W.B. Saunders. p 910–912.

6
THE MOTION ANALYSIS LABORATORY

Roy B. Davis

Clinical motion analysis is a process in which a patient's movement patterns are measured, abnormalities are identified, causes are postulated, and treatment recommendations are developed. The motion analysis laboratory is the service in the clinical setting that facilitates this process through the use of specialized measurement technology operated by a highly multidisciplinary staff. The broad base of knowledge and experience of the staff is essential in an integration of the relevant information from patient's medical history, physical examination, pertinent radiographs, and qualitative observations regarding their movement pattern with collected quantitative data, central to clinical motion analysis. Although motion analysis could potentially be applied to a wide range of clinical movement questions, its most common application at the time of this writing is the investigation and assessment of the patient's walking pattern, commonly referred to as "clinical gait analysis".

The previous chapter has described observational gait analysis. Videotape recordings of the patient walking, made in the motion analysis laboratory, augment this assessment technique and provide an overall impression of the "smoothness" or "fluidity" of the patient's gait pattern. Close-up views of a specific motion or body segments can be obtained; for example, close-up views of the feet are useful in evaluating hindfoot position and motion and forefoot clearance. The use of slow-motion replay significantly enhances the observer's ability to evaluate complex, multiplanar walking patterns.

A physical examination of the patient (also described earlier) is also performed in the lab. Measures typically include the passive lower extremity joint range of motion, joint and muscular contracture, muscle strength and tone, bony deformity and neurological assessment. Often these measurements are repeated by different staff members because of the subjective nature of these data.

Quantitative gait data constitute the primary contribution of the motion analysis laboratory to the clinical assessment of the patient's ambulatory status. The patient is instrumented and monitored by a measurement system as s/he walks along a smooth, level pathway through the laboratory. Collected data allow the motion of the patient's individual body segments and joint rotations to be quantified (i.e. kinematics) as well as the joint reactions (i.e. joint kinetics) to be computed, as described further in the next section of this chapter and in subsequent chapters. Data are also collected that indicate the activity of certain lower extremity muscles (i.e. dynamic electromyography) and the interaction between the patient's foot and the ground, e.g. a ground reaction force and the pressure distribution (i.e. pedobarography). Measures of oxygen uptake and carbon dioxide production (presented in Chapter 10 of this book) are collected in some labs and used to compute a variety of metabolic cost indices.

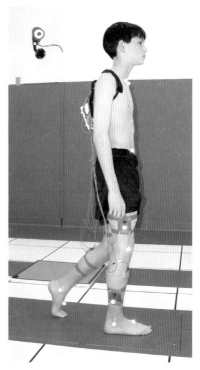

Fig. 6.1. A subject instrumented with passive reflective markers and EMG electrodes walking along the data collection pathway in a motion analysis laboratory. The subject is stepping on two force platforms and the reflective markers are being monitored by an array of motion measurement cameras (one of which is shown mounted on the wall beside the subject).

Subsequent chapters will also focus on the interpretation of quantitative gait data and its use in treatment planning. The goal of this chapter is to provide an understanding of how these data are most commonly collected and processed today, as well as to introduce the multidisciplinary team that provides support for a motion analysis laboratory.

The primary measurement systems used in the laboratory

The fundamental elements of the quantitative gait data set that are routinely provided for clinical interpretation from the motion analysis laboratory are kinematics, kinetics and electromyography (EMG). The primary measurement subsystems used in the clinical motion analysis laboratory that provide these data include motion data capture, ground force measurement, and EMG.

MOTION DATA CAPTURE

Passive reflective markers are placed on the surface of the patient's skin and aligned with specific bony landmarks and joint axes (Fig. 6.1). As the patient walks along a straight pathway in the laboratory, the locations of these markers are monitored with a three-dimensional motion data capture system comprising six, eight, twelve or more specialized video cameras, arrayed around the central walkway and interfaced to a central computer. Each camera is equipped with a cluster of light-emitting diodes that strobe the pathway and the markers on the patient with infrared or visible light. Images provided by multiple cameras of the light reflected from the markers are then processed by computer programs to determine the three-dimensional locations of the markers in space in a manner analogous to the way depth is perceived in human stereoscopic vision. These marker position data allow for the mathematical computation of the angular orientation of particular body segments as well as the angles between segments, i.e. joint angles, and are collectively referred to as "kinematics". Marker position data are also the basis of stride and temporal parameters such as walking speed, step length, stride length and cadence. The use of these marker trajectory data will be introduced in the next section with a more complete description of gait kinematics provided in the next chapter.

GROUND FORCE MEASUREMENT
Force platforms mounted in the walkway monitor the multi-component "ground reactions" (forces and torque) between the patient's foot and the ground. These reactions include vertical, medial/lateral shear and fore/aft shear forces and the torque produced about each of the three force plate axes. The point of application of the ground reaction force under the patient's foot is commonly referred to as "center of pressure". These data may be examined directly (Perry 1992a) or used to calculate loads found in and across the joints of the lower extremity. These joint reactions (referred to as joint "kinctics") are computed analytically from fundamental mechanics relationships, e.g. Newton's laws of motion, which combine the simultaneously acquired kinematic information and estimates of limb mass and inertial properties with the force platform data. A brief description of the principles and algorithms that underpin this determination is presented in a subsequent chapter.

ELECTROMYOGRAPHY
Electrodes placed on the surface of the skin (Fig. 6.1) or inserted intramuscularly as fine wires monitor muscle action potentials, again as the patient walks along the laboratory pathway, through an approach referred to as dynamic EMG. The EMG signal gives information concerning the "on-off" activity of a muscle. This information allows the relationships between the patient's neuromuscular abnormalities and joint kinematic and kinetic data to be examined. Again, a complete description of the collection of EMG data and its use is provided in other chapters of this book.

OTHER TECHNOLOGIES
Other technologies are used in varying degrees in the motion analysis laboratory. Foot switches are sometimes placed on the plantar surface of the patient's foot that indicate when different parts of the foot are in contact with the floor and used to identify the timing of the gait cycle (Perry 1992b). Alternatively, gait cycle timing may be assessed using the quantitative motion data, the force platform data, or video recordings. Increasingly, plantar pressure measurement systems (or pedobarographs) are used to monitor the loading pattern on the plantar surface of the foot. To date, this technology has most often been applied clinically at centers with expertise in the management of patients with diabetes (Cavanagh and Ulbrecht 1997). As indicated earlier, metabolic energy measurement systems are also

sometimes used to measure the energy consumption of the ambulatory patient (Thomas et al. 2001). While both of these latter two technologies have good utilization in clinical and biomechanics research, their widespread use in clinical treatment decision-making for the ambulatory patient is still developing.

The quantitative data that depicts the patient's walking pattern constitute the primary information used for clinical decision-making. The next section outlines the relationship between the collected data, i.e. marker trajectories, and those fundamental computational elements that provide the basis for the calculation of segment and joint kinematics and joint kinetics.

The connection between motion data and clinical information

It is important to have an appreciation of how the basic marker displacement and ground reaction data collected from the patient in the lab is used to calculate the kinematic and kinetic information that is presented for interpretation and clinical decision-making. With this basis, the individual or team is better prepared to address questions that arise in the interpretation session and distinguish between the patient's pathomechanics or data artifact. Consequently a brief introduction of how the marker data are used computationally will be provided here; more detailed information can be found in subsequent chapters.

The primary goal during the movement activity is the measurement of the orientation or position of the patient's body segments and joints. The methods used require that anatomically aligned axes or coordinate systems be established for each segment included in the analysis, not unlike the alignment of the arms of a plastic goniometer in the assessment of joint position during the physical examination. Since the angular motion of the segments is three-dimensional, with corresponding joint motion that is also potentially three-dimensional (depending upon particular joint constraint), these segmental axes are represented by anatomically aligned coordinate systems, referred to in this document as "anatomical coordinate systems".

To explore this further, consider the pelvis. The anatomical coordinate system for the pelvis is most often related to the plane formed by the right and left anterior superior iliac spine and the posterior superior iliac spine (Fig. 6.2). In this case, three measurement markers can be placed over these three palpable anatomical landmarks and used to mathematically compute the pelvic anatomical coordinate system. By tracking the displacement of these three markers during the walking trials, one can then compute the associated angular orientation of the pelvis.

If one is also interested in hip motion, the motion of the thigh and the pelvis must be monitored simultaneously. An anatomical coordinate system for the femur (Fig. 6.2) can be constructed as follows: a longitudinal axis from the knee center (a point midway between markers placed on the medial and lateral femoral condyles) and the hip center (a point that approximates the location of the center of the head of the femur and is computed using statistical relationships associated with the anatomy of the pelvis); a transverse axis based on markers placed on the medial and lateral femoral condyles that approximate knee flexion/extension axis and is perpendicular to the longitudinal axis; an anterior–posterior axis that is perpendicular to both the longitudinal and transverse axes. Markers placed on the medial surfaces of

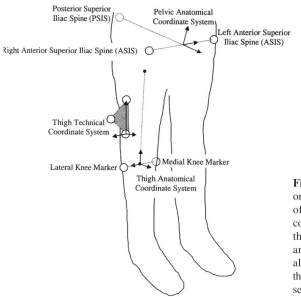

Posterior Superior
Iliac Spine (PSIS)

Pelvic Anatomical
Coordinate System

Left Anterior Superior
Iliac Spine (ASIS)

Right Anterior Superior Iliac Spine (ASIS)

Thigh Technical
Coordinate System

Lateral Knee Marker

Medial Knee Marker

Thigh Anatomical
Coordinate System

Fig. 6.2. The placement of markers on the patient defines the alignment of anatomical and technical coordinate systems of the pelvis and the thigh. The orientation of the anatomical coordinate systems allows for the computation of the three-dimensional orientation of each segment, as well as joint motion.

lower extremity segments, however, can be problematic during gait because of limited clearance between the legs as the contralateral limb swings past. Consequently, a medial knee marker that could be monitored while the patient is standing still would need to be removed before the walking trials. This means that, unlike with the pelvis, the markers on the thigh during gait do not directly represent the anatomical coordinate system for the femur. The challenge is resolved by using additional markers on the thigh during gait that are not necessarily aligned with the anatomy of the thigh, but are clearly visible to the motion data capture cameras. These additional markers are used to compute a "technical coordinate system" that is also fixed to the thigh (Fig. 6.2) along with its anatomical coordinate system. The relationship between technical and anatomical coordinate systems can be established mathematically based on data collected during static "subject calibration" when anatomically meaningful markers (such as that medial knee marker) can be placed on the patient. In this way, tracking the displacement of the technical coordinate system during the patient's movement allows a determination of the corresponding orientation and displacement of the underlying anatomical coordinate system. Now, with an anatomical coordinate system for both the pelvis and the thigh, three-dimensional hip angles can be computed as will be described in a subsequent chapter.

This brief description illustrates a number of points that provide both an introduction in preparation for material presented in forthcoming chapters as well as an opportunity to discuss some of the fundamental assumptions and limitations associated with this technology. First and foremost, it is assumed that markers placed on the skin's surface move with the underlying bones. That is, the relationship between each technical coordinate system and associated anatomical coordinate system is fixed and that both move with the underlying bone(s). The validity of this assumption varies considerably depending on the body type of the patient, e.g. the presence of excessive adipose tissue. What is more, the validity and appropriateness of a statistically based hip center location needs to be appreciated with each patient, e.g. such a model may not be appropriate for patients with significant pelvic deformity or dislocated hips. Finally, one can appreciate the importance of very careful marker placement and alignment. For example, small placement errors in relatively closely spaced markers such as the lateral and medial knee markers can result in significant angular distortion of the desired anatomical coordinate system.

It is perhaps implied by this presentation that this is the universal approach, used in all motion analysis laboratories. In reality, however, there is not universal agreement for marker placement on the patient or the alignment of these underlying anatomical coordinate systems. There are many protocols in engineering and science in which a distinction between "correct" and "incorrect" measurements can be drawn. Techniques used in clinical gait analysis cannot be so readily classified. The fundamental challenge is that there exist a number of equally valid approaches that may in fact yield comparable, although differing, results. At the same time, subtle differences in the execution of the same protocol produce significantly different results. Clearly it is essential for the proper interpretation of patient data that the details of the gait data collection protocol are well understood and careful attention be given to their systematic execution by the staff of the motion analysis laboratory.

Staff

The knowledge and skills required for the proper operation of a motion analysis laboratory are broad-based, crossing a number of traditional disciplines. As Table 6.1 indicates, the staff in the laboratory must be knowledgeable and experienced in areas ranging from the technical (e.g. measurement equipment and computer operation) to the clinical (e.g. patient assessment through a physical examination). It should be appreciated that much of this knowledge is acquired "on the job" and through continuing professional education opportunities.

In a contemporary motion analysis laboratory, the equipment can be operated and protocols executed by personnel with some system-specific training and few qualifications. That is, when the equipment has been installed and is operating normally, the simplicity of operation of the commercial systems allows data to be collected and processed. Similarly, the instrumentation of the test subject can be accomplished with very limited knowledge of anatomy and experience in the palpation of bony landmarks. In short, with today's hardware and software, data of very dubious quality can be readily collected and presented for interpretation.

This scenario can only be avoided or its frequency minimized through an awareness of data-quality issues, underpinned by knowledge and experience. Careful data collection is paramount. Usually two staff members are required to collect the movement data: one who works closely with the patient, and the other who works closely with the equipment. It is essential for these two staff members to work closely together: and it is strongly recommended that the instrumentation of the patient be a shared responsibility, with one staff member's placement or alignment of a marker or electrode checked by the other staff

TABLE 6.1
Breadth of knowledge and experience required in the motion analysis laboratory

For routine data collection
 Normal anatomy
 Abnormal anatomy*
 Patient physical examination*
 Observational gait analysis
 Gait models*
 Patient instrumentation*
 Measurement system operation*
 Computer operation*
 Database management
 Experimental measurement theory
For data interpretation and treatment recommendation (in addition to those listed above)
 Muscle physiology
 Neurological motor control
 Normal movement biomechanics
 Abnormal movement biomechanics
 Treatment efficacy, including surgery, pharmacological, bracing, physical therapy*
For ongoing laboratory development (in addition to those listed above)
 Experimental design
 Measurement instrumentation
 Sensor electronics
 Computer system integration/networking
 High level computer programming
 Database design
 Mathematics (e.g. vector algebra, statistics)
 Engineering mechanics
 Numerical analysis
 Biomechanical modeling

*Specific to the patient population(s) seen, tests performed, measurement system or software or protocols employed in the laboratory.

member. In many cases, one of the pair will have more experience in bony palpation and the other will possess a more detailed understanding of the underlying gait model. Collaboration in this way facilitates open communication and the sharing of this knowledge and experience. This teamwork will result in improved data quality and greater confidence in the data at the time of interpretation.

Clearly a multidisciplinary team is required to provide the breadth and depth of knowledge for the efficient and effective operation of a motion analysis laboratory. In the early labs (two or three decades ago), one would commonly find an engineer and physical therapist partnered with a physician. These labs were equipped to a great extent with custom hardware and software that required ongoing technical support, usually one or more engineers to ensure equipment performance and data quality. Physical therapists were tapped to work with the engineers because of their training in observational gait analysis and their patient contact experience. They were already familiar with many of the tests performed as part of the physical examination of the patient.

Today, one still commonly finds engineers and physical therapists working with physicians in clinical motion analysis laboratories. In addition, a kinesiologist or biomechanist is also quite often found in the lab as well who possesses a cross-disciplinary educational background that blends aspects of the life science training of the physical therapist with some of the "hard" science and mathematical background of the engineer. In some labs, an exercise scientist is utilized who can contribute particular expertise in physiological or metabolic energy assessment or motor control. It should be appreciated that while all of these professionals (physicians, engineers, physical therapists, etc.) may come to the motion analysis laboratory with strong academic qualifications in their respective discipline, all must receive additional "on the job" training unique to the mission of the particular motion analysis laboratory.

Given the nature of the duties in the laboratory, it is easy to understand why individual staff positions might be viewed as either being "technical" or "clinical" in nature. This division of labor was evident in the early clinical labs, with engineers fully occupied with keeping the technology in order, leaving any patient-related task to the physical therapist. This pattern of staff utilization persists in many laboratories today, with their delineation between clinical and technical responsibilities and associated staff assignments based strictly on credentialing. This compartmentalization of responsibilities can be attractive, as duties are very clearly defined, but it does not necessarily promote the highly collaborative teamwork that is required for clinical gait analysis.

An alternative to this compartmentalized staff utilization approach is cross-training and the sharing of responsibilities between staff members with different formal academic backgrounds. With this approach, engineers can be trained to assist in areas traditionally thought to be only open to physical therapists, and vice versa. A kinesiologist or biomechanist is uniquely qualified to contribute directly in all areas, again with supplementary training. The advantages of this approach are clear. Cross-training fosters teamwork, communication and respect among the staff. It is recognized that each staff member still contributes strengths to the team that are not necessarily replicated, such as the physical therapist's patient treatment experience or the engineer's mathematical skills, but all respect and appreciate that gait analysis requires constant learning in areas that readily cross traditional disciplinary boundaries.

How do these staffing considerations apply to the actual interpretation of gait data and the associated clinical decision-making? In a number of clinical labs, a patient's gait analysis information is "packaged" by the data-collection team and then turned over to one staff member, often a physical therapist or physician, who then interprets the data and formulates a treatment recommendation. This approach is time-efficient but fails to take advantage of the strength of a broad base of knowledge that is represented by the entire team. An approach that supports and promotes ongoing staff development and team building is the use of interpretation sessions attended by the entire lab staff along with the medical director of the laboratory and perhaps includes other allied health professionals such as an orthotist and clinical nurse specialist. The opportunity for learning is enhanced. One might also anticipate that the quality of the gait analysis interpretation and resulting clinical management recommendation may be improved as well.

Conclusion

The motion analysis laboratory houses both the technology and staff that support clinical gait analysis. In this facility, quantitative data are collected that pertain to the patient's kinematics (motion) as well as underlying kinetics (mechanics) and muscle activity (EMG). Often a multidisciplinary team (physicians, engineers, physical therapists and kinesiologists or biomechanists) interpret these data and formulate treatment recommendations. It is important that this team execute data collection protocols carefully and systematically. It is equally important for this team to understand the bases of these protocols so that the limitations of the patient data set can be appreciated and inappropriate interpretation can be avoided.

REFERENCES

Cavanagh PR, Ulbrecht JS. (1997) Clinical plantar pressure measurement in diabetes: rationale and methodology. *Foot* **4**: 123–135.
Perry J (1992a) *Gait Analysis: Normal and Pathological Function*. Thorofare, NJ: Slack. p 413–429.
Perry J (1992b) *Gait Analysis: Normal and Pathological Function*. Thorofare, NJ: Slack. p 431–441.
Thomas SS, Buckon CE, Melchionni J, Magnusson M, Aiona MD. (2001) Longitudinal assessment of oxygen cost and velocity in children with myelomeningocele: comparison of the hip-knee-ankle-foot orthosis and the reciprocating gait orthosis. *J Pediatr Orthop* **21**: 798 803.

7

KINEMATICS OF NORMAL GAIT

Michael Schwartz

Gait is a dynamic activity. In order to understand gait we need to understand dynamics, which is the study of objects in motion and the factors that affect these motions. These factors include force, mass, momentum and energy. Dynamics can be subdivided into kinematics and kinetics. Kinematics, the focus of this chapter, describes motion without regard to its causes. Kinetics, which will be covered in the next chapter, is concerned with the effect of forces and torques on the motions of bodies. These two chapters serve as the foundation for the study of pathological motions, their likely causes and their possible remedies.

To understand the kinematics of gait, we must first introduce some basic definitions. A *vector* is a directed line segment (an arrow), and has both a size (magnitude) and a direction (Fig. 7.1a). A *coordinate system* is a set of three mutually perpendicular vectors (x–y–z) (Fig. 7.1b). A *laboratory coordinate system* is a coordinate system that remains fixed in space (Fig. 7.2a). A *technical coordinate system* is a coordinate system derived from markers fixed to various body segments such as the pelvis or thigh. This coordinate system moves with the body segment (Fig. 7.2b). An *anatomical coordinate system* is a coordinate system derived from the technical coordinate system and subject specific alignment information. This coordinate system, which is aligned with the principal anatomical planes, also moves with the body segment (Fig. 7.2c). Finally, a *degree of freedom* (DOF) is an allowable displacement of either a linear or angular nature.

Biomechanical model

> *It is possible to be a master in false philosophy—easier, in fact, than to be a master in the truth, because a false philosophy can be made as simple and consistent as one pleases.*
> George Santayana (1863–1952)

A biomechanical model is a simplified representation of a biological system. The term "model" refers to a set of assumptions and idealizations that allow us to calculate important clinical information. Many different models are used for gait analysis; however, all of the models have certain elements in common. It is not the purpose of this chapter to provide an exhaustive discussion of the accuracy and validity of different models, but rather to focus on the kinematics that can be derived using the most common elements of standard gait models. Where appropriate, modeling limitations and their impact on the data will be discussed.

The model of the lower extremity used for this chapter consists of seven rigid bodies

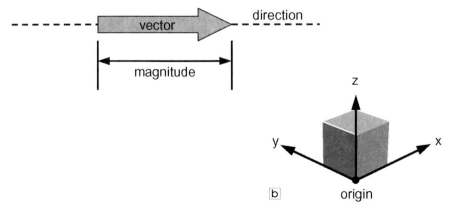

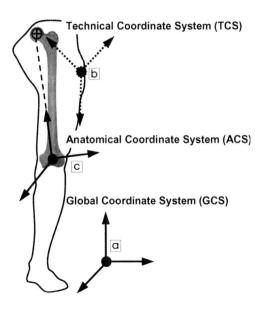

Fig. 7.1. (a) Vectors are essential elements of kinematics. Vectors are directed line segments (arrows) with a direction and a magnitude. (b) Three mutually perpendicular vectors form the basis of Cartesian coordinate systems, which are used to track the orientations of body segments in gait.

Fig. 7.2. (a) Three different types of coordinate systems are used to derive kinematics. The global coordinate system is fixed in the lab space, and (generally) oriented along the walking path. (b) A technical coordinate system is fixed to a body segment, but is not aligned with the anatomy. Technical coordinate systems are derived from observed marker positions, and as such they are sometimes referred to as marker-based coordinate systems. (c) Anatomical co-ordinate systems are attached to body segments, and aligned with the principal anatomical directions (sagittal, coronal and transverse).

(Fig. 7.3). These are the pelvis, two thighs, two shanks and two one-dimensional rigid feet. The modeling of the foot as a single, one-dimensional rigid body presents severe limitations that will be discussed further. However, due to the technical difficulties involved in measuring, analyzing and reporting the subtle and complex motions of the foot, the idealizations currently used are necessary.

The hips are modeled as ball-and-socket joints (revolute joints). These joints allow three rotational DOF. By this we mean that the hips can rotate freely in all three planes. The knees are also considered to have three rotational DOF but no translational DOF. This 3-DOF knee model does not allow for "roll-back" (the anteroposterior motion of the tibia relative

100

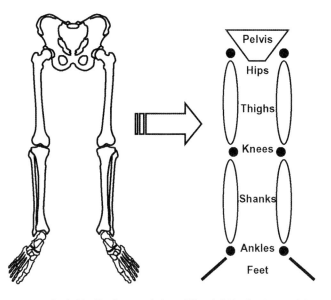

Fig. 7.3. The lower extremity is idealized as consisting of five rigid bodies (one pelvis, two thighs and two shanks) and two rigid lines (two feet). These rigid elements are considered to be connected by six 3-DOF joints (two hips, two knees and two ankles).

to the femur during flexion and extension) but does allow for screw home (the transverse-plane rotation of the tibia relative to the femur near terminal extension). The true motion of the knee joint is probably best modeled as a 1-DOF joint, where both the roll-back and screw-home mechanisms are dependent functions of the knee-flexion angle (Blankevoort et al. 1988, 1990, Lafortune et al. 1992, Piazza and Cavanagh 2000). This more sophisticated knee model is used in some areas of gait analysis but the majority of practising clinical laboratories use the simplified 3-DOF knee.

In describing ankle kinematics we are describing the motion of the foot-vector relative to the tibia. This motion incorporates talocrural, talonavicular, talocalcaneal motions as well as the other mid-foot articulations. The aforementioned joints allow for 3-DOF motions. However, using the one-dimensional foot model, only two rotations can be measured. This will be discussed further in the following sections.

In clinical gait laboratories, the most common method for deriving joint kinematics is as follows. (1) Markers are placed on the subject. (2) Alignment information is obtained (hip center, knee axis, knee center). (3) Three-dimensional marker trajectories (position vector versus time) are captured. (4) Technical marker-based coordinate systems are calculated. (5) Anatomical coordinate systems are derived (from marker-based coordinate systems and alignment information). (6) Joint angles are calculated.

Numerous references can be found in this book and elsewhere for the reader interested in the details associated with steps 1–5. For the remainder of this chapter, we will focus on the joint angles, their definition and meaning, and the patterns that they display during normal gait.

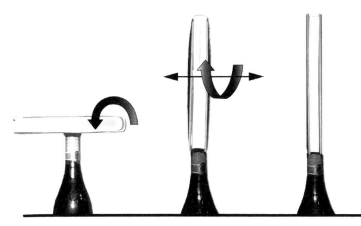

Fig. 7.4. Start with a book oriented as shown. Rotate the book by 90° about its spine, then rotate it by 90° about its face. One ends up looking at ends of the vertically oriented pages of the book.

It is fundamental (if obvious) that joints do not move. Body segments adjacent to joints move and the relative motions of these bodies are termed joint rotation. For example, the hip joint is the shared point between the pelvis and the femur. The relative motion of the femur with respect to the pelvis is interpreted as hip-joint rotation. In clinical gait analysis, it is common to report this relative motion in terms of Euler angles. Euler angles are one method, among many, which can be used to describe the position of one body segment relative to an adjacent body segment.

Euler angles are a means to describe finite sequential rotations of one body relative to another (Greenwood 1988). An important aspect of Euler angles is that *the numerical values of the angles depend on the sequence of rotations*. The sequence most commonly used is sagittal plane followed by coronal plane followed by transverse plane. Clearly, when we move our joints, we do not move them in any such sequence, but rather in a smooth manner about continuously varying axes. Nevertheless, it is mathematically necessary to define a rotation order so that we may make clinical sense and use of the data from the gait laboratory.

The sequence dependence is a consequence of a fundamental geometric theorem that *finite rotations are not conserved*. What does this theorem mean in practical terms? Imagine that you are holding a book. Rotate the book 90° about its spine, then 90° about its face. Now note the orientation of the book in space, and you will see that you are looking at ends of the vertically oriented pages of the book (Fig. 7.4). If instead you were first to rotate the book about its face and *then* about its spine, you would end up looking at the cover of the book (Fig. 7.5). The order in which the rotations are performed dictates the final position of the book in space. Now imagine that you see a book in a certain orientation. Your description of the orientation in terms of three rotations would vary depending on the order in which the rotations were carried out.

This is analogous to the situation encountered when trying to describe the orientations of bodies as measured in the gait laboratory. We observe the positions of bodies with the aid of the motion capture hardware and software. We then specify an order of rotations.

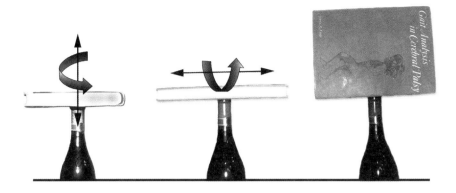

Fig. 7.5. Start with a book oriented as shown (same as in the previous case). Rotate it 90° about its face, then another 90° about the spine. One ends up looking at cover of the book.

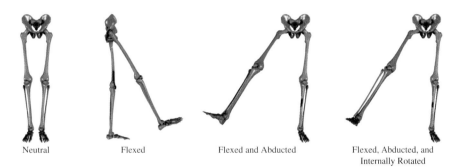

| Neutral | Flexed | Flexed and Abducted | Flexed, Abducted, and Internally Rotated |

Fig. 7.6. In order to calculate the three dimensional rotations at a joint, we must choose a default order of rotations. The standard order of rotations used in clinical gait analysis is sagittal–coronal–transverse. As an example, consider the position shown on the right. This position is decomposed into hip flexion about the pelvic ML axis, followed by hip abduction about the thigh's AP axis, followed by internal hip rotation about the mechanical axis of the thigh.

Finally, we compute the numerical values of these rotations based on the specified order. To compare kinematics between patients and laboratories, it is necessary to impose a standard rotation sequence. Some debate exists regarding which sequence makes the most sense, specifically with regard to the pelvis (Baker 2001). By far the most common sequence is sagittal–coronal–transverse (sometimes called y–x'–z"). It is this order that will be used throughout this book.

To put these abstract concepts into a clinically meaningful setting consider the following example. Begin with a reference state in which the anatomical planes of the pelvis and the thigh are in anatomical neutral position (Fig. 7.6). Consider coordinate systems, attached to each of these bodies and aligned with the principal directions. These axes are called the anatomical coordinate systems of the bodies. Rotate the thigh about the medial–lateral (M–L) pointing axis of the pelvis (proximal y-axis), by an amount called "hip flexion". This

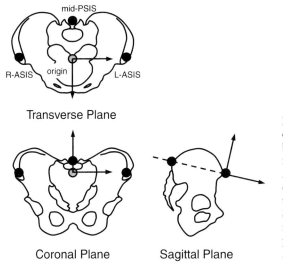

Transverse Plane

Coronal Plane   Sagittal Plane

Fig. 7.7. The pelvic anatomical co-ordinate system has an origin midway between the left and right ASIS. The mediolateral axis points from the right ASIS to the left ASIS. The AP axis points (approximately) from the midpoint of the left and right PSIS to the origin. The SI axis is mutually perpendicular to the first two. In other words, it is perpendicular to a plane containing the L/R ASIS and the PSIS.

is the first joint rotation. Next, rotate the thigh about its *current* anteroposterior axis (distal x'-axis) by the amount called "hip abduction". At this point, the longitudinal axis of the thigh is in its final orientation. Now perform a third rotation about the longitudinal axis of the thigh (distal z"). This rotation is called "hip internal rotation". Notice that while the first and third rotations occurred about physically extant axes, the second rotation occurred about an axis that is mutually perpendicular to the first and third axes, but not resident in any observable body segment. Rotations about this so-called "floating" axis are often the most difficult to interpret and extra care must be observed when considering these coronal-plane angles.

Joint-angle definitions: clinical/approximate

While the mathematical framework just described provides a method for calculation of Euler angles, it is not very useful for the clinician. However, by considering simplified scenarios we can arrive at useful, albeit approximate, angle definitions. In each of the following scenarios we assume that the initial state has all joints at 0° (anatomical position). We then assume that a uniplanar motion of the distal segment occurs to produce the final state (e.g. pure flexion). While this situation virtually never occurs, it provides a convenient framework for defining the joint angles in a way that makes the most sense clinically.

PELVIS
Pelvic anatomical coordinate system (Fig. 7.7)
The anatomical coordinate system of the pelvis is defined using the midpoint of the posterior superior iliac spine (PSIS) and the left and right anterior superior iliac spine (ASIS). The anteroposterior (AP) axis of this coordinate system points from the PSIS to the midpoint of the ASIS. The mediolateral (ML) axis points from right ASIS to left ASIS and the superoinferior (SI) axis is perpendicular to the plane formed by the AP and ML axes.

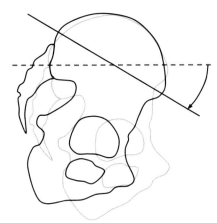

Fig. 7.8. Pelvic tilt occurs about the pelvis's ML axis. If the coronal- and transverse-plane pelvic angles are zero, pelvic tilt can be measured as the angle from horizontal to the pelvic AP axis in the sagittal plane.

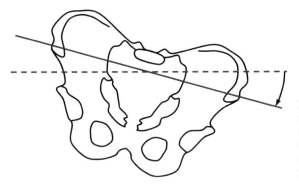

Fig. 7.9. Pelvic obliquity occurs about the pelvis's AP axis. If the sagittal- and transverse-plane pelvic angles are zero, pelvic obliquity can be measured as the angle from horizontal to the pelvic ML axis in the coronal plane.

Proximal and distal bodies

Pelvic angles are reported with respect to the laboratory. This means that the stationary laboratory coordinate system is treated as the proximal (fixed) body while the pelvis itself is considered to be the distal (moving) body.

Sagittal-plane rotation (Fig. 7.8)

The sagittal-plane rotation of the pelvis is called "pelvic tilt". Consider the pelvic anatomical coordinate system (CS) to be initially parallel to the laboratory CS. Now rotate the pelvis about its ML axis. Assume that the coronal and transverse plane angles are zero. In this case, sagittal-plane pelvic motion (anterior/posterior tilt) can be measured as the angle between the pelvic AP axis and horizontal. In a typical standing posture, the pelvic AP axis points about 10° downward, while the other two axes remain parallel to the laboratory. Thus approximately 10° of anterior pelvic tilt is present in normal standing posture.

Coronal-plane rotation (Fig. 7.9)

Again begin with the pelvic anatomical CS parallel to the laboratory CS. Now let the pelvis

105

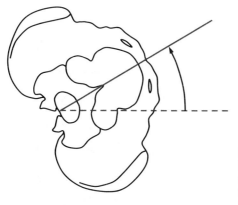

Fig. 7.10. Pelvic rotation occurs about the pelvis's SI axis. If the sagittal- and coronal-plane pelvic angles are zero, pelvic rotation can be measured as the angle from the line of progression to the pelvic AP axis in the transverse plane.

rotate about its own AP axis so that the pelvic ML axis tips relative to the horizontal plane. The angle between the pelvic ML axis and the laboratory y-axis is the pelvic obliquity. Depending on which side of the pelvis you look at, the obliquity is called either "up" or "down" (with the obvious convention).

This raises a point about the pelvis that is occasionally confusing to gait analysis neophytes. Namely, pelvic angles are typically reported using a "left" or "right" prefix. However, except for the most extraordinary cases, a person only has one pelvis! What then is the meaning of these chirognostic prefixes? As the example above makes clear, the two sides of the pelvis undergo simultaneous opposite motions in the coronal (and transverse) planes. This means that when the "left" hemi-pelvis is up, the "right" hemi-pelvis is down, and vice versa. For the pelvis, "up" is plotted as a positive number, and "down" as a negative number.

Transverse-plane rotation (Fig. 7.10)
Now consider a pelvic anatomical CS that is parallel to the horizontal plane of the laboratory[1], but has undergone a rotation about its own SI axis. For the sake of the example, imagine that the rotation was counterclockwise about this axis when viewed from above. In other words, if you were to align the thumb of your right hand with the upward pointing SI axis and wrap your fingers around the axis, the wrapping of your fingers would give the sense of the rotation. In this case, the right side of the pelvis would be rotated internally, while the left side would be rotated externally. Internal rotation is plotted as a positive number, while external rotation is plotted as a negative number.

The thumb-and-fingers method is called the "right-hand rule". A universal convention in physics and mathematics is that right-hand sense rotations, such as the one described, are algebraically positive. This convention is not particularly useful for plotting Euler

---

[1] As an aside, notice that a pelvis such as this would have "algebraic" tilt value of 0°, but would actually be posteriorly tipped relative to a normal standing posture.

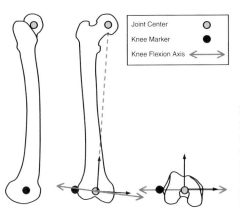

Fig. 7.11. The anatomical coordinate system of the thigh is defined from the hip center, knee center and knee-flexion axis. The longitudinal axis points from the knee center to the hip center. The coronal plane of the thigh contains the hip and knee centers and the knee-flexion axis. The AP axis is perpendicular to the plane containing the hip and knee centers and the knee-flexion axis.

angles. The widely (though not universally) adopted convention is that in the sagittal plane, "flexion" (or anterior tilt in the case of the pelvis) is positive and extension is negative. In the coronal plane, "adduction" (or up for the pelvis) is positive and "abduction" is negative and in the transverse plane "internal rotation" is positive and "external rotation" is negative. These conventions will be followed throughout this chapter.

HIP

Proximal and distal bodies

Hip angles measure the motion of the femur relative to the pelvis. The pelvis is the (mathematically) fixed body, while the femur is considered to be the moving body. This is a purely mathematical convention as motion of the hip is a purely relative effect.

Thigh anatomical coordinate system (Fig. 7.11)

The thigh's anatomical coordinate system is aligned such that the thigh SI axis is parallel to the mechanical axis of the femur (knee center-to-hip center). The ML axis is perpendicular to the SI axis in a plane containing the SI axis and the average knee-flexion axis. The thigh AP axis is perpendicular to the plane formed by the ML and SI axes, and points forward.

Sagittal-plane rotation (Fig. 7.12)

Consider a pelvis that is parallel to the laboratory coordinate system. Extend the pelvic SI axis downward (below the pelvis). As the hip flexes, the thigh's SI moves in front of the extended pelvic SI axis. Hip extension reverses this, and places the thigh's SI axis behind the extended pelvic SI axis. The angle between the SI axis of the pelvis and that of the thigh is hip flexion. At the hip (and knee), flexion is positive and extension is negative by convention.

Coronal-plane rotation (Fig. 7.13)

Hip adduction/abduction can be measured using the method just described, but viewed in the coronal plane (assuming that there is neither sagittal- nor transverse-plane hip rotation).

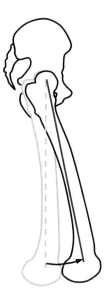

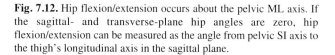

Fig. 7.12. Hip flexion/extension occurs about the pelvic ML axis. If the sagittal- and transverse-plane hip angles are zero, hip flexion/extension can be measured as the angle from pelvic SI axis to the thigh's longitudinal axis in the sagittal plane.

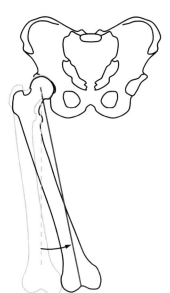

Fig. 7.13. Hip adduction/abduction occurs about the thigh's AP axis. If the sagittal- and transverse-plane hip angles are zero, hip adduction/abduction can be measured as the angle from the pelvic SI axis in the thigh's longitudinal axis in the coronal plane.

Adduction directs thigh's SI axis towards the body's midline, while abduction directs it away from the midline. Adduction of the thigh is plotted as a positive number, while abduction of the thigh is plotted as a negative number.

Transverse-plane rotation (Fig. 7.14)

Consider the pelvis and thigh viewed from above. Assume that the pelvis has undergone no rotations relative to the laboratory, and that the hip is in a neutral position in the sagittal

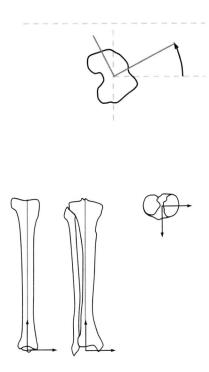

Fig. 7.14. Hip internal/external rotation occurs about the thigh's longitudinal axis. If the sagittal- and coronal-plane hip angles are zero, hip rotation can be measured as the angle from the pelvic AP axis to the thigh AP axis in the transverse plane.

Fig. 7.15. The anatomical coordinate system of the shank (tibia) is defined from the knee center, ankle center and either the knee-flexion axis or an approximated ankle-flexion axis. The longitudinal axis points from the ankle center to the knee center. The coronal plane of the tibia contains the hip and knee centers and either the knee-flexion axis or the ankle-flexion axis.

and coronal planes. Now let the hip undergo a pure internal rotation (rotation about the long axis of the thigh). We can measure internal or external hip rotation as the angle between the AP axes of the pelvis and the thigh.

It is important to reiterate that all joint angles describe the relative motions of proximal and distal bodies. Thus we could have achieved the same hip angles (in the above examples) with a "fixed" thigh and an externally rotating pelvis. This issue is especially important to keep in mind when interpreting hip angles.

KNEE
Proximal and distal bodies
Knee angles measure the motion of the shank moving relative to the thigh.

Shank coordinate system (Fig. 7.15)
The shank anatomical CS is analogous to that of the thigh. The ankle-flexion axis, ankle-joint center and knee-joint center replace the knee-flexion axis, knee center and hip center

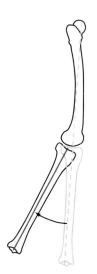

Fig. 7.16. Knee-flexion/extension occurs about the thigh's ML axis. If the sagittal- and transverse-plane knee angles are zero, knee-flexion/extension can be measured as the angle from the thigh's longitudinal axis to the shank's longitudinal axis in the sagittal plane.

respectively. The ML axis of the shank points along an approximate ankle-flexion axis. There is a considerable divergence of opinion about exactly how this axis should be defined. In some laboratories, a bimalleolar axis is used. In others, the knee axis and a tibial torsion measurement are used to specify the ankle axis. Yet others simply use the unmodified knee-flexion axis. As noted above, while these technical details are important, to dwell on them here would be an unnecessary distraction from the primary goal of this chapter.

Knee motion is primarily in the sagittal plane. It is well established that the out of plane knee motions are coupled to the sagittal-plane rotations. In this sense, the knee has only one true DOF. However, as with the hip, we will consider scenarios in which the three planes of motion are considered to be independent. This assumed independence does not compromise the accuracy or validity of the measured knee angles.

Sagittal-plane rotation (Fig. 7.16)
As before, the proximal segment (in this case the thigh) is parallel to the laboratory coordinate system. Also, as before, assume that both coronal and transverse plane motions are zero. Knee flexion/extension is then measured as the angle between the longitudinal thigh axis and the longitudinal shank axis.

Coronal-plane rotation (Fig. 7.17)
Knee varus/valgus is measured using these same vectors viewed in the coronal plane. Varus motion directs the shank axis toward the midline, while valgus directs it away from the midline.

Transverse-plane rotation
In the case where knee flexion/extension and knee varus/valgus are zero, knee rotation can measured as the angle between the thigh AP axis and the shank AP axis, as viewed from above.

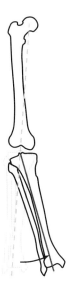

Fig. 7.17. Knee varus–valgus (adduction–abduction) occurs about the shank's anterior–posterior axis. If the sagittal and transverse plane knee angles are zero, knee varus–valgus can be measured as the angle from the thigh's longitudinal axis in the shank's longitudinal axis in the coronal plane.

ANKLE AND FOOT

Proximal and distal bodies

Ankle angles measure the motion of the foot vector relative to the shank.

Anatomical coordinate system (Fig. 7.18)

The anatomical coordinate system of the foot is greatly simplified for reasons mentioned above. The foot is typically modeled as a one-dimensional vector, directed from the middle of the calcaneus to the midpoint of the second and third metatarsal joints. Only sagittal- and transverse-plane rotations are measured due to the foot's one-dimensional approximation. Unlike the other joints in the lower extremity, the rotations of the foot and ankle are not Euler angles.

Sagittal-plane rotation (Fig. 7.19)

Consider a shank that is parallel to the laboratory CS. The angle between the foot vector and the AP axis of the shank is ankle dorsi/plantarflexion.

Transverse-plane rotation (Fig. 7.20)

The transverse-plane motion of the foot is generally reported as a foot-progression angle. The foot-progression angle is the angle between projection of the foot vector on to the laboratory horizontal plane, and the line of progression. This can be thought of as the orientation of the shadow cast by the foot from a light directly overhead.

WARNING

It is worth reiterating here that these clinical/approximate angle definitions are only strictly applicable in the exact scenarios described: namely that the proximal segment is fixed in

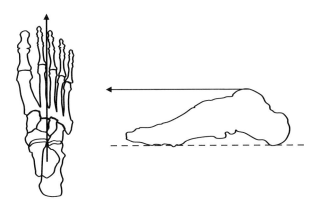

Fig. 7.18. The foot is modeled as a one-dimensional vector rather than a three-dimensional body. The vector is directed from the middle of the calcaneus to the middle of the forefoot, parallel to the plantar surface of the foot.

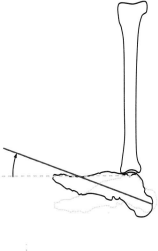

Fig. 7.19. Dorsiflexion and plantarflexion are measured as the angle between the shank's AP axis and the foot vector, projected on to the sagittal plane.

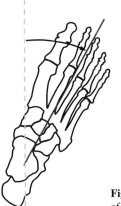

Fig. 7.20. Foot progression is the angle between the foot vector and the line of progression, projected on to the laboratory's transverse plane.

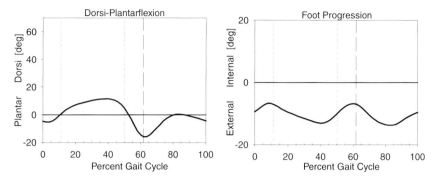

Fig. 7.21. Kinematic graphs of the ankle and foot in the sagittal and transverse planes, respectively. In the sagittal plane, dorsiflexion and plantarflexion of the foot are referenced to the segment above (the shank). However, at Gillette Children's Hospital, foot progression is referenced to the axes of the laboratory.

a neutral position, and the motion is only occurring in a single plane. It is extremely rare that these circumstances occur in normal or pathological gait. Thus the true three-dimensional kinematics, as reported by the gait analysis system, are indispensable.

Kinematics of normal gait

We now turn our focus from the definitions of angles, to the values of these angles in the gait of persons with no orthopedic or neurologic impairments. We will refer to these as "able-bodied" gait patterns. It is important to point out that even among the population without any impairment, modest variations in gait patterns exist.

It is convenient to break the gait cycle down into different phases, and examine the kinematics on a phase-by-phase basis. These phases promote the understanding of the functional roles played by active muscle forces, body weight and inertial forces. These influences will be made even clearer in Chapter 8. We will consider the following seven phases of the gait cycle: (1) loading response, (2) mid-stance, (3) terminal stance, (4) pre-swing, (5) initial swing, (6) mid-swing, and (7) terminal swing. It should be remembered that the end of terminal-swing phase for one gait cycle is equivalent to initial contact of the subsequent gait cycle. The functional purposes and qualitative descriptions of these phases are covered in Chapter 4.

For the descriptions that follow, please refer to the kinematic graphs provided. These graphs contain the data from the Gillette Children's Specialty Healthcare Motion Analysis Laboratory. These graphs are meant for instructive purposes only, and are not intended for use in gait laboratories. It is imperative that individual laboratories derive a set of control gait curves using their own equipment, personnel and biomechanical model.

ANKLE (Fig. 7.21)

Sagittal-plane dorsiflexion/plantarflexion

Loading response begins at initial contact. At this instant, the ankle is slightly plantarflexed (~−5°). It is common, however, to see values ranging from a few degrees of plantarflexion

113

to a few degrees of dorsiflexion. A common mistake made in observational analysis is to presume that the ankle is dorsiflexed at initial contact. This misconception generally arises from viewing the foot relative to the floor, and noting its upward pointing orientation. However, as discussed above, ankle dorsiflexion/plantarflexion motion is measured by from the foot relative to the tibia.

Following initial contact, the ankle plantarflexes until the foot is flat on the floor. This motion is sometimes referred to as "first rocker". This plantarflexion occurs under the eccentric control of the anterior tibialis, which lowers the foot to the floor and thereby prevents foot-slap. First rocker occurs during the phase of the gait cycle known as loading response.

The ankle then begins to dorsiflex ("second rocker") while the momentum of the body carries the leg and torso forward. The ankle continues to dorsiflex through mid stance. The rate of this dorsiflexion is controlled by the soleus, which plays a pivotal role in maintaining knee joint behind the progressing center of pressure. The ankle reaches a peak dorsiflexion around 10°–15° at the end of second rocker. Second rocker occurs during the phase of the gait cycle known as *mid-stance*.

Heel-lift ends the dorsiflexion phase for the ankle. Heel-lift results from a number of factors including: passive stretching and tensioning of the gastrocsoleus complex, forward momentum of the body, active plantarflexion of the gastrocnemius and knee flexion. Heel-lift ("third rocker") initiates the phase of the gait cycle known as *terminal stance*. The ankle continues to actively plantarflex until toe-off, where it reaches its maximum value of ~25° plantarflexion. The terminal-stance/pre-swing phase accounts for the majority of propulsion during gait.

Early swing is characterized by a rapid dorsiflexion of the ankle necessary for foot clearance. The ankle comes all of the way back to neutral under the action of the anterior tibialis by mid-swing, and then drops into a slight amount plantarflexion in terminal swing. This places the ankle/foot into their initial contact position for the next gait cycle.

Coronal-plane inversion/eversion
The simplified foot model (one-dimensional) described earlier in this section does not allow coronal-plane foot rotations to be measured. As noted earlier the omission of these angles is largely due to technical difficulties involved in tracking foot-mounted markers.

Transverse-plane internal/external foot progression
The foot progression angle at initial contact is slightly external ($\sim -10°$). In healthy subjects, this angle is strongly influenced by the amount of tibial torsion present. In cases where pathology is present, mid-foot and forefoot deformities can also have a considerable impact on this measurement. There is very little transverse-plane motion of the foot relative to the floor in the during stance phase. What little range of motion (ROM) does exist ($-5°$) occurs primarily from initial contact through foot-flat, and from heel-lift through toe-off.

In swing phase, foot progression remains nearly constant. There tends to be a slight external rotation in early swing, followed by an internal rotation in late swing (~5° ROM). Keeping in mind that foot progression is plotted relative to the laboratory, it can be understood that the source of this rotation could be the ankle, knee, hip or pelvis. In any case, the motion tends to be quite subtle, and not of great consequence in a population that does not have any pathology. In children with foot-clearance problems this is no longer the case. In these subjects the swing-phase foot-progression angle is used primarily to assess compensatory mechanisms.

KNEE (Fig. 7. 22)

Sagittal-plane flexion/extension

At initial contact, the knee is slightly flexed (~10°) anticipating the imminent onset of contact. During loading response, the knee flexes from its initial value to about 20°. This *controlled buckling* is critical for accepting the body's weight in a manner that spares the joints from unnecessarily large impact loads.

During mid-stance the knee actively extends to around 5° of flexion. The knee, like all of the other joints, does not reach the end of its range of motion during gait. This spares the passive structures from bearing significant chronic-cyclic loads.

In terminal-stance the knee begins to flex. There is a synergism between heel lift and knee flexion. This is a natural consequence of the closed-chain limb geometry. The knee continues to flex through pre-swing, up to and beyond toe off. At toe-off, the knee is typically flexed between 40° and 50°. During the latter half of stance phase, the thigh develops significant translational and rotational momentum that will be used to carry the leg through swing-phase. The appropriate conditions at toe-off are crucial to normal swing-phase leg mechanics, which are largely passive.

Swing-phase knee flexion is an essential mechanism for ground clearance. In early swing, the momentum of the thigh promotes continued knee flexion, up to a peak of around 60°. At this point the knee undergoes a large, rapid extension to a terminal swing value around 5° of flexion (again, avoiding the extreme extension range). Just prior to terminal swing/initial contact the knee flexes slightly to prepare for landing. This flexion is caused by the hamstrings, which are simultaneously preparing to extend the hip.

Coronal-plane varus/valgus

In normal gait, the coronal-plane motion of the knee is primarily dictated by the geometry of the knee and the angle of flexion. In its unloaded, slightly flexed state, the knee tends to be nearly neutral in the coronal plane. Very little coronal-plane knee motion occurs in early and mid-stance. The motion that does occur is too small and variable for it to be measured reliably by standard gait laboratory hardware. From late stance through swing phase, when the knee is undergoing ~60° ROM of flexion, there is a passive varus motion of the knee up to ~10°[2].

The knee-varus angle is the source of significant debate and discussion in the gait-analysis community (Baker et al. 1999). There is evidence that true coronal-plane knee motion is

---

[2] Strictly speaking, the motion should be termed adduction, resulting in a varus position of the knee. The modest misuse of the terms varus and adduction used herein is quite typical of clinical gait analysis, and is therefore adopted for this chapter.

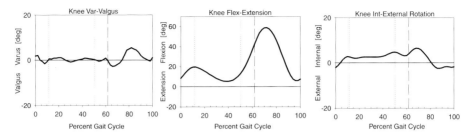

Fig. 7.22. Kinematic graphs of the knee in the coronal, sagittal and transverse planes, respectively. In each case, motion of the shank is referenced to the thigh.

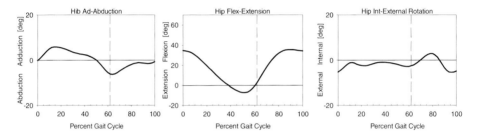

Fig. 7.23. Kinematic graphs of the hip in the coronal, sagittal and transverse planes, respectively. In each case, motion of the thigh is referenced to the pelvis.

coupled to knee flexion. On the other hand, it is well known that a slight transverse-plane malalignment of the knee-flexion axis can cause rotational artifacts that amplify this coupled motion. It is hoped that recent analytical developments will aid in resolving these issues in the near future.

Transverse-plane internal/external rotation
The transverse-plane motion of the knee is primarily due to the screw-home mechanism that occurs near full extension. The total range-of-motion of the knee in the transverse plane is relatively small (< 10°). There are concerns about the ability of standard motion-analysis equipment and methods to measure this angle accurately. For both of these reasons, the transverse-plane knee motion is interpreted cautiously. There are situations, such as in cases of ligamentous laxity, or in the assessment of orthotics for patients with myelomeningocele, where internal/external knee rotation (as well as knee varus/valgus) can be an important and useful clinical tool.

HIP (Fig. 7.23)
Sagittal-plane flexion/extension
At initial contact, the hip is flexed to ~35°. During loading response, active hip extension occurs via the gluteus maximus and hamstrings. This is followed by a primarily passive

(or even restrained) extension through mid-stance. The hip passes into extension at the beginning of terminal stance, and continues to a maximally extended position of $-5°$ to $-10°$. The hip then begins to flex during pre-swing in unison with the rapidly flexing knee. This "pull-off" mechanism is critical for proper swing-phase mechanics. At toe-off the hip is roughly neutral.

During early and mid-swing the hip continues to flex, reaching a maximum value of ~35°. During terminal swing, the hip-flexion angle remains nearly constant, with a slight tendency to extend a few degrees just before initial contact.

Coronal-plane adduction/abduction
At initial contact the hip is neutrally positioned in the coronal plane. During loading response the hip adducts ~5°. The primary source of this adduction is the lowering of the contralateral side of the pelvis as the contralateral limb unloads and flexes at the knee and hip. During mid-stance, abduction back to a neutral position is actively achieved through lateral hip musculature such as the gluteus medius. In terminal-stance and pre-swing the hip abducts to a toe-off value ~ $-5°$. This occurs in a largely passive manner through the unloading and flexing of the ipsilateral limb. Keep in mind that pre-swing on the ipsilateral limb corresponds to loading response on the contralateral limb. From its maximally abducted position near toe-off, the hip abducts back to a neutral position at terminal swing. The mechanism for this is primarily passive. Specifically, the active abduction of the contralateral hip during stance phase raises the pelvis to a level position. In doing so, the ipsilateral swing leg, which is hanging nearly vertically, is effectively adducting.

Transverse-plane internal/external rotation
The normal range of motion for internal/external hip rotation is <10°. The subtle motion of the hip in this plane is difficult to measure reliably since it is quite sensitive to skin-motion artifact and other modeling compromises like the knee-alignment device. Nevertheless, some general trends can be observed.

The hip is neutral at initial contact. The hip then internally rotates ~5° during loading response and remains there throughout stance. During mid-swing and terminal swing, the hip first internally then externally rotates a few degrees in each direction. These dynamic motions are somewhat inconsistent, difficult to measure and hold unclear meaning. It is again important to recognize that transverse-plane hip rotation can occur by means of transverse-plane pelvic rotation acting around a fixed thigh.

The *mean value* of the hip-rotation angle is an important value, especially in pathological gait. The reason for this is that the mean hip rotation angle is strongly indicator of the amount of anteversion present in the femur. Recall the definition of hip internal/external rotation (Figs 7.10, 7.11). The angle between the knee axis (essentially the bicondylar axis) and the pelvic ML axis is the essential component of the hip rotation. The more anteversion present, the larger this angle becomes. Of course it is possible for a person to externally rotate their hip actively, thereby neutralizing the dynamic effect of anteversion. This will be discussed further in later chapters.

117

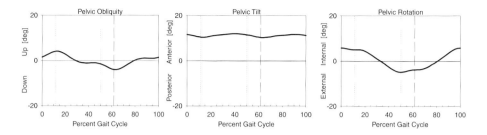

Fig. 7.24. Kinematic graphs of the pelvis in the coronal, sagittal and transverse planes. In each case, motion of the pelvis is referenced to the coordinates (axes) of the laboratory.

PELVIS (Fig. 7.24)
Sagittal-plane flexion/extension
There is little motion of the pelvis in the sagittal plane. The total ROM during normal gait is only ~5°. At initial contact, the pelvis is anteriorly tilted ~10°. During the first half of stance the pelvis tilts first posteriorly, then anteriorly a few degrees, to the initial contact value at the time of contact on the contralateral side. The pattern then repeats while the contralateral leg is in stance phase. The mean value of pelvic tilt is ~10°. Both the mean value, and the range of motion, can be dramatically altered by hip-flexor tightness/spasticity, lumbar lordosis and other pathologies typical of cerebral palsy. Therefore, while sagittal-plane pelvic motion is quite unremarkable in normal gait, it is important to study so that the deviations commonly seen in pathological gait can be better understood.

Coronal-plane obliquity
The coronal-plane motion of the pelvis follows a pattern very similar to the coronal-plane motion of the hip. At initial contact, the ipsilateral side of the pelvis is nearly level to slightly "up". During loading response the contralateral limb unloads and flexes causing the contralateral side of the pelvis to drop. During this drop, the ipsilateral side of the pelvis gains ~5° of additional upwards obliquity. Notice that this "upward" obliquity is not necessarily linked to upward motion of the pelvis, but instead is a consequence of "downward" motion of the contralateral side. Following loading response, the pelvis drops to a level position by mid-stance. The pelvis drops very slightly from this time until initial contact on the contralateral side, at which point the pattern just described repeats, but in reverse.

Transverse-plane internal/external rotation
At initial contact the ipsilateral pelvis is slightly internally rotated (~5°) due to the forward position of the limb terminus at contact. There is a gradual external rotation to a value of ~5° of external rotation by the time of contralateral limb contact. The pattern then reverses. Once again, while these motions are quite subtle in normal gait, they can be greatly amplified in pathological gait as a direct or compensatory result of orthopedic and neuromuscular impairment.

Summary

This chapter has discussed gait kinematics under three general headings: technical details, biomechanical modeling and patterns observed in normal gait. With a thorough understanding of these elements, the reader is prepared to begin the study of pathological gait. In terms of technical details and biomechanical modeling, we have intentionally kept the discussion to the minimum. Nevertheless, a myriad of important and subtle elements are embodied in these details, and the advanced reader is strongly encouraged to seek more information.

The elements of normal gait described herein attempt to stress the most relevant issues. A complete set of kinematic graphs is included for reference. It is important to stress that these graphs/tables are the result of a single laboratory's implementation of a single biomechanical model. The reader is cautioned against using these data in their own laboratory until s/he is certain that the biomechanical model, activity in question and population under investigation conforms to those used in the acquisition and processing of the reference data.

To gain the most value from gait analysis, one should also become proficient with the elements of kinetics, since kinematics and kinetics are inextricably linked. The next chapter provides the information necessary to fulfil this goal.

REFERENCES

Baker R. (2001) Pelvic angles: a mathematically rigorous definition which is consistent with a conventional clinical understanding of the terms. *Gait Posture* **13:** 1–6.

Baker R, McDowel B, Finney L, Cosgrove A (1999) A new approach to determining the hip rotation profile during clinical gait analysis. *Gait Posture* **9:** 134.

Blankevoort L, Huiskes R, de Lange A. (1988) The envelope of passive knee joint motion. *J Biomech* **21:** 705–720.

Blankevoort L, Huiskes R, de Lange A. (1990) Helical axes of passive knee joint motions. *J Biomech* **23:** 1219–1229.

Greenwood DT. (1988) *Principals of Dynamics*. Englewood Cliffs, NJ: Prentice Hall.

Lafortune MA, Cavanagh PR, Sommer HJ 3rd, Kalenak A. (1992) Three-dimensional kinematics of the human knee during walking. *J Biomech* **25:** 347–357.

Piazza SJ, Cavanagh PR. (2000) Measurement of the screw-home motion of the knee is sensitive to errors in axis alignment. *J Biomech* **33:** 1029–1034.

8
KINETICS OF NORMAL GAIT

Roy B. Davis and Sylvia Õunpuu

As stated in the previous chapter, kinematics is a quantitative description of motion presented principally for clinical gait analysis as time histories of angular displacement, i.e. segment and joint angles over the gait cycle. The availability of "joint kinetics" (principally joint moments and powers) for clinical gait analysis allows one to examine mechanisms that either control or produce that motion, thus potentially developing a more comprehensive understanding of the motion. It is important to appreciate joint kinetic results in the context of the corresponding gait kinematic and electromyographic data. These three types of information provide different perspectives on the same gait events. Ideally, their simultaneous interpretation provides an opportunity for the corroboration of evidence that supports a specific finding or resolution of apparently conflicting observations.

A fundamental challenge in the interpretation of joint kinetic data is that, unlike kinematic quantities such as a knee flexion angle, these quantities cannot be directly observed. As described further below, joint kinetic results are computed through a combination of segmental kinematics, ground reaction loads, and estimates pertaining to the mass distribution of the subject. Fundamental relationships from physics, i.e. equations and principles provided by Newton, Euler and d'Alembert provide the theoretical basis for the calculation of joint kinetics.

The aim of this chapter is to provide a cursory review of the theoretical concepts that underpin the determination of joint kinetics and a description of the hip, knee and ankle kinetics for a group of children who are without neuromuscular impairment. It is hoped that this background in normal gait kinetics will better prepare the reader for other chapters in this text that deal with the interpretation of pathological gait data. Readers who require a more substantial presentation of the computational details associated with joint kinetics are referred to other publications (e.g. Winter 1990, Õunpuu et al. 1996, Davis and Palladino 2000). The classic early contributions of Elftman (1939) and Bresler and Frankel (1950) are also highly recommended.

Fundamental concepts

One can appreciate the relatively unrestricted passive motion of the hip, knee and ankle joints during the physical examination of the normally developing child. To control this free joint motion and segment position during any activity such as gait, contractile forces are produced in the muscles that cross each of these joints. Muscles actively produce tension by either concentric (shortening) or eccentric (lengthening) contractions. In addition, they experience passive elastic forces, most notably during passive elongation. These muscle forces are produced along a muscle line of action which is generally displaced some distance

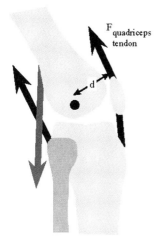

Fig. 8.1. This sketch depicts knee flexor and extensor muscle tendons that cross the knee. The magnitude of the muscle moment produced by the force in the quadriceps tendon that passes some distance "d" (i.e. moment arm) anterior to the knee center of rotation is simply the product of these latter two quantities, i.e. force times distance.

away from the associated joint (Fig. 8.1). In this way, the effectiveness of the force of the muscle is amplified by the relative magnitude of this moment arm or lever arm. This simple concept of the lever, first described by Archimedes, is the basis for understanding joint moments. Put very simply, the moment of muscle force is the product of the magnitudes of muscle force and the length of the associated muscle moment arm.

It would be ideal to have quantitative data associated with the internal moment produced by individual muscles during an activity such as gait as it would provide direct evidence of insufficient (e.g. weakness) or excessive (e.g. spasticity) muscle involvement. Unfortunately there is no practical way of measuring the force produced by individual muscles during gait. Analytical techniques have been proposed to estimate force in individual muscles. For example, Chao and Rim (1973) and Crowninshield (1978) proposed that forces are optimally distributed between the several muscles that cross a joint, based on the premise that individual muscles crossing a joint work no harder than is required for the task. Despite the potential of this analytical technique and others, it is unlikely that the muscles of the patient with motor control pathology or pain obey such a governing relationship. Currently there is no practical, reliable and noninvasive method for estimating individual muscle forces or moments in the patients seen for clinical gait analysis.

This quandary is partly resolved by measuring the external forces and moments that are applied to the body during gait and that are countered by the internal muscle moments. The application of Newton's laws of motion then allows one to relate these external forces and moments with internal reactions, i.e. joint reaction forces and moments. A simple example will illustrate this approach, referred to as "inverse dynamics", and some important points regarding its limitations.

The foot shown in Figure 8.2 is held in a horizontal position above the floor. The weight of the foot produces an *external* joint moment that tends to plantar flex the ankle. To counterbalance this tendency, an *internal* moment is produced by the combined effort of some undetermined number of the several ankle dorsiflexor muscles, e.g. tibialis anterior,

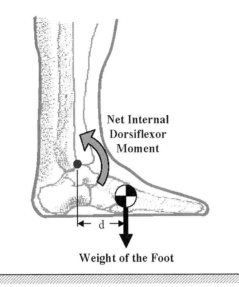

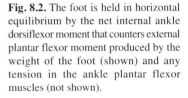

Fig. 8.2. The foot is held in horizontal equilibrium by the net internal ankle dorsiflexor moment that counters external plantar flexor moment produced by the weight of the foot (shown) and any tension in the ankle plantar flexor muscles (not shown).

extensor digitorum longus, or extensor hallucis longus. It must be noted that these dorsiflexor muscles are also counterbalancing all other forces that would tend to plantar flex the ankle, such as any force (active or passive) in the ankle plantar flexor muscles, e.g. gastrocnemius, soleus, or tibialis posterior. This example illustrates an important limitation of the inverse dynamics approach. The ankle moment shown in Figure 8.2 represents a *net* internal moment that includes all of the moments of force produced actively or passively by all structures (muscle tendons, ligaments) that cross the joint. In this case, one can refer to the net internal ankle moment as a *dominant* dorsiflexor moment, but it would be absolutely incorrect to refer to the moment as a tibialis anterior muscle moment.

The preceding discussion cites segment weight as an external load that is incorporated into Newton's laws of motion to compute the net joint reaction. Two other external loads are included in this calculation as well. During gait, a load is applied to the plantar surface of the foot from the ground. Simply put, the force of gravity pulls the individual down, producing a "ground reaction" that pushes upward. Muscles propel the individual forward (or retard forward motion) by producing a friction force under the foot that pulls the ground backward and the body forward (or tends to push the ground away and slows the forward motion of the body). This is realized in an anterior–posterior shear ground reaction force component. Similarly, a mediolateral shear ground reaction force component is seen that prevents the individual's foot from slipping laterally during single support. A vertical torque is also applied to the foot as a result of friction that restricts the tendency of the foot (and individual) from rotating freely about a vertical axis.

In addition to these ground reaction forces and torque, forces arise in response to changes in motion. In throwing a baseball, a force is required to accelerate that ball forward. A heavier ball, i.e. with more mass, would require more force to be accelerated in the same way. In this way, the mass of the ball reflects its resistance to a change in linear velocity or acceleration. The ball has inertia. In this same way, as will be described further in the next section, the lower extremity requires a joint moment to both initiate a swing forward and to control the deceleration of the swing. This resistance to a change in rotational or angular velocity is reflected in the mass moment of inertia of the limb, a quantity that reflects both its mass as well as how that mass is distributed about a point or axis of rotation, such as the hip joint.

The next section will describe both the joint moments and joint powers that are produced during gait. Joint power is derived from the mechanical definition of power. Consequently, this quantity combines the magnitude of the joint moment with the simultaneous angular velocity of the joint (or the speed at which the joint is being flexed or extended). When the direction of the joint motion coincides with the direction of the joint moment, the joint is said to be generating power. When the direction of the joint motion is opposite to the direction of the joint moment, the joint is said to be absorbing power. For example, an internal ankle plantar flexor moment that is coincident with a plantar flexing motion is seen as power generation. It is important to keep in mind that the magnitude of joint power is influenced equally by both the magnitude of the joint moment and the magnitude of the joint angular velocity. For example, low joint power generation can be seen when the joint moment is significant, but the joint is moving slowly.

Normal kinetic patterns
The data described in this section represent average values for a group of 27 children (17 females, 10 males, mean age 9.9 ± 3 years, mean mass 33 ± 12 kg, mean height 137 ± 17 cm) who were evaluated in 1988 and 1989 at Newington Children's Hospital (Newington, Connecticut). All children were free of neuromuscular and orthopaedic impairment and walked at self-selected speed (119 ± 14 cm/sec) and cadence (130 ± 13 steps/min) during the data collection session. Reflective markers were placed on the children and tracked using an optoelectronic motion measurement system similar to that described in an earlier chapter. Force platforms embedded in the walkway provided ground reaction force data. Note that the joint moment and power results that are presented below have been normalized with respect to the individual subject's body mass. Readers are advised to be careful to appreciate this display convention as there is no set standard within the literature. Other investigators include leg length or height as well as body mass in the normalization of the joint kinetic trace. Readers are referred to Õunpuu et al. (1991) for more complete descriptions of the protocols and methods used for this data collection and analysis.

Joint-moment and power patterns are computed from kinematic data combined with estimates of the subject's anthropometry and measured ground reactions. As indicated above, this poses a challenge in developing an understanding of joint moment and power patterns as these quantities cannot be observed directly. An understanding of the sagittal plane moments and power at the ankle is probably most accessible and will be presented first in the discussion which follows. Hip kinetics are presented next because of their relative importance in supporting the stance limb and propelling the body and lower extremities forward. Finally, the sagittal plane kinetics of the knee are described. The sagittal plane

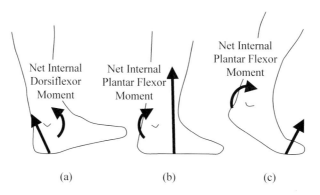

Fig. 8.3. These "free body diagrams" of the foot during the first (a), second (b) and third rocker (c) intervals depict the relationship between the external loading of the ground reaction force and the net internal ankle moment. Note the external loading associated with the weight and inertia of the foot are not shown for simplicity.

presentation is followed by a brief description of the coronal plane kinetics of the hip and knee. Although they are computed as part of a full three-dimensional analysis, the transverse plane kinetics are not included in this discussion as they are not currently used in clinical decision-making, unlike the results associated with the other two planes.

ANKLE – SAGITTAL PLANE OF THE TALOCRURAL JOINT

The ankle is a good starting-point for this discussion because the predominant external load applied to the foot during gait is the ground reaction force. The mass of the foot is small relative to the other segments of the body and consequently the contribution of segment weight and segment inertia to the joint moment can be considered negligible in most cases. Consequently (Fig. 8.3), "free body diagrams" of the foot during the first, second and third rocker intervals, depicts only external loading of the ground reaction force for simplicity.

At initial contact, the foot lands with the ankle slightly plantar flexed. Initially, during the first-rocker interval, there is a very brief plantar flexing ankle motion (Fig. 8.4, point A). At this point, the ground reaction force is applied to the heel and passes behind the ankle. This external load (along with the weight of the foot) produces an external moment that would tend to further plantar flex the ankle and encourage the foot to "slap" the ground. This external load is countered by a small net internal dorsiflexor moment (produced by the pretibial muscles) that controls the lowering of the forefoot to the ground. Following this brief plantar flexion motion, the ankle begins to dorsiflex as the tibia continues forward advancement over the now plantigrade foot. The dorsiflexing motion combined with the small dorsiflexor moment results in a small power generation wave.

During second rocker (point B), the tibia continues to advance over the plantigrade foot, resulting in ankle dorsiflexion. The magnitude of ground reaction force grows to approximately 100%–125% of body weight during this interval. More importantly (with respect to the external moment associated with this force), the point of application of the ground reaction force, commonly referred to as the "center of pressure", moves rapidly forward under the plantigrade

124

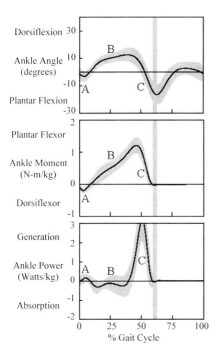

Fig. 8.4. These graphs present the ankle kinematics, internal moment and power for the sagittal plane of the joint. The solid line represents the mean curve for 31 able-bodied children (i.e. without neuromuscular or orthopaedic impairment). The gray band represents the first standard deviation about the mean. The vertical gray bar at approximately 60% of the gait cycle delineates the end of stance and the beginning of swing phase (i.e. toe-off).

foot. This results in a relatively rapid increase in the magnitude of external dorsiflexor moment associated with the ground reaction force. The internal plantar flexor moment balances the external load and counters its tendency to dorsiflex the ankle. Clearly this plantar flexor moment does not plantarflex the ankle, but it does control the forward advancement of the shank (that dorsiflexes the ankle). Some limited ankle power absorption is realized during this interval associated with eccentric contraction of the ankle plantar flexors. One might expect greater power magnitude, i.e. coincident with the increasing ankle moment amplitude. One is reminded that power is the combination of the joint moment and the speed of the joint motion. Over this interval, ankle dorsiflexion slows as evidenced by the flattening of the slope of the ankle angle curve. For an instant at about 40% of the gait cycle, the speed or angular velocity of the ankle is zero (i.e. the slope is zero), resulting in zero ankle power despite the relatively large amplitude of the ankle moment. To reiterate, to understand joint power, observe both the joint moment and the joint angular velocity (the slope of the joint angle plot). Joint power amplitudes reach significant levels only when there is rapid joint motion in the presence of substantial joint moment, as seen in the next rocker interval.

During third rocker (point C), the heel has left the ground, the ankle center has begun to accelerate forward, and the ground reaction force is still applied under the forefoot with its associated center of pressure still moving forward. The external load produces an external moment that would tend to further dorsiflex the ankle. However, this external load is countered by a net internal plantar flexor moment that plantar flexes the dorsiflexed ankle with increasing speed through concentric contraction of the ankle plantar flexors. The

125

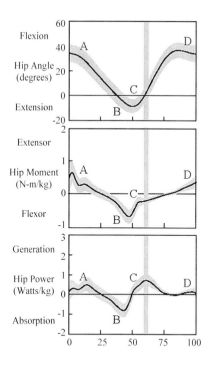

Fig. 8.5. These graphs present the hip kinematics, internal moment and power for the sagittal plane of the joint. The solid line represents the mean curve for 31 able-bodied children (i.e. without neuromuscular or orthopaedic impairment). The gray band represents the first standard deviation about the mean. The vertical gray bar at approximately 60% of the gait cycle delineates the end of stance and the beginning of swing phase (i.e. toe-off).

plantar flexor ankle moment peaks at about 50% of the gait cycle, at the end of the single support phase and the beginning of the second double support phase. This combines to produce a significant burst of ankle power generation which begins at approximately 40% of the gait cycle, peaks at 50% of the gait cycle and then rapidly falls off as the ankle moment decreases. This power generation burst is often cited as evidence of the importance of the role of the plantar flexors in powering the stance limb into swing, i.e. pushing off. The significance of the timing of this ankle power generation burst will be discussed further below.

HIP – SAGITTAL PLANE OF THE THIGH (AS DEFINED BY THE ORIENTATION OF THE MEDIAL AND LATERAL FEMORAL CONDYLES)

Early in stance (Fig. 8.5, point A), a hip extensor moment is produced through concentric contraction hip extensors, allowing the hip to extend to pull the body forward (and upward). Through this action, the generated hip power elevates the center of gravity of the body to its highest point in mid-stance while producing forward momentum. Later in single support (point B), the center of gravity of the body falls from its highest point while continuing to move forward. Consequently the hip continues to extend, powered by gravity. A hip flexor moment is produced as the hip flexor musculature is stretched passively, absorbing power.

The hip begins to flex at 50% of the gait cycle, at the end of single support and the beginning of the second double support. This marks the beginning of a hip power generation burst (point C) that continues to increase in magnitude until toe-off and is maintained at a reducing level for the first third of swing phase. This power propels the lower extremity into swing. It is noted that the timing of its onset (50% of the gait cycle) is closely aligned with peak ankle power generation and the reduction of electrical (electromyographic) activity in the ankle plantarflexors (Perry 1992). It appears that the ankle initiates the propulsion of the stance limb into swing in terminal stance and then the hip assumes that responsibility in pre-swing and into swing phase.

Just as the hip flexor moment (point C) accelerates the lower extremity into swing, the hip extensor moment in the second half of swing (point D) serves to decelerate the lower extremity in preparation for the next foot contact. The power amplitude is small in late swing because of relative immobility of the hip. This coordinated hip flexor moment/acceleration followed by hip extensor moment/deceleration mechanism also results in efficient control of the knee, as will be described in the next section.

KNEE – SAGITTAL PLANE OF THE JOINT (AS DEFINED BY THE ORIENTATION OF THE MEDIAL AND LATERAL FEMORAL CONDYLES)

Eccentric contraction of the knee extensors produces the net knee extensor moment (point A in Fig. 8.6), which supports and controls knee flexion during loading response in response primarily to the external ground reaction force which tends to flex the knee. Since the knee is flexing in the presence of a knee extensor moment, power is absorbed. It is thought that this power absorption acts to dissipate the shock load that propagates upward in the body following foot contact. Aside from this knee extensor moment during loading response, the magnitude of the load developed across the knee with respect to joint moment is remarkably small (point B). It is impressive that this highly mobile joint maintains a position of 5°–10° of knee flexion throughout much of single support without a supporting knee extensor moment. Moreover, given the rapid knee flexion that is developed in late stance and maintained into swing, one might anticipate the presence of a corresponding knee flexor moment to power this motion. The further examination of the kinetics of the ankle and hip helps explain these apparent inconsistencies.

During single support, knee stability is provided by a plantar flexion/knee-extension couple, i.e. the increasing internal ankle plantar flexor moment seen during second rocker. That is, excessive flexion of the knee is prevented by the internal ankle moment control of the forward advancement of tibia over the plantigrade foot. The same eccentric contraction of the gastrocnemius muscle during this interval produces a small knee flexor moment as it crosses both the ankle and the knee.

The swing-phase knee flexion wave begins in stance at 40% of the gait cycle. Recall that this also marks heel rise when the ankle center accelerates upward and forward as well as the onset of the ankle power generation wave. This suggests that ankle power generation in late stance not only promotes ankle plantar flexion, but the initiation of swing-phase knee flexion. The speed of the knee flexion motion noticeably increases at 50% of the gait cycle as the thigh is accelerated forward by the onset of hip flexion/power generation. The response at the knee to the influence of the hip can be explained by thinking of the thigh and shank as a double pendulum. In other words, as the thigh is rotated (accelerated) forward by the hip power, the knee center is linearly accelerated forward. The proximal end of the

127

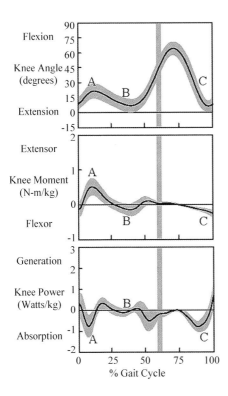

Fig. 8.6. Graphs showing the knee kinematics, internal moment and power for the sagittal plane of the joint. The solid line represents the mean curve for 31 able-bodied children (i.e. without neuromuscular or orthopaedic impairment). The gray band represents the first standard deviation about the mean. The vertical gray bar at approximately 60% of the gait cycle delineates the end of stance and the beginning of swing phase (i.e. toe-off).

shank translates with the knee center, but the mass and inertia of the shank resist a change in rotational orientation of the segment. Consequently, as the thigh is rotated in space, the shank merely translates. This change in relative orientation results in the production of knee flexion in swing. Knee flexion in swing appears to be passively generated, a by-product of ankle plantar flexor power and hip flexor power.

Peak knee flexion in swing is achieved at the end of the first third of swing phase. This is followed by rapid extension of the knee in preparation for the next foot contact. Coincident with the rapid knee extension, one might anticipate that a net knee extensor moment might be seen during this interval, but actually a knee flexor moment is present (Fig. 8.6, point C). The explanation for this apparent inconsistency is found in the hip kinetics. At the point of peak knee flexion in swing, the hip flexion motion has begun to decelerate. The hip extensors (including the hamstrings) produce the hip extensor moment that decelerates the forward rotation of the thigh. As thigh rotational velocity abates, the knee center and the proximal end of the shank decelerate. The forward momentum of the shank, however, encourages continued forward displacement of the distal shank. That is, as the proximal end slows, the distal end continues forward, thus rotating the shank and extending the knee passively. The knee flexor moment serves to control the rate of knee extension to avoid injury to the ligamentous structures that comprise the posterior knee capsule. Elegantly, the hamstrings, in crossing both the hip and the knee, aid in producing both a hip extensor moment that promotes knee extension and a knee flexor moment that slows and controls that motion.

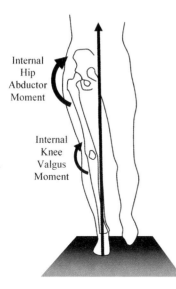

Internal
Hip
Abductor
Moment

Internal
Knee
Valgus
Moment

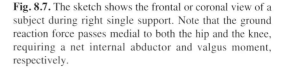

Fig. 8.7. The sketch shows the frontal or coronal view of a subject during right single support. Note that the ground reaction force passes medial to both the hip and the knee, requiring a net internal abductor and valgus moment, respectively.

HIP – CORONAL PLANE OF THE JOINT

An abductor moment is produced at the hip in stance to counter the effects of gravity and support the pelvis and upper body. As Figure 8.7 demonstrates, the weight line of the subject is medial to the hip center. Consequently one can anticipate that, during single support, gravity would tend to pull the swing side of the pelvis down. To control this motion, a hip abductor moment is produced through eccentric contraction of the hip abductors. Figure 8.8a shows that the abductor moment increases in magnitude during the first double support phase as load is transferred from the contralateral limb to the stance limb and reaches a peak at the beginning of single support. The amplitude of the moment is maintained through single support and falls off rapidly during the second double support phase.

Hip power absorption is seen early in stance as the abductor moment controls hip adduction (that arises through the drop of the contralateral pelvis). Later in stance, low-amplitude power generation is realized as the hip abductor moment aids in elevating the depressed contralateral pelvis and moving the hip from its adducted position back toward neutral (i.e. an abducting motion).

KNEE – CORONAL PLANE OF THE JOINT

The coronal plane moments of the knee (Fig. 8.8b) and the hip follow a similar pattern. The external moment applied to the knee would tend to produce a varus displacement of the knee. Internal structures at the knee (ligaments, tendons, and bony topography of the joint) resist this tendency through the production of an internal knee valgus moment. It is noted that the amplitude of this moment in single support is less than the hip abductor moment because the moment arm of the ground reaction force is reduced at the knee. Since the coronal plane motion of the knee in stance is slight, the power associated with this valgus moment can be considered negligible.

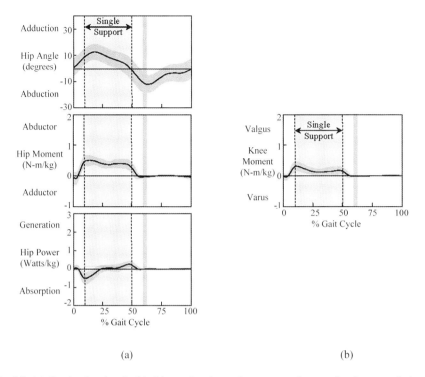

Fig. 8.8. (a) Graphs showing the hip kinematics, internal moment and power for the coronal plane of the joint. The solid line represents the mean curve for 31 able-bodied children (i.e. without neuromuscular or orthopaedic impairment). The gray band represents the first standard deviation about the mean. The vertical gray bar at approximately 60% of the gait cycle delineates the end of stance and the beginning of swing phase (i.e. toe-off). (b) Graph showing the internal knee moment for the coronal plane of the joint. The solid line represents the mean curve for 31 able-bodied children (i.e. without neuromuscular or orthopaedic impairment). The gray band represents the first standard deviation about the mean. The vertical gray bar at approximately 60% of the gait cycle delineates the end of stance and the beginning of swing phase (i.e. toe-off).

Influence of trunk position on lower extremity joint kinetics

There is a tendency in the clinical interpretation of internal joint moment and power results to focus too intently on the musculotendinous structures that cross the lower extremity joints, i.e. to formulate explanations simply in terms of the dominance of agonist and antagonist muscle groups. One needs to also remain mindful that the internal joint kinetics reflect the body's response to external loads, in that they are reactions to external moments. Consequently, when presented with abnormal internal kinetic patterns it is important to consider possible aberrations in the external loading as well as internal neuromuscular pathology.

For example, consider the influence of trunk position on lower extremity joint kinetics. Because of the large mass of the trunk segment, small changes in trunk position can have a significant effect on the lower extremity moments. Trunk motion modifies the location of the center of mass of the body which, in turn, alters the direction of the ground reaction force and thus the external moments applied to the lower extremities. In this way, trunk

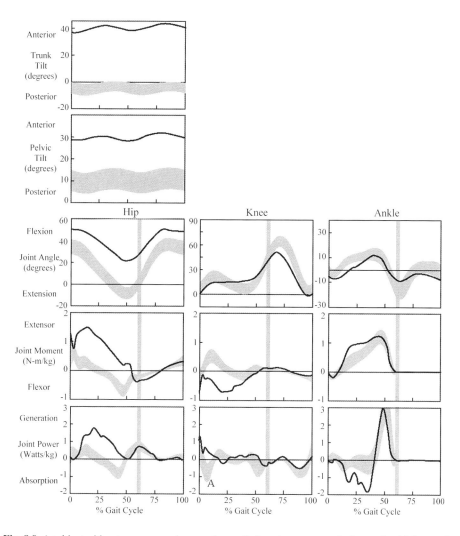

Fig. 8.9. A subject without neuromuscular or orthopaedic impairment was asked to walk with her trunk leaning forward. The solid lines shown in these graphs represent the kinematic and kinetic changes associated that trunk attitude while the gray band represents the first standard deviation about the mean results for a group of 31 able-bodied children.

position and movement during gait may function to reduce the lower extremity joint moments as a compensation for lower extremity muscle weakness. Optimally, the muscle (internal moment) response can be reduced or eliminated through trunk position/motion if muscle weakness is present.

The impact of trunk position on joint kinetics can be seen in the gait data of a subject (without neuromuscular or orthopaedic impairment) who was asked to walk with her trunk leaning forward (Fig. 8.9). With the increased forward trunk lean, there is a corresponding rotation of the pelvis anteriorly and shift in hip motion toward flexion. This position of the trunk brings the body center of gravity forward and increases the external load that tends to flex the hip joint. The body's response to this increased external moment is an increased internal hip extensor moment or increased demand on the hip extensors, required to support the trunk. This increased moment is also prolonged (i.e. the cross-over from extensor to flexor is delayed) in comparison with the typical curve. There is an associated increase in hip power generation and delay in the cross-over from power generation to absorption. Similarly, at the knee the increased anterior position of the body center of gravity increases the external load that tends to extend the knee further. The body's response to this increased load is an increased knee flexor moment. At the ankle, the anterior shift in the body center of gravity results in a more rapid forward displacement of the center of pressure under the foot. This results in a subtle increase in the plantar flexor moment required to support the increasing external load that tends to dorsiflex the ankle. Also seen is an associated increase in ankle power absorption. Note that all of these kinetic anomalies are directly attributed to the forward trunk lean and no underlying neuromuscular problem. This example illustrates the importance of considering upper body or trunk position in the clinical interpretation of lower extremity joint kinetic data.

Conclusion

This chapter has provided a cursory review of the theoretical underpinning of joint kinetics and described the lower extremity patterns for a group of children free of gait-related pathology. Through the examination of the change in these normal kinetic patterns associated with forward trunk lean, the authors sought to reinforce the point that it is essential to appreciate more than the structures that cross the joint when interpreting pathological joint kinetic details. Just as with other gait quantities, care must be taken in the interpretation of pathological joint kinetic data to consider all aspects of their collection (e.g. consideration of possible equipment malfunction or walking aberrations) and computation (e.g. modeling simplifications and limitations). The patient's stride-to-stride repeatability of a particular kinetic pattern or phenomena should be evaluated before definitive conclusions are drawn. Readers are referred to the literature to further substantiate their understanding of joint kinetics, including the influence of walking velocity on joint moments and power (Winter 1991).

The use of joint kinetics information in clinical gait analysis provides an opportunity to further substantiate one's understanding of a patient's gait pattern (as obtained through a review of their kinematic and electromyographic data). Moreover, joint kinetics can help elucidate a subtlety in or clarify confusion about the patient's gait. Joint kinetic patterns provide an alternative perspective on the patient's gait pattern that can complement an understanding provided by an observation of their gait, their clinical examination, and the quantitative gait kinematic and electromyographic findings. Ultimately, a further understanding of joint kinetics may provide the most direct basis for treatment decision-making as most intervention strategies, including orthopaedic surgery, endeavor to alter the mechanics of the patient's movement.

REFERENCES

Bresler B, Frankel JP. (1950) The force and moments in the leg during level walking. *Trans Am Soc Mech Eng* **72:** 27–52.

Chao EY, Rim K. (1973) Application of optimization principles in determining the applied moments in human leg joints during gait. *J Biomech* **6:** 497–510.

Crowninshield RD. (1978) Use of optimization techniques to predict muscle force. *J Biomech Engr* **100:** 88-92.

Davis RB, Palladino J. (2000) Biomechanics. In: Enderle J, Blanchard S, Bronzino J, editors. *Introduction to Biomedical Engineering*. San Diego: Academic Press. p 411–465.

Elftman H. (1939) Force and energy—changes in the leg during walking. *Am J Physiol* **125:** 339–356.

Õunpuu S, Gage JR, Davis RB. (1991) Three-dimensional lower extremity joint kinetics in normal pediatric gait. *J Pediatr Orthop* **11:** 341–349.

Õunpuu S, Davis RB, DeLuca PA. (1996) Joint kinetics: methods, interpretation and treatment decision-making in children with cerebral palsy and myelomeningocele. *Gait Posture* **4:** 62–78.

Perry J. (1992) *Gait Analysis: Normal and Pathological Function*. Thorofare, NJ: Slack. p 51–87.

Winter DA. (1990) *Biomechanics and Motor Control of Human Movement*. New York: John Wiley and Sons.

Winter DA. (1991) *The Biomechanics and Motor Control of Human Gait: Normal, Elderly and Pathological*. Waterloo, Ontario: University of Waterloo Press.

133

9
DYNAMIC ELECTROMYOGRAPHY

Henry G. Chambers and Jessica Rose

Many elements combine to determine the gait of a child with cerebral palsy. Neural impulses, ground reaction forces, angles of muscle action determined by skeletal alignment, static ligamentous structures and muscle activity all contribute to the forces in gait. Although the action of the muscles may be inferred from watching a patient walking, or by ascribing muscle activity to kinetic data, it is often difficult to determine which muscles are active or inactive during a particular motion. This knowledge may be important in determining which therapeutic intervention will correct the problem. For example, if a muscle transfer is planned, electromyographic (EMG) data may help to determine which muscles should be used as a "motor" for the muscle transfer.

Muscle structure and function

The dynamic EMG recorded during gait represents the sum of signals from multiple motor-unit action potential (MUAP) trains. As the muscle contraction strengthens, the EMG signal increases in both amplitude and density. This reflects an increase in both the average firing rate of active motor-units as well as in the number of active motor-units. Thus the dynamic EMG record during gait reveals information on the timing and intensity of muscle activity. However, there are limitations that apply to the interpretation of dynamic EMG in cerebral palsy due to changes in muscle structure and function. Understanding muscle structure and function provides an essential foundation for interpretation of dynamic EMG.

THE MOTOR-UNIT

The motor-unit is the basic functional unit of the motor system and consists of a single motor neuron, the neuromuscular junction, and the muscle fibers innervated by the motor neuron (Fig. 9.1). An example of the important relation between muscle structure and function is that the number of muscle fibers innervated by a single motor neuron varies, depending on the function of the muscle. In muscles that control fine movements of the hand, motor units have only three to six muscle fibers. In comparison, motor units in a typical gross motor muscle, such as gastrocnemius, have about 2000 muscle fibers (Rowland 1991). The motor endplate at the neuromuscular junction is responsible for electrochemical communication between the neuron and muscle fiber.

The motor endplate contains microscopic vesicles in the axon terminal that, upon electrical stimulation, fuse with the presynaptic membrane and release the neurotransmitter acetylcholine (Ach) (Fig. 9.2). Contraction is initiated when Ach binds with the postsynaptic membrane of the muscle and initiates an action potential in the sarcolemma, the excitable

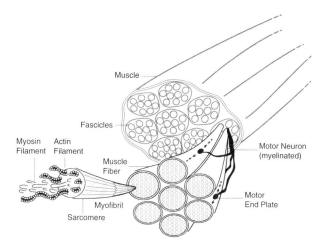

Fig. 9.1. The hierarchical structure of skeletal muscle. Muscle fascicles are composed of many muscle fibers. The motor-unit consists of the motor neuron, the motor endplate and the muscle fibers innervated by the motor neuron. Each muscle fiber is composed of interdigitating contractile proteins, actin and myosin, structured as sarcomeres that are arranged in a series.

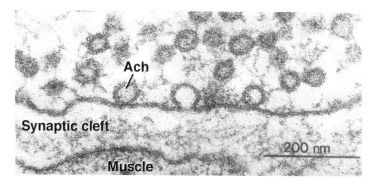

Fig. 9.2. An electromicrograph of the motor endplate and neuromuscular junction showing acetylcholine vesicles fused with presynaptic membrane (Carnack, 1987).

membrane surrounding each muscle fiber. The signal propagates into the fiber, through the transverse tubular system, releasing calcium ions from the sarcoplasmic reticulum into the sarcomere, allowing the proteins—actin and myosin—to interact (Fig. 9.1) (Gamble 1988, Ghez 1991, Lieber 2002). Depolarization of the sarcolemma creates a detectable voltage change that is recorded by EMG electrodes placed in or over the muscle.

SIGNAL PROPAGATION

The motor neuron innervates the central region of the muscle fiber and the signal propagates through the sarcolemma, along the length of the muscle fiber. An EMG recording of a single action potential from a motor-unit reflects the time required for the signal to propagate

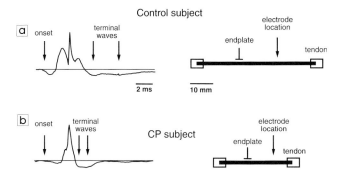

Fig. 9.3. (a) Estimation of muscle-fiber length from the duration of the motor-unit action potential (MUAP). Left: MUAPs recorded using a monopolar needle electrode from the medial gastrocnemius muscles of a child with CP and non-disabled control. The onset, spike and terminal waves of the MUAP indicate the times at which the action potential leaves the motor endplate, passes the electrode, and reaches the muscle–tendon junction. (b) From the latencies of the MUAP features, the lengths of the muscle fibers were estimated, assuming a normal muscle-fiber conduction velocity of 4m/s. The child with CP has shorter durations, indicating shorter fiber lengths.

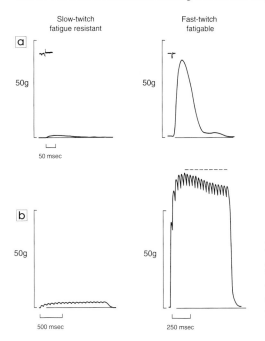

Fig. 9.4. Muscle-fiber twitch and tetanic force generation illustrating the relatively low (a) twitch and (b) tetanic force generated by the type 1, slow-twitch, fatigue-resistant fiber as compared to the type 2 fast-twitch, fast-fatigable fiber. (Adapted from Burke et al. 1973.)

along the length of the fiber. Thus, based on a known conduction velocity, an EMG recording of a single action potential can be used to quantify fiber length (Fig. 9.3) (Lateva et al. 1996, Lateva and McGill 2001).

When a single action potential reaches the muscle fiber there is a brief latency period (5ms), followed by contraction and relaxation of that muscle fiber (100ms) (Fig. 9.4). The latency period represents depolarization of the sarcolemma, as well as the mechanics of initiating the actin and myosin interaction. The twitch contractile duration represents the twitch response, or fiber contraction and relaxation. It includes the time required to actively pump calcium back into the sarcoplasmic reticulum as the contraction subsides (Ghez 1991). Sustained muscle contraction results from temporal summation of multiple motor-unit action potential impulses and results in tetanic or fused contraction and sustained force generation (Ghez 1991, Lieber 2002) (Fig. 9.4b).

MUSCLE COMPOSITION AND ARCHITECTURE

Muscle fibers can vary in several characteristics including twitch-contraction speed and force generation, fatigue resistance, and oxidative capacity. In general, slow-twitch (type 1) fibers generate lower peak tension, are fatigue-resistant and rely on oxidative metabolism, whereas fast-twitch (type 2) fibers generate more tension, are faster to fatigue and rely on oxidative and glycolytic metabolism (Saltin and Gollnick 1983, Gollnick and Hodgeson 1986). A functional match exists between the electrical properties of motor neurons and the mechanical behavior of the muscle fibers they innervate. Slow-twitch (type 1) fibers are recruited at lower firing-rates than are fast-twitch (type 2) fibers (Pinter 1990). Muscles that are used phasically for strength activity, such as gastrocnemius contain approximately equal proportion of slow-twitch (type 1) and fast-twitch (type 2) fibers. Tonic postural muscles, such as soleus, contain a higher proportion of slow-twitch fibers (Gollnick and Hodgeson 1986, Lieber 2002).

Muscles are composed of fibers arranged in fascicles, sharing common aponeurotic sheaths, tendon attachments and fiber pennation. Muscle architectural characteristics such as pennation angle, fiber length to muscle length ratio and physiological cross-sectional area, vary between muscles and influence muscle function. Larger-fiber pennation angles generate more power at the expense of excursion (Lieber 2002). For example, muscles with smaller pennation angles, higher fiber length to muscle-length ratio and smaller cross-sectional area, such as those found in hamstrings and tibialis anterior, provide larger excursion and higher contractile velocity. In contrast, muscles with larger pennation angles, smaller fiber length to muscle length ratio and larger cross-sectional area, such as those found in gastrocnemius and quadriceps, generate increased force at the expense of contractile velocity (Lieber 2002) (Fig. 9.5).

CHANGES IN MUSCLE STRUCTURE AND FUNCTION IN CEREBRAL PALSY

Skeletal muscle is known to adapt to changes in habitual exercise by alterations in both structure and function (Lieber 2002). In children with cerebral palsy, it appears that spastic muscle receives a prolonged but weaker signal and in response develops structural changes in the muscle fibers. Evidence from dynamic EMG indicates that spastic muscles in children with cerebral palsy routinely experience prolonged contraction during movement (Perry et al. 1974, Csongradi et al. 1979, Rose et al. 1999). In addition, evidence from muscle biopsies has shown that spastic muscle from children with cerebral palsy has structural abnormalities that are similar to changes seen with experimental chronic low-frequency stimulation (Castle et al. 1979, Rose et al. 1994, Ito et al. 1996). The structural abnormalities that have been identified in biopsies of spastic muscle from children with cerebral palsy include a

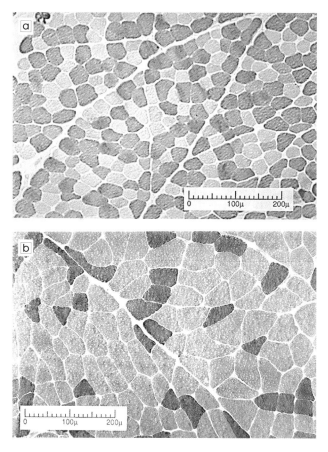

Fig. 9.5. Cross-sections of (a) normal skeletal muscle stained with ATPase pH 9.4 showing type 1 fibers stain light and type 2 fibers stain dark, and (b) muscle from a child with CP showing type 1 fiber predominance and abnormally increased fiber-size variation (Rose, 1994).

predominance of type 1 fibers and marked fiber-size variation including type 1 and type 2 hypertrophy and atrophy (Castle et al. 1979, Rose et al. 1994, Ito et al. 1996). The degree of fiber-size variation ranged from relatively minor to large variations associated with extreme fiber-type predominance, endomysial fibrosis and fatty replacement. Substantial muscle atrophy and fatty replacement in cerebral palsy may result in smaller sampling targets in the muscle and may disturb the signal-to-noise ratio, making EMG recording and analysis more difficult.

Muscle function in cerebral palsy has been studied in terms of maximal voluntary contraction torque and was found to be reduced by approximately 50% in cerebral palsy (Brown et al. 1991, Damiano et al. 1995, 2001, Rose and McGill 2002). Muscle weakness in cerebral palsy has also been examined by testing maximal voluntary muscle activation defined as the ratio of maximal voluntary EMG amplitude to M-wave amplitude (all available motor units activated through electrical stimulation) and by analyzing motor-unit

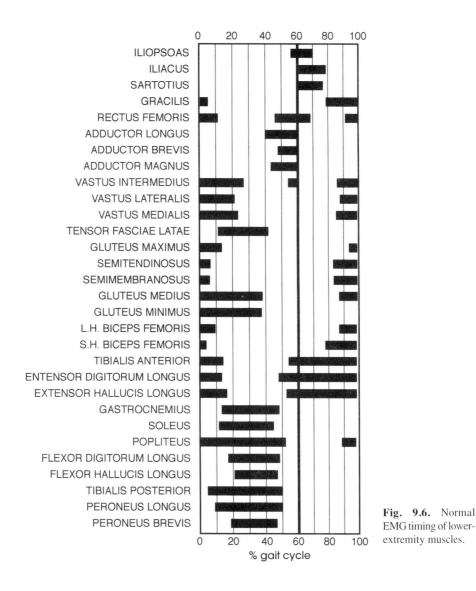

Fig. 9.6. Normal EMG timing of lower-extremity muscles.

firing characteristics (Rose and McGill 2002). Maximal voluntary activation of the gastrocnemius and tibialis anterior was found to be reduced to approximately 30% of normal in children and adults with cerebral palsy (Rose and McGill 2002). Motor-unit firing rate and recruitment were found to be normal at lower levels of contraction (Rose and McGill 2002). This suggests that in cerebral palsy there is an inability to drive motor-units to achieve higher levels of muscle contraction. The substantially reduced levels of maximal muscle activation in cerebal palsy indicate an inability to fully activate the muscle. Therefore the maximal voluntary contraction (MVC) EMG values recorded during gait analysis are not comparable to normal values and reflect a lower level of muscle activation. This limitation must be considered when interpreting dynamic EMG amplitude that has been normalized relative to the patient's MVC values.

EMG interpretation

The dynamic EMG signal is interpreted primarily in terms of timing. It is reported in relation to a percentage of the gait cycle, the stance and swing phases of gait and the functional phases of gait.

NORMAL EMG PATTERNS

The normal EMG patterns of the lower-extremity muscles during gait are illustrated in Figure 9.6. In general, timing of muscle activity during the gait cycle depends on muscle action. For example, muscles that cross anterior to the hip joint are generally active during the transition from stance to swing phase, whereas muscles that cross posterior to the hip or knee are active during the transition from swing to stance phase. Similarly, muscles that cross anterior to the ankle are active in swing and early stance, whereas muscles crossing posterior to the ankle are active during stance.

The precise onset and termination of the EMG signal is commonly reported as a percentage of the gait cycle and is determined by hand or by computer processing. Quantification of EMG timing requires a definition of what constitutes significant EMG signal. An EMG duration of at least 5% of the gait cycle, with an amplitude of at least 5% of maximal voluntary EMG amplitude is commonly used (Perry 1992). Manual designation of the onset and cessation of EMG timing has been shown to be variable, with intra-examiner variability as high as 51%. In contrast, computer processing has been found to be 100% repeatable and is therefore recommended (Perry 1992). Detrembleur and colleagues (1997) demonstrated that there is a velocity-dependent change in the normal time-pattern of muscle activation. They noted that it is important for the clinician to differentiate EMG modification due to pathology versus those due to slow walking.

Normal EMG patterns have been determined for toddlers, children and adults (Sutherland et al. 1988). In very young children, 1 year old, stance phase is increased and there is prolongation of medial hamstrings and tibialis anterior during stance phase. The onset of vastus medialis in swing occurs early and the onset of tibialis anterior in swing is delayed. The EMG timing of other muscles was not found to be different from mature patterns and generally the EMG timing of lower-extremity muscles matures by 2 years of age. The exception was that approximately 25% of children between the ages of 2 and 7 years were found to have premature firing of the ankle plantarflexors in swing and early stance phase (Sutherland et al. 1988), which has implications for interpreting plantarflexor EMG patterns during gait in children up to age 7.

Dynamic EMG provides information on the timing and relative intensity of muscular action during gait. However, the intensity of the EMG signal can only be interpreted relative to an individual's maximum voluntary activation, which has been found to be compromised in cerebral palsy (Rose and McGill 2002). Thus, based on dynamic EMG alone, the absolute intensity or strength of muscle activation cannot be interpreted or compared between individuals with cerebral palsy. Interpreting absolute intensity in relation to normal values requires additional EMG data on the full potential for activation of a muscle, as measured by M-wave amplitude.

INTERPRETATION OF COMMON EMG PATTERNS AND TREATMENT IMPLICATIONS IN CEREBRAL PALSY

Comparison of gait EMG patterns of children with cerebral palsy to normal gait EMG patterns requires consideration of both the normal, average values and variability of EMG patterns as well as stride characteristics during gait. Dynamic gait EMG patterns are generally described as premature, prolonged, out-of-phase, continuously active, curtailed, delayed or absent.

Surface or fine-wire EMG can be used to measure the muscle activity. When one is interested in group muscle activity, such as the gastrosoleus or adductors, then surface electrodes suffice. However, there may be a problem with recording electrical activity from adjacent muscles or "cross-talk", but this does not usually alter clinical decisions. In deep, buried muscles (iliacus, tibialis posterior, flexor hallucis longus, and flexor digitorum longus) or superficial muscles with potential cross-talk (rectus femoris), fine-wire electrodes must be placed within the muscle to obtain any meaningful information. One must weigh the information gained from fine-wire EMG data with the discomfort the patient may experience in its placement. Young children often are not able to cooperate with this technically demanding procedure. Fine wire measurements may also be inconsistent as there can be variability in the activity within each muscle as well. For example, a fine wire placed proximally in one muscle may not represent the activity of the entire muscle.

Foot-switches or similar timing devices are utilized to report the EMG data in relation to the gait cycle. These data can also be used to verify gait events during the gait analysis. The raw data obtained may be presented as raw data or manipulated via computer programs as an ensemble average.

THE STIFF-KNEE GAIT

One of the primary patterns of gait abnormalities at the knee is the stiff-knee gait (Gage et al. 1987, Perry 1987, Sutherland et al. 1990). It is manifest by problems in foot clearance during the swing phase of gait. There is a diminished and delayed peak knee flexion in sagittal knee kinematics. The EMG pattern of the rectus femoris demonstrates abnormal activity during the swing phase of gait, a time in which the rectus femoris does not normally work (Fig. 9.7). In some cases there is also activity of the other quadriceps muscles as well as the hamstring muscles. Miller et al. (1997) demonstrated three patterns of rectus EMG in stiff-knee gait. One group had predominant swing-phase activity, one group had constant rectus activity through the entire gait cycle, and one group had normal rectus activity. They noted the greatest improvement in swing-phase knee flexion in the group with predominant swing-phase rectus activity. Chambers et al. (1998) demonstrated that there was improvement in the peak knee flexion after rectus femoris transfer even when there was cocontraction of the other quadriceps muscles. In patients who have spasticity of the quadriceps and hamstring muscles, there is less predictability of the rectus femoris transfer. This is often present in stroke patients who may also have rigidity as a component of their neurologic injury.

141

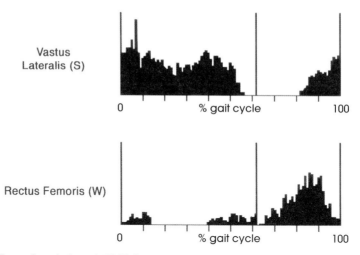

Vastus
Lateralis (S)

0   % gait cycle   100

Rectus Femoris (W)

0   % gait cycle   100

Fig. 9.7. Rectus femoris dynamic EMG demonstrating swing-phase activity of the rectus femoris muscle.

THE VARUS FOOT

In children with cerebral palsy, particularly spastic hemiplegia, there is often a varus positioning of the foot. This can occur during swing phase in which the prerequisite of gait is not satisfied (pre-position of the foot at initial contact) because of the varus present at foot strike. It can also occur during stance phase leading to weightbearing on the lateral aspect of the foot with painful callosities and shoe-wear problems. Often varus occurs in both phases and may be associated with equinus at the ankle. Three main muscles are the cause of this disorder: the gastrocsoleus complex, the tibialis anterior, and the tibialis posterior muscles. Although the phase in which the varus occurs can be evaluated during routine kinematic evaluation, little information on which muscles contribute to the varus can be gained from kinetics or from simply observing the patient and/or reviewing the videotape. The use of EMG (both surface and fine-wire) enables one to determine the etiology of the varus deformity (Barto et al. 1984, Skinner and Lester 1986, Sutherland 1993). Surface electrodes are placed over the gastrosoleus group and the tibialis anterior muscle. A fine-wire technique must be used for the tibialis posterior muscle. Figure 9.8 demonstrates two of the possible combinations of EMG that can be obtained in a child with equinovarus. Each of these children had identical physical examinations, kinematics and kinetics. Once the offending muscles have been identified, there may still be controversy as to the correct surgery that should be performed, but without the EMG data, a completely informed surgical plan cannot be made.

RECURVATUM KNEE

Recurvatum at the knee in children with cerebral palsy can occur for many reasons. Dynamic or fixed equinus at the ankle can lead to an overactive ankle plantarflexion/knee-extension

142

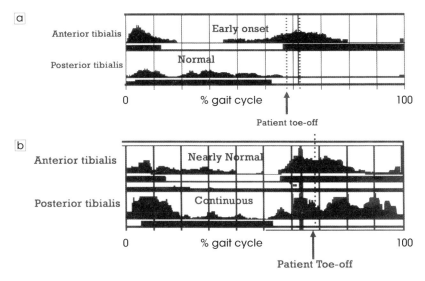

Fig. 9.8. (a) Early-onset activity of the anterior tibialis muscle in child with varus foot. (b) Full-cycle activity of the posterior tibialis muscle in child with varus foot.

couple that, in turn, leads to recurvatum. Overactivity of the rectus femoris or the entire quadriceps mechanism also can contribute to recurvatum. Surgical overlengthening and/or severe weakness of the hamstrings can contribute to the recurvatum as well. EMG plays an important role in the evaluation of this gait disorder as each of the possible offending muscles can be studied throughout the gait cycle. Treatment can then be directed at the correct level. Often the problem cannot be determined by observation, kinematics and/or kinetics.

CLINICAL IMPLICATIONS OF SPASTIC MUSCULATURE
Many younger children with cerebral palsy do not have fixed contractures that contribute to their gait abnormalities. For example, the problems of a jump-type gait with increased hip flexion, hip adduction, knee flexion and equinus may all result from dynamic as opposed to static muscle contracture. The use of dynamic EMG in these muscles may provide additional data to determine which muscles are contributing to the deformity. This information can be useful in deciding which muscles or muscle groups would benefit from chemo-denervation such as phenol or botulinum toxin injections.

Conclusion
Electromyography is an important component of gait analysis. It provides additional information about the timing and action of muscles that are the prime movers of body segments and bones. Understanding the activity of the muscle as well as the other forces acting on a moving body is critical to understanding the root causes of a gait abnormality. While there are limitations to the use of EMG, these mainly relate to sampling errors. There is a risk of overinterpreting EMG data as well. A muscle may have electrical activity, but

143

it may not be generating significant force. Thus future research will be necessary to correlate electrical activity with force generation. Ultimately, when combined with the kinematic and kinetic data, EMG data can provide significant information on which critical clinical recommendations can be made.

REFERENCES

Barto PS, Supinski RS, Skinner SR. (1984) Dynamic EMG findings in varus hindfoot deformity and spastic cerebral palsy. *Dev Med Child Neurol* **26:** 88–93.

Brown J, Rodda J, Walsh E, Wright G. (1991) Neurophysiology of lower-limb function in hemiplegic children. *Dev Med Child Neurol* **33:** 1037–1047.

Burke RF, Levine DN, Tsairis P, Za jac FE. (1973) Physiological types and histochemical profiles in motor units of the cat gastrocnemius. *J Physiol (Lond)* **234:** 723–748

Castle M, Reyman T, Schneider M..(1979) Pathology of spastic muscle in cerebral palsy. *Clin Orthop* **142:** 223–233.

Chambers H, Lauer A, Kaufman K, Cardelia J, Sutherland DH. (1998) Prediction of outcome after rectus femoris surgery in cerebral palsy: the role of cocontraction of the rectus femoris and the vastus lateralis. *J Pediatr Orthop* **18:** 70–712.

Csongradi J, Bleck E, Ford W. (1979) Gait electromyography in normal and spastic children with special reference to quadiceps femoris and hamstring muscles. *Dev Med Child Neurol* **21:** 738–748.

Damiano D, Vaughn G, Abel M. (1995) Muscle response to heavy resistance exercise in children with spastic cerebral palsy. *Dev Med Child Neurol* **37:** 731–739.

Damiano DL, Martellotta TL, Quinlivan JM, Abel MF. (2001) Deficits in eccentric versus concentric torque in children with spastic cerebral palsy. *Med Sci Sports Exerc* **33:** 117–122

Detrembleur C, Willems P, Plaghki L. (1997) Does walking speed influence the time pattern of muscle activation in normal children? *Dev Med Child Neurol* **39:** 803–807.

Gage JR, Perry J, Hicks RR, Koop S, Werntz JR. (1987) Rectus femoris transfer to improve knee function of children with cerebral palsy. *Dev Med Child Neurol* **29:** 159–166.

Gamble J. (1988) *The Musculoskeletal System: Physiological Basics*. New York: Raven Press. p 116–137.

Ghez C. (1991) Muscles: effectors of the motor system. In: Jessel T, editor. *Principles of Neural Science*. Amsterdam: Elsevier. p 244–245.

Gollnick P, Hodgeson D. (1986) The identification of fiber types in skeletal muscle: a continual dilemma. *Exerc Sport Sci Rev* **14:** 81–104.

Ito J, Araki A, Tanka T, Cho K, Yamazaki R. (1996) Muscle histopathology in spastic cerebral palsy. *Brain Dev* **18:** 299–303.

Lateva ZC, McGill KC. (2001) Estimating motor-unit architectural properties by analyzing motor-unit action potential morphology. *Clin Neurophysiol* **112:** 127–135.

Lateva ZC, McGill KC, Burgar CG. (1996) Anatomical and electrophysiological determinants of the human thenar compound muscle action potential. *Muscle Nerve* **19:** 1457–1468.

Lieber R. (2002) *Skeletal Muscle Function and Plasticity. The Physiological Basis of Rehabilitation. Implications for Rehabilitation and Sports Medicine*. Baltimore: Williams and Wilkins. p 13–250

Miller F, Cardoso Dias R, Lipton G, Albarracin J, Dabney K, Castagno M. (1997) The effect of rectus EMG Patterns on the outcomes of rectus femoris transfers. *J Pediatr Orthop* **17:** 603–607.

Perry J. (1987) Distal rectus femoris transfer. *Dev Med Child Neurol* **29:** 153–158.

Perry J. (1992) *Gait Analysis: Normal and Pathological Function*. New York: McGraw Hill. p 381–411.

Perry J, Hoffer M, Giovan P, Antonelli D, Greenberg R. (1974) Gait analysis of the triceps surae in cerebral palsy. *J Bone Joint Surg Am* **56:** 511–520.

Pinter MJ. (1990) The role of motorneuron membrane properties in the determination of recruitment order. In: Binder MD, Mednell ZM. *The Segmental Motor System*. New York: Oxford University Press. p 165–181.

Rose J, McGill K. (2002) Neuromuscular activation and motor-unit firing characteristics in cerebral palsy. *Dev Med Child Neurol* **44** (suppl. 91): 34–35.

Rose J, Haskell W, Gamble J, Hamilton R, Brown D, Rinsky L. (1994) Muscle pathology and clinical measures of disability in children with cerebral palsy. *J Orthop Res* **12:** 758–768.

Rose J, Martin J, Torburn L, Rinsky L, Gamble J. (1999) Electromyographic differentiation of diplegic cerebral palsy from idiopathic toe walking: involutary co-activation of the quadriceps and gastrocnemius. *J Pediatr Orthop* **19:** 677–682.

Rowland P. (1991) Diseases of the motor unit. In: Jessel T, editor. *Principles of Neural Science*. Amsterdam: Elsevier. p 548–563.

Saltin B, Gollnick P. (1983) Skeletal muscle adaptability: significance for metabolism and performance. In: Adrian R, editor. *Handbook of Physiology*. Bethesda, Maryland: American Physiologic Society. p 555–631.

Skinner SR, Lester DK. (1986) Gait electromyographic evaluation of the long-toe flexors in children with spastic cerebral palsy. *Clin Orthop* **207:** 70–73.

Sutherland DH. (1993) Varus foot in cerebral palsy: an overview. *Instr Course Lect* **42:** 539–543.

Sutherland D, Olshen R, Biden E, Wyatt M. (1988) *The Development of Mature Walking*. London: Mac Keith Press. p 154–162.

Sutherland DH, Santi M, Abel MF. (1990) Treatment of stiff-knee gait in cerebral palsy: a comparison by gait analysis of distal rectus femoris transfer versus proximal rectus release. *J Pediatr Orthop* **10:** 433–441.

10
ENERGY EXPENDITURE IN CEREBRAL PALSY

Jean Stout and Steven Koop

Human walking is a method of moving the body from one location to another. In the best circumstances, walking is done with the smallest energy expense. While it is generally acknowledged that children with cerebral palsy (CP) walk inefficiently, energy expenditure is not routinely measured when performing gait analysis in most laboratories. However, when the goal of surgical intervention in walking is to improve function or ease the effort of the task, energy assessment provides a unique but important assessment. Most families consider that it is essential to have adequate information about functional gains when making treatment decisions, and it is difficult to counsel families about the risks and benefits of treatment for gait deviations if information about the functional outcomes, including energy expenditure, is not available. Routine energy assessment in the Gillette laboratory and elsewhere has proved to be an effective and time-efficient tool that is a valuable contribution to the evaluation of abnormal gait (Koop et al. 1989, 2001, Duffy et al. 1996, Boyd et al. 1999).

Energy assessment as an outcome tool
Energy expenditure can be considered an objective tool for assessment of functional ability. It is an objective tool because it does not rely on parental report, patient report, perceived exertion or perceived fatigue. It is a functional tool because its interpretation provides an indication of endurance, fatigue, and ability to accomplish the routine daily task of locomotion. Gage (1991) included energy conservation as one of the five attributes of normal gait and states that variation in this attribute encompasses the deviations of the other four. Energy assessment helps to span the gap between a laboratory "technical" outcome and a community "functional" outcome and demonstrate their interconnectivity. Recent work has demonstrated this interconnectivity through moderate correlation to both gait outcome measures and functional outcome measures (Novacheck et al. 2000, Schwartz 2001, Tervo et al. 2002).

Methods of energy-expenditure assessment
The energy generated by the body to accomplish cellular activity can be determined by direct or indirect calorimetry or by mathematical models that estimate the energy required for limb-segment movement during walking.

CALORIMETRY
The basis of direct calorimetry is the fact that all cellular processes in the body result in the production of heat. Heat produced by the human body can be measured directly by placing

a person in an airtight thermally insulated chamber that acts as a calorimeter. This method is sensitive but impractical for most studies of walking or running.

Indirect calorimetry is based on the fact that all energy metabolisms in the body depend on the utilization of oxygen. Skeletal muscle may be considered a machine that is fueled by the chemical energy of substrates derived from food stored as carbohydrates, lipids, and proteins in the body. These substrates are used to form high-energy compounds, predominantly creatine phosphate and adenosine triphosphate (ATP), from which energy in the terminal phosphate bond can be made available for cellular reactions involved in muscle contraction. The formation of these high-energy bonds is dependent on oxygen: in the presence of adequate amounts of oxygen a molecule of glucose yields 36 molecules of ATP while anaerobic metabolism of the same glucose molecule yields only two molecules of ATP. Thus by measuring oxygen uptake at rest and during exercise conditions it is possible to obtain an indirect estimate of energy expense.

Indirect calorimetry by measuring oxygen uptake is relatively simple compared to direct calorimetry and can be accomplished by closed- or open-circuit spirometry. During closed-circuit spirometry a subject breathes and re-breathes from a pre-filled container of oxygen (or spirometer). Such devices are usually bulky and stationary, and resistance to breathing is substantial during significant exercise. Removal of carbon dioxide may not be adequate.

During open-circuit spirometry a subject inhales ambient air. Because oxygen is consumed and carbon dioxide is produced during energy-yielding reactions, the exhaled air contains less oxygen and more carbon dioxide than the inhaled air. Analysis of the difference reflects the body's production of energy. In early studies of oxygen utilization by open-circuit spirometry, expired air was collected by a modified Douglas Bag system. This was cumbersome and often required support from an assistant. Recent studies have obtained breath-by-breath measurements of oxygen uptake, carbon dioxide output, ventilation volumes, respiratory rate and heart-rate from a portable computer equipped with a pneumotachograph and oxygen and carbon dioxide analyzers sampling more than 100 times per second. These systems can be mounted on a cart and pushed alongside a child during walking. A self-molding facemask and lightweight connecting tubing ensure accurate gas collection and do not require support. Data are instantly displayed on a monitor and are visible during the test process (Fig. 10.1).

Oxygen utilization is most often expressed by two indices, oxygen consumption and oxygen cost. Oxygen consumption is a calculation of the rate of oxygen uptake normalized by body mass. It is most commonly expressed in milliliters of oxygen per minute per kilogram of body mass (ml/min/kg). Oxygen cost describes the amount of energy needed to walk a standard unit of distance also normalized by body mass (ml/kg-meter) (Fig. 10.2). Oxygen cost is equivalent to normalized oxygen consumption divided by velocity. Oxygen consumption indicates the intensity of physical effort during exercise and is time-dependent. Oxygen cost is not time-dependent, and is a measure of gait efficiency.

HEART-RATE AND SPEED
Known as either the Physiological Cost Index (PCI) (Butler et al. 1984) or the Energy

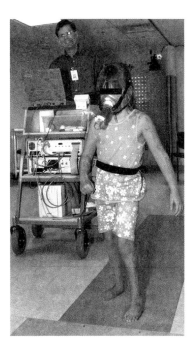

Fig. 10.1. Patient during an open-circuit spirometry test using a pneumotachograph, and a self-molding facemask attached to a mobile cart.

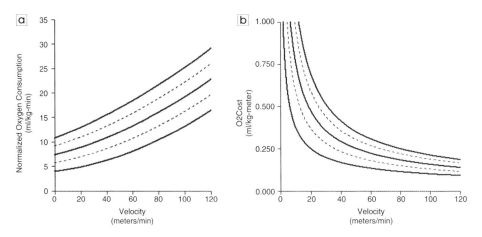

Fig. 10.2. Typical oxygen consumption (a) and oxygen cost (b) graphs normalized for body weight versus velocity. The mean and ±1 and ±2 S.D. are displayed.

Expenditure Index (EEI) (Rose et al. 1990, 1991a), this is calculated by the formula ((walking heart-rate – resting heart rate)/walking velocity). Its use is based on a known linear relationship between heart-rate and oxygen uptake within a range of heart-rates during certain workloads in a typical population (Bar-Or 1983, Astrand and Rodahl 1986). The reliability of the PCI as a tool to measure the impact of treatment in children with CP is in doubt. Recent

148

investigations have shown that the PCI is unreliable compared to metabolic measurements (Boyd et al. 1999). Also, as a group, children with CP tend to have a higher resting heart-rate. Their lower mechanical efficiency results in high submaximal heart-rates, making submaximal heart-rate a poor predictor of aerobic capacity (Bar-Or 1983). Reconditioning may also play a role (Bar-Or et al. 1976).

MATHEMATICAL/MECHANICAL ENERGY ESTIMATION

Two primary "mechanical" estimations of energy are found in the literature. Both are based on data typically available though gait analysis. One relies on inverse dynamics, the other on the work-energy theorem.

Inverse dynamics

Calculation of the mechanical work required for walking can be done using inverse dynamics. This method requires the magnitude and direction of the ground reaction force in all three planes, complete kinematic measurements, and an anthropometric model of the lower extremities. Mathematical integration of power curves over a given amount of time yields the amount of mechanical work at a particular joint for the plane of motion being considered. This method has been used to estimate the work performed in affected limbs of individuals with disabilities including children with hemiplegia (Mansour et al. 1982, Olney et al. 1990, Winter 1990). The advantage of this type of mechanical energy estimation is that the energy requirements of individual joints can be calculated. However, unless this calculation is based on the data from all three planes of the lower extremities, the head and trunk, and the upper extremities, the method will underestimate the energy cost of walking. Another disadvantage, particularly in the assessment of pathologic gait, is that the use of external loads to judge the work associated with walking does not measure the body's ability to efficiently respond to those loads. This may also lead to underestimation of the energy expense of the gait deviations. Examples of underestimation include simultaneous contraction of antagonistic muscle groups (such as the quadriceps and hamstring muscles) and muscles working in an isometric fashion (Rose et al. 1991b, Frost et al. 1997).

Work-energy theorem

Another method of mechanical power estimation is based on mathematical segment analysis and kinetic and potential energy exchange using the work-energy theorem (Cavagna et al. 1983, Frost et al. 1997, Unnithan et al. 1999). This approach has been used to determine the amount of energy required to move the center of mass through space. The body is divided into segments for which the mass and moments of inertia are estimated. The velocity, kinetic and potential energy changes of every segment are calculated for each instant in time. The method has been used to assess the differences noted in the energy expenditure between children and adults, based on body size and proportions. Energy-expense calculations using the work-energy theorem require assumptions about the potential and kinetic energy components in the system, such as allowing complete exchange between potential and kinetic energy components in the system, allowing no transfers of energy, or variable transfers of energy between adjacent segments of the same limb or between the limbs and

149

trunk. These assumptions may incorrectly estimate true total mechanical energy expense by overestimation or underestimation, depending on the assumptions used. This method measures only the external work of walking without consideration of internal work (the work to move the limbs). This also underestimates energy expense. Like mechanical models using inverse dynamics, the energy-exchange method does not account for the effects of stored elastic energy, coactivation of antagonist muscles, any isometric work or changes in neuromotor development and maturation which may influence energy expenditure.

Energy expenditure in walking

Energy expenditure in walking has been studied since the 1950s (Passmore and Durnin 1955, Ralston 1958, Coates and Meade 1960). The mechanisms that the body uses to conserve energy are optimizing the excursion of the center of mass, control of momentum, and active and passive transfer of energy between body segments. The vertical and horizontal displacements of the center of mass are almost sinusoidal and are equal and opposite during typical walking (Winter 1990). The body accomplishes this through control of pelvic rotation, tilt and obliquity and coordinated knee and ankle motion. Inman and colleagues (1981) demonstrated that without pelvic rotation, and with stiff limbs, the center of mass of the body would be lifted approximately 9.5 cm with each step, compared to typical vertical excursion of 4.5 cm. Energy transfers have been identified as power-conserving mechanisms in walking (Asmussen 1953, Pierrynowski et al. 1980, Williams and Cavanagh 1987), although recent studies are less clear, especially in children who are the least economical (Martin et al. 1993, Frost et al. 1997). Control of momentum occurs through the action of eccentric muscles, such as the soleus in midstance. Ralston (1958) hypothesized that individuals naturally select a walking speed that minimizes energy expenditure. His research suggested that energy expenditure during walking is directly proportional to the square of velocity.

Expense of walking in typically developing children

The major attributes of normal walking (stability in stance, sufficient foot clearance during swing, appropriate swing-phase pre-positioning of the foot, and adequate step length) are absent when a child first achieves the ability to stand independently. The stiff, broad-based, unstable gait of a toddler evolves into gait with most of the characteristics of an adult by 4 years of age, with very fine skills such as foot placement on uneven terrain improving all the way through adolescence. It is not surprising that energy conservation, the fifth major attribute of normal walking, matures throughout the growth years.

Research into energy expenditure specifically in children has revealed that younger children consume more energy than teenagers and adults (Astrand 1952, Cavagna et al. 1983, Rowland and Green 1988, Waters et al. 1988, Ebbeling et al. 1992, Frost et al. 1997, DeJaeger et al. 2001). Data from our own laboratory substantiate these results, indicating that preschool children are less efficient than either school-aged children or teenagers (Koop et al. 1989, 2001) (Fig. 10.3). Despite the fact that children and adults walk in geometrically and kinematically similar ways, size, changes in morphology, muscular efficiency, and motor skill during growth have an effect on the energy cost of locomotion. Smaller children

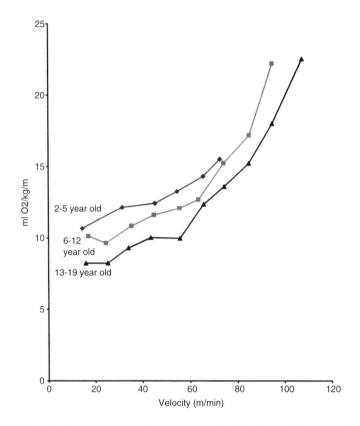

Fig. 10.3. Normalized oxygen consumption versus velocity. Preschool children are noted to demonstrate a higher oxygen-consumption rate for the same velocity than school-aged children or teenagers. The age categories are 2–5 years, 6–12 years, and 13–19 years. All data were collected at the Center for Gait and Motion Analysis of Gillette Children's Specialty Healthcare.

perform a greater amount of work per unit mass and per unit time to maintain a given walking speed than larger children. Because of this, a given walking speed is not functionally equivalent at different ages, as it requires differing amounts of power to move the center of mass (Cavagna et al. 1983). Consistent with the hypothesis of Ralston (1958), it has been shown an optimal speed of walking exists at which transfer between gravitational potential energy and kinetic energy is maximal and the weight-specific work necessary to move the center of mass for a given distance is at a minimum. Until approximately 9 years of age, the younger the child, the slower the optimal walking speed. After that age, the optimal speed of walking typically matches the free-walking speed chosen by an individual. The minimum cost of walking also decreases with age (DeJaeger et al. 2001).

Waters studied the oxygen uptake of 260 individuals walking on an outdoor track with a modified Douglas bag. The subjects were analyzed in four groups: children (6–12 years

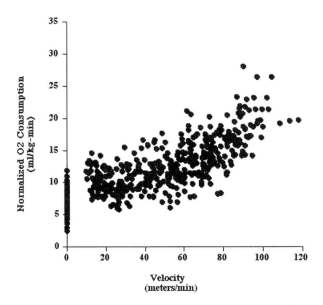

Fig. 10.4. Normalized oxygen consumption versus velocity, including standing (zero velocity) data for children between the ages of 2 and 19 years walking at slow, free, and fast self-selected velocities. The data demonstrate that at velocities below 40 m/min the characteristic is no longer linear.

old), teens (13–19 years old), adults (20–59 years old), and seniors (60–80 years old). Because no differences were found among adults, their data was pooled. However, the authors failed to include data on velocities below 40 meters/min or a reference (zero velocity) (Waters et al. 1988). Regardless of age, oxygen consumption and cost were found to vary with walking speed. Oxygen consumption increased with speed in a linear relationship while oxygen cost diminished with speed in a logarithmic relationship. No gender difference was found for oxygen consumption or cost but heart rate was higher for female subjects than male subjects in all age-groups. The linear regression equations for oxygen consumption in the three age-groups seem to converge on a single value of 2.6 ml/kg/min at zero velocity (standing in place).

Data collected at our laboratory are consistent with the results reported by Ralston (1958), and demonstrate that the rate of oxygen consumption normalized by body weight varies with the square of velocity (Koop et al. 1989, 2001). Our data differ from those of Waters and colleagues (1988), however, in that they include standing, zero-velocity resting values, and walking velocities below 40 meters/min (Fig. 10.4).

DeJaeger and colleagues (2001) confirmed the nonlinear relationship between oxygen consumption and walking speed in a study of children between 3 and 12 years of age and also showed that oxygen consumption diminished with age. They believed that younger children were less efficient, in part due to differences in body proportions. Children under 5 years of age typically have more lean body mass and a greater surface area to body mass ratio. For young children, therefore, basal energy expense is a disproportionately high component of the cost of walking. In DeJaeger's work the decrease in walking energy expense for children aged 5 years and above correlated with the smaller component of basal energy expense as their body size increased. However, others suggest that developmental changes in neuromotor organization that occur around age 6 may also be contributing factors in energy expense efficiency (Shumway-Cook and Woollacott, 1985).

Energy expenditure in cerebral palsy

Alterations of the central nervous system, which produce the characteristic features of CP such as reduced selective muscle control, dependence on patterned movements, abnormal muscle tone, imbalance between muscle agonists and antagonists across joints, and/or deficient equilibrium reactions, result in gait deviations that require greater energy expense than typical walking. Campbell and Ball (1978) documented that children with CP can expend up to three times the energy of their able-bodied counterparts. Considerable new work is now available on the physiological effects of exercise and walking in children with CP and children born preterm which adds new insight into the mechanisms behind the increased expenditure (Bar-Or et al. 1976, Bar-Or 1983, Unnithan et al. 1996, 1998, 1999, Hebestreit and Bar-Or 2001). An increasing number of clinicians are also investigating the mechanical roles specific to cerebral palsy, which may add to understanding (Westwell-O'Connor et al. 2001).

While the altered neurologic function of CP is the primary cause of walking that is energy-expensive, there are additional factors at work. Alterations in tone may lead to contractures of muscles that impair the movement of limb segments during walking. Tone and contractures may induce torsional deformity in the femur and tibia, coxa valga, hip subluxation, and/or malalignment of foot-bone structure that further worsens gait. Multiple physiologic reasons exist for increased energy as well. These include fiber-type make-up of muscles, using a greater percentage of VO_2 max, history of hyaline membrane disease, compensation for musculoskeletal deviations with energy-inefficient mechanisms, increased co-contraction of muscles and/or greater dependence on upper-extremity work for those who use assistive devices. What becomes important in the combination of the clinical and physiological perspectives regarding energy is that if the reasons for the increased energy expenditure are more clearly understood, then treatment can be more specific to avenues that will result in decreased energy use. However, because of their interdependent nature, differentiating between the sources of energy expense has been difficult. Schwartz (2001) has attempted to bridge this gap of understanding by distinguishing the energy expenditure of children who are primarily tone-dominant (spastic) versus those who are gait pathology dominant (lever-arm dysfunction and/or contractures). This may suggest differences in treatment (Fig.10.5). Several of the physiologic reasons for increased energy expenditure in CP will now be discussed.

Physiologic reasons for increased energy in cerebral palsy

ALTERNATIONS IN UPTAKE CAPACITY

Maximal aerobic capacity (VO_2 max) is the highest rate of oxygen consumed by the body in a given period of time during exercise of a significant portion of body muscle mass

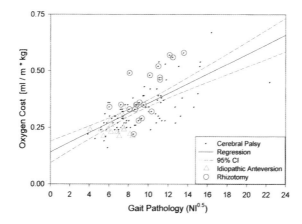

Fig. 10.5. Oxygen cost versus square root of the Normalcy Index (Schutte et al. 2000) as an index of gait pathology (higher index = greater gait pathology). Data demonstrate some distinctions between gait that is "tone-dominant" (rhizotomy) and gait that is more dominated by malalignments (idiopathic anteversion).

(Krahenbuhl et al. 1985, Wasserman et al. 1987). The main criterion for indicating that VO_2 max has been achieved during a progressive test is an increase in power load, which is not accompanied by an increased rate of oxygen uptake. The VO_2 max is typically normalized for body weight and increases throughout childhood. VO_2 max is known to be 10%–15% higher for children age 6–12 years than for a 20-year-old adult (Astrand 1952, Braden and Strong 1990). In children and adolescents with cerebral palsy, the maximal aerobic capacity has been measured to be 10%–30% less than able-bodied children of the same age (Lundberg et al. 1967, Bar-Or et al. 1976, Lundberg 1978, Hoofwijk et al. 1995). Pathophysiologic factors that may limit VO_2 max include central mechanisms of the cardiopulmonary system (stroke volume, heart-rate, etc.), but also peripheral mechanisms (controlling bloodflow, excitation processes in the muscle fiber, local fatigue and enzyme availability) (Green and Patla 1992, Saltin and Strange 1992, Sutton 1992). One possible physiological mechanism for the lower VO2 max values in CP may be the influence of high muscle-tone that reduces venous return and inhibits muscle lactate clearance during exercise, which thereby increases local muscle fatigue (Lundberg 1978). A central mechanism that might contribute to the lower VO2 max in children with CP (and therefore early fatigue at decreased exercise levels) may be history of lung dysfunction related to preterm birth. A review of the exercise capacity of non-disabled children born preterm suggests that some children with a history of bronchopulmonary dysplasia have been noted to have impaired lung function including impaired gas transfer at rest and during exercise (Hebestreit and Bar-Or 2001).

In addition to the fact that VO_2 max is reduced in children with CP, it has also been demonstrated that they perform using a higher percentage of their VO_2 max during exercise than their non-disabled peers (Unnithan et al. 1996). The implication is that they would fatigue more easily during prolonged exercise, and that local muscle factors probably represent the single most important reason for the elevated O_2 cost of walking in children with CP. Children with CP walking at moderate speeds have been demonstrated to exhibit exhaustion when blood lactate levels reached levels typically noted at 50%–60% VO$_2$ max (Dahlback and Norlin 1985).

ANAEROBIC POWER AND MUSCLE-FIBER TYPE

While important, it is unlikely that maximal aerobic power is a limiting factor in the capacity of a child with CP to perform daily activities. One of the difficulties for children with CP to complete a 6-minute level-walk exercise test is often related to decreased endurance, that is, the inability to walk for that duration of time without stopping. In many children with CP, motion is often a series of "bursts of activity" that would be consistent with this inability to maintain walking without stopping. Performance requiring activation of the short-term energy system can be defined as those activities that require substantial anaerobic power, which may be more consistent with the energy-system children with CP use to complete tasks. In children with CP and other neuromuscular diseases, therefore, anaerobic power could be considered a better measure of functional capacity than aerobic power.

It has been demonstrated that children with CP have peak anaerobic power and muscular endurance (mean power) in the range of 2–4 standard deviations below the values of able-bodied, age-matched peers. Differences within subgroups of children with CP have been demonstrated as well (Parker et al. 1992). Because tests of anaerobic power represent the assessment of function of primarily type II muscle fibers, low anaerobic performance in children with CP may represent a difference in the muscle-fiber type make up of muscles (Bar-Or et al. 1980, Bar-Or 1996).

Although not all studies of muscle histopathology in children with CP have demonstrated a consistent picture, Rose and colleagues (1994) demonstrated that children with CP who had a predominance of type I fibers (in total area compared with type II) expended more energy and had more prolonged EMG activity during walking than children exhibiting a predominance of type II fibers. Spasticity may produce structural changes in the muscle that could result in metabolic insufficiency and fatigue. Type I fiber predominance and type IIB fiber deficiency has been reported in the gastrocnemius muscle in children with CP. This is one example in which loss of fiber type in a predominantly "power producer" muscle could have dramatic effects on energy expenditure (Ito et al. 1996). This is significant, especially when one considers that in normal gait, greater than 40% of the power production for walking comes from the plantarflexors (primarily the gastrocnemius) in terminal stance. The adductor muscles (magnus, longus and gracilis) have also been shown to exhibit selective type IIB fiber atrophy and type I hypertrophy (Castle et al. 1979) and, in children with CP, the adductors represent a group of muscles that often are used as accessory hip-flexors. Because children with CP have better selective motor control at the hip than at the ankle, hip-flexor power generation is another dominant source of power generation for the walking cycle.

MUSCLE MECHANICS, CO-CONTRACTION AND MECHANICAL POWER

Because mechanical properties associated with spastic muscles may require increased coactivation and co-contraction to perform the same amount of external work, in CP

155

anaerobic power production is essential to a discussion of energy expenditure. Unnithan and colleagues (1996) demonstrated that lower-extremity co-contraction indexes (between vastus lateralis and hamstrings and anterior tibialis and soleus) explained almost 43% of the variance in energy cost in a group of children with CP. This is probably related to the early fatigue of skeletal muscle.

Compromised muscle mechanics because of increased muscle stiffness or the presence of hypersensitive stretch reflexes may also limit the contractile force capabilities of a muscle. Observation that greater passive force was required per unit of external stretch in children with CP compared with able-bodied peers has suggested that spasticity, in part, may be caused by altered viscoelastic properties within muscles, which results in increased passive stiffness (Berger et al. 1982, Dietz and Berger 1983). It is postulated that added stiffness necessitates greater muscle activation to overcome resistance. Because more work may be required to produce the same movement, energy expenditure increases. Premature firing of a stretch reflex during the second rocker phase of the gait cycle can be differentiated from a volitional vaulting mechanism for clearance of the opposite extremity by the fact that the former has been shown to exhibit different characteristics of dynamic joint stiffness (Davis and DeLuca 1996). These differences in stiffness characteristics may also be reflective of "energy-efficient" versus "energy-inefficient" gait mechanisms. Estimates of total body mechanical power have been found to be significantly higher in children with CP compared to age-matched peers, and that a substantial amount of the variance in metabolic cost (87%) could be explained by one of the estimates of mechanical power (Unnithan et al. 1999). If one desires to understand the mechanisms of increased energy expenditure in children with CP, therefore, mechanical properties of muscles and mechanical power estimates cannot be ignored.

Clinical metabolic energy data in children with cerebral palsy
As mentioned earlier, clinical measurement of metabolic energy expenditure for children with CP has been studied for decades. Assessment during walking represents a submaximal energy assessment, so no indication of maximal aerobic capacity or maximal anaerobic capacity is determined. The value lies in the fact that the assessment is functional tool with known correlation to other gait parameters (Novacheck et al. 2000, Schwartz 2001, Tervo et al. 2002). Baseline assessment of energy can provide a context within which a child's disability can be measured. Follow-up assessment can provide critical evaluation of the effectiveness of a particular treatment and has been used as a clinical tool to evaluate the outcome of surgical intervention (Dahlback and Norlin 1985, Duffy et al. 1996, Boyd et al. 1999, Novacheck et al. 2002). Therefore it is important to understand how energy expenditure varies within subgroups of children with CP, among children who do or do not use assistive devices for ambulation, and the effect of orthotic use on energy expenditure. The influence of surgical intervention on energy expenditure is also an important topic, but is beyond the scope of this chapter.

Because there is a variety of methodologies and testing equipment available to assess metabolic energy it is often difficult to compare results. For this reason, the data presented here was collected at the Center for Gait and Motion Analysis at Gillette Children's Specialty

Healthcare. We use a MedGraphics CPX-D system (MedGraphics Corporation, St Paul, MN 55127) to collect and analyze breath by breath data of oxygen uptake, carbon dioxide output, breathing rate, tidal volume and heart rate. Custom software calculates variables of interest. Metabolic measurement of energy expenditure has been a routine aspect of a typical gait analysis at our facility since 1988. The data represent the average of 3 minutes of breath by breath information collected during steady-state walking (a physiologic plateau of oxygen uptake, heart-rate, respiratory rate and other parameters at a level sufficient to meet the energy demands of the tissues while at a constant workload). Other details of methodology can be found elsewhere (Koop et al. 1989). The two common indices of energy expenditure are typically determined: oxygen consumption (the rate of oxygen uptake normalized for body weight, typically ml/kg-min) and oxygen cost (ml/kg-meter). Gross oxygen consumption and cost are used without subtraction of resting values.

Energy expenditure within subtypes of cerebral palsy
Between 1987 and 2000, over 700 ambulatory children with a diagnosis of CP who had not received intramuscular medications for tone reduction within 6 months or undergone lower-extremity or tone-reducing surgery were evaluated in the motion laboratory at Gillette Children's Specialty Healthcare. Boys and girls demonstrated heights between the 10th and 25th percentiles. However, their weights were near the 50th percentile. This increased mass to size ratio in itself could be responsible for some of their increased energy consumption. Walking velocity was reduced across all age groups. Thirty-two per cent of the children walked in the community without an orthosis or assistive device (cane, crutch or walker); 43% walked in the community with only an orthosis whereas another 12% required an assistive device. The remaining 13% walked only in their household or during therapy sessions. Although a high percentage were community ambulators, their parents report that only 20% of them did so without difficulty and were able to keep up with their peers. The likely reason for this was that approximately 80% of this group as a whole demonstrated a normalized oxygen consumption and oxygen cost that was more than 2 standard deviations above the expected value for a child of the same age without disability (Koop et al. 2001) (Fig.10.6). These data are consistent with the data of Parker and colleagues (1992), who also assessed anaerobic power and muscle endurance among the subgroups of children with CP, in that children with greater disability expend more energy. The distribution of neurological involvement in the children seen in our laboratory was as follows: 25% hemiplegia, 50% diplegia, 10% triplegia and 15% quadriplegia.

To summarize, four subtypes of *hemiplegia* have been previously described based on increasing involvement as indicated in three-dimensional kinematics using gait analysis (Winters et al. 1987). Data on energy expenditure also demonstrate progressively greater energy requirements among the four types of hemiplegia (Stout et al. 1994). Children with type I hemiplegia typically have energy expenditure within 2 standard deviations of normal. Children with type IV hemiplegia expend the greatest amount of energy, typically in the range of 1.6 times that of their able-bodied peers. Minimal distinction is noted between type II and type III, both based on velocity as well as the percentage of energy expenditure increase above normal (Fig.10.7a). While children with hemiplegia clearly consume less

157

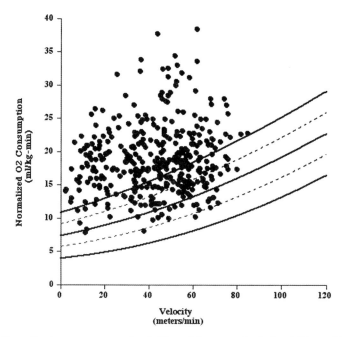

Fig. 10.6. Normalized oxygen consumption (ml/kg-min) versus velocity for children with cerebral palsy in reference to children without a disability.

energy than children with other forms of CP (*diplegia*, *triplegia* and *quadriplegia*) there is little predictive value in the other traditional topographic subgroups within CP. Children with diplegia walk faster than those with triplegia or quadriplegia, but all have a similar rate of oxygen consumption. Because of the faster walking velocity, children with diplegia are more efficient than those with triplegia or quadriplegia. All expend more energy to walk than the typical child with type IV hemiplegia (Fig. 10.7b).

Subtypes based on function and contractures

Better separation or division can be made between those children who use assistive devices (such as crutches or a walker) and those who do not. The greater energy expenditure for children who use assistive devices is likely to reflect a greater level of disability as well as the greater energy expense when performing upper-extremity work (Fig.10.8a). The primary differentiation in energy expenditure between these groups is related to walking velocity rather than a clear difference in the rate of oxygen consumption per unit of body weight. The energy requirement of a child with diplegia who uses assistive devices, for example, is roughly equivalent to the energy requirement of a non-disabled person climbing stairs.

A similar separation appears in the presence of hip or knee contracture: those without contractures are more efficient than those with a contracture who walk without an assistive device, and both groups are much more efficient than those with contractures who rely upon an assistive device to walk. Putting this in perspective, children without contracture who

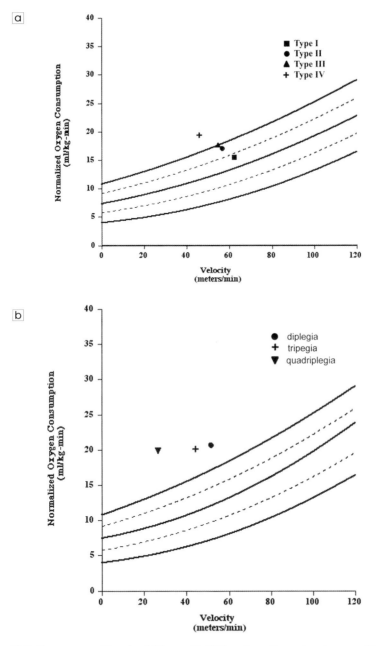

Fig. 10.7. Energy expenditure in children with CP based on diagnosis subgroups. Each diagnostic category is depicted as a percentage above the expected value for age related peers at the chosen velocity. (a) Increased energy expenditure is noted with increased involvement among the four subtypes of hemiplegia. Minimal distinction is noted between types II and III. (b) For children with diplegia, triplegia and quadriplegia, each subgroup by diagnosis is equally inefficient although some differences in velocity exist.

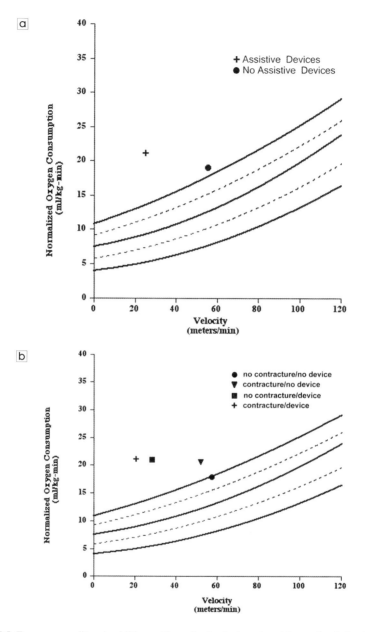

Fig. 10.8. Energy expenditure in children with cerebral palsy based on (a) use of assistive devices or (b) presence of contractures with or without an assistive device.

walk without an assistive device expend approximately 1.43 times that of their able-bodied peers; those with contracture and require use of an assistive device for ambulation expend 2.41 times more than their non-disabled peers (Fig. 10.8b).

Orthoses and energy expenditure

Studies have suggested an improvement in energy expenditure with the use of selected orthoses for children with both hemiplegia and diplegia (Buckon et al. 2001, Maltais et al. 2001). Our clinical database has data for children with and without orthotics, but the numerous types of orthoses, the different subtypes of children with CP, and the differing amounts of time within a particular orthosis make it difficult to present these data in a concise fashion.

ENERGY EXPENDITURE AS A GUIDE FOR TREATMENT PLANNING

These data suggest that the traditional patient groups (based on topographic description or function levels) may not be sufficient to create groups that guide effective treatment. The strong correlation between walking speed, contractures, the need for assistive device, and excessive energy use suggests that the severity of gait deviations does influence energy expense. Use of the Normalcy Index has demonstrated a strong linear correlation between an increased Normalcy Index and increased oxygen cost in children with CP (Schutte et al. 2000, Schwartz 2001) (Fig.10.5). This correlation suggests two ways in which the Normalcy Index and oxygen cost might be used to guide treatment. First, an oxygen cost value that is disproportionately high for a specific elevated normalcy index (when compared to other children with CP) suggests excessive oxygen utilization by muscles; that observation might direct treatment towards tone reduction. Secondly, if a correlation between specific deformities (contractures or bone malalignment) and elevations in the normalcy index can be found, it might point towards specific decisions regarding correction of muscle contractures and/or bone deformity. In either case the Normalcy Index, combined with oxygen cost measurement, has potential as a tool for quantifying treatment outcomes.

Conclusion

This purpose of this chapter has been to provide information regarding the multiple factors that contribute to the increased energy expenditure in children with CP, as well as to give an updated review of what our clinical experience has shown regarding the differences in energy expense among children with CP. As stated at the beginning of the chapter, energy assessment helps to span the gap between a laboratory "technical" outcome and a community "functional" outcome, and as such becomes an important aspect of critical evaluation of any treatment outcome. Certainly, knowledge that energy is increased does not explain the mechanisms of the increase. That is the area where clinical research and scientific research come together. However, understanding how a particular child is functioning in relation to his peers with CP does become important as a guide to future expectations, treatment planning, and the timing of that treatment. Knowledge of the effect of treatment interventions on energy is important to guide expectations of potential benefit. Both are invaluable when counseling a family about their child's current function and future function with or without treatment intervention.

REFERENCES

Asmussen E. (1953) Positive and negative muscular work. *Acta Physiol Scand* **28**: 364–382.
Astrand P. (1952) *Experimental Studies of Physical Working Capacity in Relation to Sex and Age*. Copenhagen:

Ejnar Munksgaard.

Astrand PO, Rodahl K. (1986) *Textbook of Work Physiology*. Singapore: McGraw Hill.

Bar-Or O. (1983) *Pediatric Sports Medicine for the Practioner*. New York: Springer. p 227–249.

Bar-Or O. (1996) Role of exercise in the assessment and management of neuromuscular disease in children. *Med Sci Sports Exerc* **28:** 421–427.

Bar-Or O, Inbar O, Spira R. (1976) Physiological effects of a sports rehabilitation program on cerebral palsied and poliomyelitic adolescents. *Med Sci Sports Exerc* **8:** 157–161.

Bar-Or O, Dotan R, Inbar O. (1980) Anaerobic capacity and muscle fiber distribution in man. *Int J Sports Med* **1:** 89–92.

Berger W, Quintern J, Dietz V. (1982) Pathophysiology of gait in children with cerebral palsy. *Electroencephalogr Clin Neurophysiol* **53:** 538–548.

Boyd R, Fatone S, Rodda J, Olesch C, Starr R, Cullis E, Gallagher D, Carlin JB, Nattrass GR, Graham K. (1999) High- or low- technology measurements of energy expenditure in clinical gait analysis? *Dev Med Child Neurol* **41:** 676–682.

Braden DS, Strong WB. (1990) Cardiovascular responses to exercise in childhood. *Am J Dis Child* **144:** 1255–1260.

Buckon CE, Thomas SS, Jakobson-Huston S, Sussman M, Aiona M. (2001) Comparison of three ankle-foot orthosis configurations for children with spastic hemiplegia. *Dev Med Child Neurol* **43:** 371–378.

Butler P, Engelbrecht M, Major RE, Tait JH, Stallard J, Patrick JH. (1984) Physiological cost index of walking for normal children and its use as an indicator of physical handicap. *Dev Med Child Neurol* **26:** 607–612.

Campbell J, Ball J. (1978) Energetics of walking in cerebral palsy. *Orthop Clin North Am* **9:** 374–377.

Castle ME, Reyman TA, Schneider M. (1979) Pathology of spastic muscle in cerebral palsy. *Clin Orthop* **142:** 223–232.

Cavagna GA, Franzetti P, Fuchimoto T. (1983) The mechanics of walking in children. *J Physiol* **343:** 323–339.

Coates JE, Meade F. (1960) The energy demand and mechanical energy demand in walking. *Ergonomics* **3:** 97–119.

Dahlback GO, Norlin R. (1985) The effect of corrective surgery on energy expenditure during ambulation in children with cerebral palsy. *Eur J Appl Physiol* **54:** 67–70.

Davis RB, DeLuca PA. (1996) Gait characterization via dynamic joint stiffness. *Gait Posture* **4:** 224–231.

DeJaeger D, Willems PA, Heglund NC. (2001) The energy cost of walking in children. *Pflugers Arch* **441:** 538–543.

Dietz V, Berger W. (1983) Normal and impaired regulation of muscle stiffness in gait: a new hypothesis about muscle hypertonia. *Exp Neurol* **79:** 680–687.

Duffy CM, Hill AE, Cosgrove AP, Corry IS, Graham HK. (1996) Energy consumption in children with spina bifida and cerebral palsy: a comparative study. *Dev Med Child Neurol* **38:** 238–243.

Ebbeling CJ, Hamill J, Freedson PS. (1992) An examination of efficiency during walking in children and adults. *Pediatr Exerc Sci* **4:** 36–49.

Frost G, Dowling J, Bar-Or O, Dyson K. (1997) Ability of mechanical power estimates to explain differences in metabolic cost of walking and running among children. *Gait Posture* **5:** 120–127.

Gage JR. (1991) *Gait Analysis in Cerebral Palsy*. London: MacKeith Press. p 61–95.

Green HJ, Patla AE. (1992) Maximal aerobic power: neuromuscular and metabolic considerations. *Med Sci Sports Exerc* **24:** 38–46.

Hebestreit H, Bar-Or O. (2001) Exercise and the child born prematurely. *Sports Med* **31:** 591–599.

Hoofwijk M, Unnithan VB, Bar-Or O. (1995) Maximal treadmill performance of children with cerebral palsy. *Pediatr Exerc Sci* **17:** 305–313.

Inman VT, Ralston HJ, Todd F. (1981) *Human Walking*. Baltimore: Williams & Wilkins.

Ito J, Araki A, Tanaka H, Tasaki T, Cho K, Yamazaki R. (1996) Muscle histopathology in spastic cerebral palsy. *Brain Dev* **18:** 299–303.

Koop S, Stout J, Starr R, Drinken W. (1989) Oxygen consumption during walking in normal children and children with cerebral palsy. *Dev Med Child Neurol* **31** (suppl. 59): 6. (Abstract.)

Koop SE, Stout JL, Luxenberg M. (2001) A comparison of the energy expense of normal walking and walking affected by cerebal palsy. *Proceedings of the American Orthopaedic Association,* Palm Beach, FL, June.

Krahenbuhl GS, Skinner JS, Kohrt WM. (1985) Developmental aspects of maximal aerobic power in children. *Exerc Sport Sci Rev* **13:** 503–538.

Lundberg A. (1978) Maximal aerobic capacity of young people with spastic cerebral palsy. *Dev Med Child Neurol* **20:** 205–210.

Lundberg A, Ovenfors CO, Saltin B. (1967) Effect of physical training on school-children with cerebral palsy. *Acta Paediatr Scand* **56:** 182–188.

Maltais D, Bar-Or O, Galea V, Pierrynowski M. (2001) Use of orthoses lowers the O_2 cost of walking in children with spastic cerebral palsy. *Med Sci Sports Exerc* **33:** 320–325.

Mansour JM, Lesh MD, Nowak MD, Simon SR. (1982) A three dimensional multi-segmental analysis of the energetics of normal and pathological human gait. *J Biomech* **15:** 51–59.

Martin PE, Heise GD, Morgan DW. (1993) Interrelationships between mechanical power, energy transfers, and walking and running economy. *Med Sci Sports Exerc* **25:** 508–515.

Novacheck T, Stout J, Tervo R. (2000) Reliability and validity of the Gillette Functional Assessment Questionnaire as an outcome measure in children with walking disabilities. *J Pediatr Orthop* **20:** 75–81.

Novacheck T, Trost J, Schwartz M. (2002) Intramuscular psoas lengthening improves dynamic hip function in children with cerebral palsy. *J Pediatr Orthop* **22:** 158–164.

Olney SJ, MacPhail HE, Hedden DM, Boyce WF. (1990) Work and power in hemiplegic cerebral palsy gait. *Phys Ther* **70:** 431–438.

Parker DF, Carriere L, Hebestreit H, Bar-Or O. (1992) Anaerobic endurance and peak muscle power in children with spastic cerebral palsy. *Am J Dis Child* **146:** 1069–1073.

Passmore R, Durnin GA. (1955) Human energy expenditure. *Physiol Rev* **35:** 801–839.

Pierrynowski MR, Winter DA, Norman RW. (1980) Transfers of mechanical energy within the total body and mechanical efficiency during treadmill walking. *Ergonomics* **23:** 147–156.

Ralston HJ. (1958) Energy-speed relation and optimal speed during level walking. *Zeitschrift fur Angewandte Physiol* **17:** 277–283.

Rose J, Gamble JG, Burgos A, Medeiros J, Haskell WL. (1990) Energy expenditure index of walking for normal children and for children with cerebral palsy. *Dev Med Child Neurol* **32:** 333–340.

Rose J, Gamble JG, Lee J, Lee R, Haskell WL. (1991a) The energy expenditure index: a method to quantitate and compare walking energy expenditure for children and adolescents. *J Pediatr Orthop* **11:** 571–578.

Rose SA, Õunpuu S, DeLuca PA. (1991b) Strategies for the assessment of pediatric gait in the clinical setting. *Phys Ther* **71:** 961–980.

Rose J, Haskell WL, Gamble JG, Hamilton RL, Brown DA, Rinsky L. (1994) Muscle pathology and clinical measures of disability in children with cerebral palsy. *J Orthop Res* **12:** 758–768.

Rowland TW, Green GM. (1988) Physiological responses to treadmill exercise in females: adult-child differences. *Med Sci Sports Exerc* **20:** 474–478.

Saltin B, Strange S. (1992) Maximal oxygen uptake: "old" and "new" arguments for a cardiovascular limitation. *Med Sci Sports Exerc* **24:** 30–37.

Schutte LM, Narayanan U, Stout JL, Selber P, Gage JR, Schwartz MH. (2000) An index for quantifying deviations from normal gait. *Gait Posture* **11:** 25–31.

Schwartz M. (2001) The effects of gait pathology on the energy cost of walking. *Gait Posture* **13:** 260. (Abstract.)

Shumway-Cook A, Woollacott M. (1985) The growth of stability: postural control from a developmental perspective. *J Mot Behav* **17:** 131–147.

Stout JL, Gage JR, Bruce R. (1994) Joint kinetic patterns in spastic hemiplegia. *Dev Med Child Neurol* **70** (Suppl): 8–9. (Abstract.)

Sutton JR. (1992) VO2max—new concepts on an old theme. *Med Sci Sports Exerc* **24:** 26–29.

Tervo RC, Azuma S, Stout J, Novacheck T. (2002) Correlation between physical functioning and gait measures in children with cerebral palsy. *Dev Med Child Neurol* **44:** 185–190.

Unnithan VB, Dowling JJ, Frost G, Bar-Or O. (1996) Role of cocontraction in the O_2 cost of walking in children with cerebral palsy. *Med Sci Sports Exerc* **28:** 1498–1504.

Unnithan VB, Clifford C, Bar-Or O. (1998) Evaluation by exercise testing of the child with cerebral palsy. *Sports Med* **26:** 239–251.

Unnithan VB, Dowling JJ, Frost G, Bar-Or O. (1999) Role of mechanical power estimates in the O_2 cost of walking in children with cerebral palsy. *Med Sci Sports Exerc* **31:** 1703–1708.

Wasserman K, Hansen JE, Sue DY, Whipp BJ. (1987) *Principles of Exercise Testing and Interpretation.* Philadelphia: Lea & Febiger.

Waters RL, Lunsford BR, Perry J, Byrd R. (1988) Energy-speed relationship of walking: standard tables. *J Orthop Res* **6:** 215–222.

Westwell-O'Connor M, Õunpuu S, DeLuca P. (2001) Energy analysis of the lower extremity during swing phase in individuals with cerebral palsy. *Gait Posture* **13:** 272–273. (Abstract.)

163

Williams KR, Cavanagh PR. (1987) Relationship between distance running mechanics, running economy, and performance. *J Appl Physiol* **63:** 1236–1245.

Winter DA. (1990) *Biomechanics and Motor Control of Human Movement*, 2nd edn. New York: John Wiley.

Winters TF, Jr, Gage JR, Hicks R. (1987) Gait patterns in spastic hemiplegia in children and young adults. *J Bone Joint Surg Am* **69:** 437–441.

11
THE ROLE OF MUSCULOSKELETAL MODELS IN PATIENT ASSESSMENT AND TREATMENT

Allison S. Arnold and Scott L. Delp

The management of gait abnormalities in persons with cerebral palsy is a challenging task. Theoretically, gait abnormalities can be diminished by first identifying the biomechanical factors that contribute to abnormal movement and then either decreasing the muscle forces that disrupt normal movement (e.g. via muscle-tendon lengthenings or botulinum toxin injections), and/or increasing the muscle and ground reaction forces that have the potential to improve movement (e.g. via strengthening exercises, orthoses, or derotational osteotomies). However, different patients with cerebral palsy exhibit varying degrees of neurologic impairment, spasticity, weakness, muscle contracture and bone deformity, suggesting that gait deviations arise from a variety of sources, each requiring a different treatment. Treatment planning is further complicated because there is currently no scientific basis for determining how patients' neuro-musculoskeletal impairments contribute to abnormal movement. The static muscle tests performed during a patient's physical exam (Chapter 5) and the kinematic, kinetic, and electromyographic (EMG) data obtained from gait analysis (Chapters 6–9) are not always sufficient to identify the biomechanical source of a patient's abnormal gait or to predict the consequences of treatments. This limitation exists, in part, because the transformation from EMG patterns to motion is extremely complex (Fig. 11.1) and because the effects of common surgical procedures on muscle-tendon mechanics and musculoskeletal geometry are not easily measured. This chapter describes how computer simulations of the musculoskeletal system can be used, in combination with gait analysis, to enhance our understanding of movement abnormalities and to provide a theoretical basis for planning treatments.

Imagine the following hypothetical scenario. A child with a troublesome gait abnormality visits a cerebral palsy clinic. The child undergoes a routine physical exam, a gait analysis, and perhaps a medical imaging study. A computer model of the child's musculoskeletal system is created that characterizes the force generating capacity of the muscles, the geometric relationships between the muscles, tendons and bones, the kinematics of the joints, and the inertial properties of the body (see the shaded region of Fig. 11.1). The model is driven by a set of muscle excitation signals, and the resulting motion of the model is governed by mathematical equations that describe the activation dynamics of muscle, the contraction dynamics of muscle, and the multi-joint dynamics of the body during walking. The muscle excitation signals are specified such that the computer model "walks"

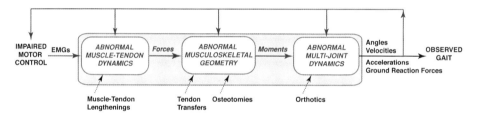

Fig. 11.1. Many factors contribute to movement abnormalities in persons with cerebral palsy. Gait analysis is used routinely to record EMG patterns, joint angles, and ground reaction forces during walking, but the transformation between EMG patterns and coordinated multi-joint movement (shaded region) is complicated. Furthermore, to make treatment decisions clinicians must try to predict how the motions induced by muscles might change after treatment. Typically, treatments alter the muscle-tendon dynamics or the musculoskeletal geometry, and these changes are not easily measured. Computational models that characterize patients' muscle-tendon dynamics, musculoskeletal geometry, multi-joint dynamics of the body during walking may enhance interpretation of motion analysis studies and improve the planning of treatments.

in a way that resembles the child's abnormal gait. Analysis of the motions produced by muscles identifies the specific causes of the child's abnormal movements. The model is used to evaluate several possible treatments and a comprehensive surgical plan and/or physical therapy regimen is designed, based on the child's clinical exam, the gait analysis and the modeling study. The child returns for a postoperative gait analysis one year after treatment. As predicted by the model, the child's walking ability has improved dramatically.

This scenario offers one vision of how musculoskeletal simulations might someday be used to improve the treatment of gait abnormalities in persons with neuromuscular disorders. However, creating biomechanical models that enable accurate prediction of treatment outcomes remains a formidable, multifaceted challenge. Most biomechanical studies of muscle function to date have relied on "generic" models, based on measurements of muscle architecture, musculoskeletal geometry, neuromuscular excitation patterns, and multi-joint movement kinematics from a relatively small number of unimpaired subjects. Only a few investigators have attempted to characterize the bone geometry or the muscle force generating properties of children with deformities, spasticity or contracture (Tardieu and Tardieu 1987, Rose et al. 1994, Lundy et al. 1998, Arnold and Delp 2001). Dynamic simulations that resemble normal gait, driven by as many as 54 muscle-tendon actuators, have been created (Yamaguchi and Zajac 1990, Taga 1995, Gerritsen et al. 1998, Anderson and Pandy 2001, Neptune et al. 2001). However, no simulation has been developed that can explain how a particular child's impairments contribute to abnormal gait, or can predict how an individual will ambulate following orthopaedic surgery. Furthermore, constructing a patient specific model for every child with a gait abnormality would be costly and labor intensive. Given these difficulties, is the hypothetical scenario outlined above realistic, or overly optimistic? What is the role of musculoskeletal modeling in patient assessment and treatment?

We believe that musculoskeletal simulations have tremendous potential to enhance the management of movement abnormalities in persons with cerebral palsy. However, models that are used to guide treatment decisions must be formulated, tested, and interpreted with care, being cognizant of the underlying limitations of the models and the conditions that determine when, and for which patients, the results of a simulation are applicable. Models do not need to include patient specific representations of all the neuromuscular and musculoskeletal elements involved in the production of movement to be valuable. Rather, we envisage that many of the insights needed to improve treatment outcomes will come from analyses of models with varying complexity.

Models of the musculoskeletal system can facilitate the assessment and treatment of gait abnormalities in several ways. First, models can provide information about a range of biomechanical parameters that are not easily measured, such as the lengths and moment arms of muscles, the force and moment generating capacities of muscles, and the multi-joint accelerations produced by muscles during movement. A relatively simple model that characterizes musculoskeletal geometry, for example, can be used in conjunction with joint angles obtained from gait analysis to estimate the lengths of muscles during normal and pathologic gait (Hoffinger et al. 1993, Delp et al. 1996, Schutte et al. 1997, Thompson et al. 1998). Knowledge of the muscle-tendon lengths may be useful because a "short" muscle that restricts movement can often be surgically lengthened or injected with botulinum toxin. Analyses of the muscle-tendon lengths during movement may help to distinguish patients who walk with abnormally short muscles from those who do not walk with short muscles, and thus may provide a basis for identifying patients who would benefit from treatment. Studies to test this hypothesis are under way.

Second, musculoskeletal models enable users to pose "what if?" questions, introduce changes to a model, and quantify the biomechanical consequences. For instance, a model that describes muscle-tendon mechanics and musculoskeletal geometry can be used to determine how the moment generating capacities of muscles are altered by tendon lengthenings (Delp and Zajac 1992, Delp et al. 1995), tendon transfers (Dul et al. 1985, Delp et al. 1994, Lieber and Friden 1997), and other musculoskeletal procedures. These surgeries are often performed on persons with cerebral palsy in an effort to produce a more normal balance of the moments about the joints during movement, but are not always successful. A model that allows surgical effects to be quantified may help investigators to design more effective orthopaedic procedures. Without a model, evaluating the outcome of a treatment is often difficult, if not impossible, because of the many uncontrolled parameters of clinical trials.

Third, musculoskeletal simulations provide a powerful theoretical framework for examining cause-and-effect relationships between the excitation patterns of muscles and the multi-joint accelerations of the body during movement. Clinical assessments of muscle function during walking are often based upon a muscle's EMG activity and the joint moments to which the muscle contributes. However, these are not the only factors that determine the actions of a muscle on the body. A muscle that crosses one joint has the potential to accelerate other joints, and biarticular muscles can produce angular accelerations of the joints that oppose their applied moments (Hollerbach and Flash 1982, Zajac and Gordon 1989). For example, the soleus exerts only an ankle plantarflexion moment, yet Zajac and Gordon (1989) demonstrated that the soleus can accelerate the knee into extension more than it accelerates the ankle into plantarflexion. To identify which muscles may produce abnormal movement, therefore, a model that characterizes the coupled dynamics of the limb segments, the muscle-tendon mechanics, and the musculoskeletal geometry is needed.

The remainder of this chapter reviews several studies in which biomechanical models of varying complexity have been used to enhance the analysis of a particular gait abnormality or improve the design of a treatment plan. Each example first introduces the clinical question that motivated the development of a model and then describes selected simulation results. The chapter concludes with a brief discussion of some of the limitations of current musculoskeletal simulations. Consideration of these limitations suggests areas for future research.

Analysis of hip muscle moment arms during internally rotated gait

Children with cerebral palsy frequently walk with excessive internal rotation of the hip. Spastic medial hamstrings or adductors, among other factors, are thought to contribute to the excessive internal rotation in many patients based on EMG evidence that the muscles are active during walking, and on the presumption that these muscles generate an internal hip rotation moment (Sutherland et al. 1969, Chong et al. 1978). Surgical lengthening of these muscles is often expected to decrease excessive internal rotation (Hoffer 1986, Root 1987, Tachdjian 1990). However, the extent to which the hamstrings and adductors contribute to hip internal rotation is unclear, and the changes in hip rotation following surgery are inconsistent. The rotational moment arm of a muscle about the hip determines whether the muscle has the potential to produce an internal or an external hip rotation moment. Therefore knowledge of the muscle moment arms is needed to establish a scientific rationale for muscle-tendon surgeries intended to reduce internal rotation moments.

Determination of hip rotation moment arms in patients with cerebral palsy is difficult for two main reasons. First, rotational abnormalities of the hip are often accompanied by excessive anteversion of the femur (Bleck 1987), a torsional bone deformity that may alter the lines of action and moment arms of muscles about the hip. Second, the muscle moment arms must be evaluated over the range of limb positions assumed by persons with cerebral palsy during walking; this frequently includes exaggerated flexion of the hips and knees in addition to increased internal rotation of the hip. We have performed a series of studies to determine which muscles have the greatest potential to rotate the hip in children with femoral deformities who walk with a crouched, internally rotated gait (Arnold et al. 1997, 2000, Delp et al. 1999, Arnold and Delp 2001). These studies have provided new guidelines for the treatment of excessive hip internal rotation.

In one study, we evaluated the hip rotation moment arms of the medial hamstrings and adductors using highly accurate musculoskeletal models of three individuals with cerebral palsy that we constructed from magnetic resonance images (Fig. 11.2). Analysis of these models, at the limb positions corresponding to each subject's internally rotated gait, revealed that the semimembranosus, semitendinosus, adductor brevis, adductor longus and gracilis had *external* rotation moment arms or very small internal rotation moment arms throughout the gait cycle in all three subjects (Arnold et al. 2000). Hence, none of these muscles could have generated a substantial hip internal rotation moment in these subjects, whose gait abnormalities and femoral deformities might be considered typical of patients who walk with excessive internal rotation of the hip.

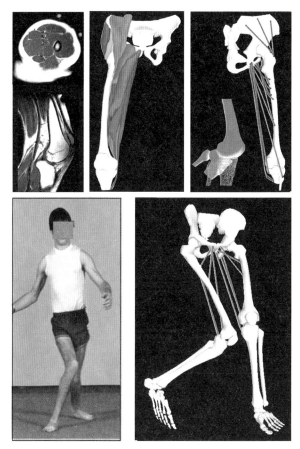

Fig. 11.2. Determination of hip rotation moment arms during crouched, internally rotated gait. Musculoskeletal models of subjects with cerebral palsy were created from magnetic resonance images. For each subject, three-dimensional surface representations of the muscles and bones were generated from two-dimensional contours segmented manually from each of approximately 200 images (top left). Surfaces from overlapping series of images were registered to obtain an accurate representation of each subject's anatomy at the "scanned" limb position (top center). Kinematic models of the hip and the knee were implemented, and the muscle lines of action were defined (top right). The rotational moment arms of the medial hamstrings, adductors, and other muscles were evaluated at the body positions corresponding to each subject's internally rotated gait (bottom).

Based on these observations, we hypothesized that the rotational moment arms of the medial hamstrings and adductors are shifted toward external rotation by excessive femoral anteversion and/or by exaggerated hip flexion, knee flexion or hip internal rotation. We tested this hypothesis using a model of the lower extremity with a "deformable" femur that estimates the moment arms at the body positions of patients who walk with crouched, internally rotated gait (Arnold et al. 2001). We determined that the semimembranosus, semitendinosus and gracilis muscles in our model had negligible or external rotation moment arms when the hip was internally rotated or when the knee was flexed—the body positions

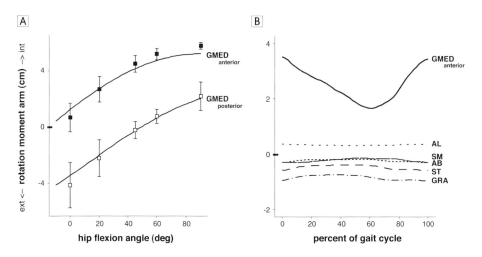

Fig. 11.3. Hip rotation moment arms of the gluteus medius versus hip-flexion angle (A) and gait cycle (B). Rotational moment arms of the anterior (filled squares) and posterior (open squares) compartments of the gluteus medius determined experimentally (mean ± 1 S.D. for four specimens) and calculated with a musculoskeletal model (solid lines) increase dramatically with hip flexion (A). This suggests that internally rotated gait may be a result of excessive hip flexion, which shifts the rotational moment arms of the gluteal muscles toward internal rotation. Internal rotation moment arms of the anterior compartment of the gluteus medius during walking, computed with an image-based model of a subject with cerebral palsy, are approximately four times larger than the rotational moment arms of the medial hamstrings or adductors (B).

that children with cerebral palsy commonly assume during walking. When the femur was excessively anteverted, the rotational moment arms of the adductor brevis, adductor longus, pectineus and proximal compartments of the adductor magnus in our model shifted toward external rotation. These results indicate that neither the medial hamstrings nor the adductors are likely to contribute substantially to excessive internal rotation of the hip and that other causes of internal rotation should be considered with planning treatments for these patients.

We used our musculoskeletal models to examine other potential causes of excessive hip internal rotation (Arnold et al. 1997, Delp et al. 1999). Our experimental studies of hip rotation moment arms in cadavers have shown that the rotational moment arms of the gluteus medius and gluteus minimus increase dramatically with hip flexion (Delp et al. 1999). The moment arms computed with our musculoskeletal models are consistent with this observation (Fig. 11.3). Since excessive flexion of the hip frequently accompanies internally rotated gait (Bleck 1987, Gage 1991), and since the gluteal muscles are typically active and play an important role in walking (Perry 1992), we suggest that the excessive hip flexion of patients, which increases the internal rotation moment arms of the gluteus medius and minimus, is more likely than the hamstrings or adductors to cause internal rotation. We have further observed that the gluteus maximus has a large capacity for external rotation when the hip is extended (Delp et al. 1999); thus strengthening or enhancing activation of the gluteus maximus in persons with crouched, internally rotated gait may help to correct both the excessive hip flexion and internal rotation. These studies of hip muscle moment arms highlight the need for musculoskeletal models that can account for altered bone geometry and abnormal joint kinematics when hypothesizing the causes of gait abnormalities and planning treatments.

Analysis of muscle moment generating capacity after tendon surgery

Persistent plantarflexion of the ankle, termed equinus gait, is one of the most common movement abnormalities among cerebral palsy patients. Equinus gait is frequently caused by contracture (i.e. shortening of the fibers) of the triceps surae. Either isolated contracture of the gastrocnemius or combined contracture of the gastrocnemius and soleus may be present. When only the gastrocnemius is contracted, surgical lengthening of the gastrocnemius aponeurosis is usually successful in restoring the normal range of ankle motion while maintaining plantarflexion strength (Rose et al. 1993). However, tendo-Achilles lengthening, the procedure commonly performed to treat combined contracture of the gastrocnemius and soleus, is less effective. If the Achilles tendon is not lengthened enough, passive plantarflexion moment continues to cause ankle equinus after surgery (Sharrard and Bernstein 1972, Lee and Bleck 1980). By contrast, if the Achilles tendon is lengthened too much, the active force generating capacity of the muscles can be compromised, resulting in disabling muscle weakness (Sutherland and Cooper 1978, Segal et al. 1989).

The force generating capacity of a muscle after tendon surgery is influenced by the architecture of the muscle-tendon complex (i.e. the lengths and arrangement of the muscle fibers). Since the gastrocnemius and soleus exhibit different architectures, one might expect these muscles to respond differently to tendon lengthening (Delp and Zajac 1992). These effects are difficult to quantify in clinical studies because individual muscle forces cannot be measured without invasive techniques. However, a musculoskeletal model that accounts for differences in the muscle architectures can be used to evaluate how tendon lengthening affects the muscles' force and moment generating characteristics.

We have used a musculoskeletal model to examine the trade-off between restoring range of ankle motion and maintaining plantarflexion strength in cases of combined contracture of the gastrocnemius and soleus (Delp et al. 1995). We first developed a model that represents the normal force and moment generating characteristics of the major muscles crossing the ankle. We then altered the model to represent contracture of the gastrocnemius and soleus. The force length properties of each muscle-tendon complex were derived by scaling a dimensionless model of muscle and tendon by four parameters: peak isometric muscle force, optimal muscle fiber length, tendon slack length, and pennation angle (Zajac 1989). Values of these parameters were specified based on experimental data published in the literature (Wickiewicz et al. 1983, Friederich and Brand 1990). To represent contracture of the gastrocnemius and soleus, the optimal fiber lengths of the muscles were decreased by 45% (Ziv et al. 1984). This decrease in the fiber lengths caused a substantial increase in the passive moments generated by the muscles, which is consistent with clinical observations (Bleck 1987, Tardieu and Tardieu 1987). We simulated the effects of tendo-Achilles lengthening by elongating the tendons of both the contracted gastrocnemius and the contracted soleus. The effects of gastrocnemius aponeurosis lengthening were simulated by elongating

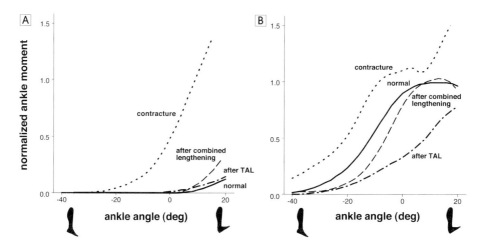

Fig. 11.4. Passive ankle moment (A) and total ankle moment (B) generated by a model of the triceps surae versus ankle angle. After simulated tendo-Achilles lengthening, the passive plantarflexion moment developed by the contracted triceps surae is restored approximately to normal (A), but the total moment-generating capacity of the triceps surae is substantially less than normal (B). After combined tendo-Achilles lengthening and gastrocnemius aponeurosis lengthening, the passive moment developed by the triceps surae is greater than normal (A); however, the total moment-generating capacity of the triceps surae is nearly normal (B). Muscles were assumed to be at their maximum level of activation when the total moments were calculated, and the moments were normalized by the maximum active moment of the normal triceps surae.

the tendon of the gastrocnemius while the soleus tendon remained unaltered. The theoretical effectiveness of the simulated surgeries was evaluated based on the potential of each procedure to reproduce normal passive and active moment generating characteristics of the triceps surae about the ankle.

In the simulations, neither tendo-Achilles lengthening nor gastrocnemius aponeurosis lengthening alone was an effective treatment for combined contracture of the gastrocnemius and soleus. Lengthening of the gastrocnemius aponeurosis did not diminish the excessive passive moment developed by the contracted soleus. Lengthening of the Achilles tendon by 2 cm restored the passive moment of the contracted muscles to near normal (Fig. 11.4A); however, this change in tendon length decreased the total moment generating capacity of the triceps surae substantially (Fig. 11.4B).

The moment generating characteristics of the triceps surae could be restored more effectively in the model if the contracted gastrocnemius and the contracted soleus were corrected independently. After simulated lengthening of both the Achilles tendon and the gastrocnemius aponeurosis by 1 cm, the total moment generating capacity of the triceps surae was slightly less than normal (Fig. 11.4B), but greater than after a 2 cm lengthening of the Achilles tendon alone (Fig. 11.4B, dashed and dot-dashed curves). These results suggest that independent lengthening of the gastrocnemius and soleus can account for differences in the architectures of these muscles, and theoretically could provide a more efficacious means for correcting equinus gait and preserving plantarflexion moment generating capacity in cases of combined contracture. Although independent adjustment of the muscles is slightly more complicated than tendo-Achilles lengthening, Saraph and colleagues (2000) reported favorable outcomes in a 2 year follow up of 22 patients. This example illustrates how a model of musculoskeletal geometry and muscle-tendon mechanics can help explain and enhance our understanding of the biomechanical effects of treatments.

Analysis of muscle actions during stiff knee gait

Many individuals with cerebral palsy walk with insufficient knee flexion during the swing phase, or stiff knee gait. This movement abnormality is often attributed to excessive activation of the rectus femoris (Gage et al. 1987, Perry 1987, Sutherland et al. 1990), a biarticular muscle that generates both hip flexion and knee extension moments. Stiff knee gait is commonly treated by rectus femoris transfer, a procedure in which the distal tendon of the muscle is detached from the patella and reattached to one of several sites posterior to the knee. However, the surgical outcomes are inconsistent and sometimes unsuccessful, in part because the biomechanical factors that contribute to stiff knee gait have not been adequately characterized. Analysis of the multi-joint motions produced by the rectus femoris is complex; the hip flexion moment it generates has the potential to increase knee flexion while the knee extension moment it generates acts to decrease knee flexion. We have developed forward dynamic simulations of the swing limb to identify factors that influence peak knee flexion during normal gait, and to determine how abnormal forces generated by the rectus femoris during swing affect knee flexion.

We calculated the accelerations of the swing limb from muscle excitation patterns. A model of the lower extremity with five segments (pelvis, thigh, patella, shank and foot), three degrees of freedom (flexion/extension of the hip, knee and ankle), and 12 muscle-tendon actuators was created (Piazza and Delp 1996). Each muscle-tendon actuator generated force as a function of its activation, length, and velocity (Zajac 1989). The excitation patterns of the muscles, the motions of the pelvis, and the angles and angular velocities of the joints at toe off were specified as inputs to the simulation. The resulting kinematics of the swing limb were calculated by numerically integrating the equations of motion of the model forward in time. A simulation of the swing phase of normal gait was developed using muscle excitation patterns that were derived from published intramuscular EMG recordings (Perry 1992). Other simulations were conducted using an exaggerated excitation input to the rectus femoris (i.e. excitation of the rectus femoris at 30% of its maximum level throughout the swing phase) to clarify the dynamical actions of the rectus femoris at the knee.

Our simulations confirmed that overactivity of the rectus femoris inhibits knee flexion during swing, and thus may cause stiff knee gait (Fig. 11.5). Additionally, our analyses revealed that several other factors, such as weakened hip flexors or stance phase factors that diminish the angular velocity of the knee at toe off, may also be responsible for decreased knee flexion during the swing phase (Piazza and Delp 1996).

To gain more insight into the biomechanical factors that contribute to stiff knee gait, we have begun to develop and analyze simulations that reproduce the swing limb trajectories of individual patients. In one case study, for example, we created a dynamic model of a

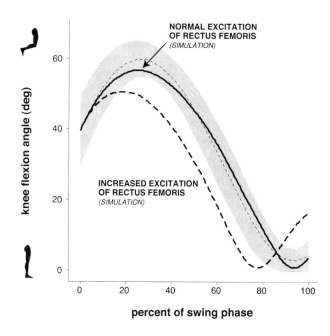

Fig. 11.5. Knee-flexion angle versus percentage of swing phase, generated from muscle-actuated, forward dynamic simulations of the swing limb. The knee angle for the nominal simulation, in which all of the muscle-tendon actuators were supplied with normal excitations (solid curve) compares favorably with experimental measurements of knee flexion during normal gait (mean ± 1 S.D. for 10 unimpaired subjects, shaded region). When the excitation input to the rectus femoris was exaggerated (dashed curve), knee flexion during the swing phase was limited. This result confirms that overactivity of the rectus femoris may cause stiff-knee gait.

subject with stiff knee gait who walked with excessive and prolonged activity of the rectus femoris (Goldberg et al. 2001). We used an inverse dynamics formulation, in combination with kinematic data from gait analysis, to calculate the subject's muscular joint moments during the swing phase. We then used these calculated moments to drive a forward dynamic simulation. When we prescribed the initial kinematic conditions for the simulation based on the subject's measured joint angles and angular velocities at toe off, the knee motions of the model reproduced the subject's stiff knee gait. However, when normal kinematic conditions at toe off were input into the simulation, without changing the muscular joint moments, the peak flexion of the knee during swing was greater than during normal gait (Fig. 11.6). These data suggest that abnormal muscular moments were not the primary cause of diminished knee flexion in this subject, and may explain why this subject's knee flexion did not improve following rectus femoris transfer surgery.

In summary, we believe that kinematic conditions at toe off should be considered along with rectus femoris activity before surgery is performed on the rectus femoris in an attempt to correct stiff knee gait. This study emphasizes the need for rigorous, dynamics based analyses of the actions of muscles when attempting to determine the causes of a patient's gait

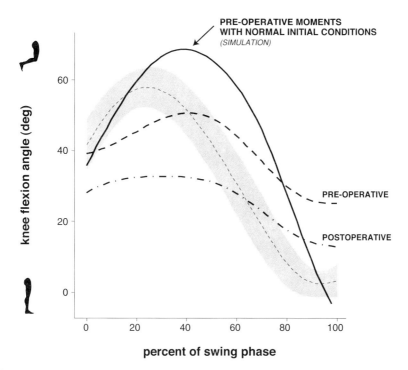

Fig. 11.6. Knee-flexion angle versus percentage of swing phase, generated from patient-specific, forward dynamic simulations of the swing limb. When the initial kinematic conditions for the simulation (i.e. knee angle, knee velocity, and hip velocity at toe-off) were prescribed based on the subject's measured joint angles and angular velocities, the knee motions of the model reproduced the subject's stiff-knee gait (dashed lines). When normal kinematic conditions at toe-off were input into the simulation, without changing the subject's muscular joint moments, the resulting knee motion resembled normal gait (solid line and shaded region). This result suggests that abnormal muscular moments were not the primary cause of the subject's diminished knee flexion.

abnormality.

Discussion and future directions

Musculoskeletal simulations can provide clinically useful insights into the pathomechanics of gait abnormalities and the functional consequences of treatments, as evidenced by the examples presented in this chapter. However, the limitations of current models must be reduced, and the accuracy with which models represent individuals with neuro-musculoskeletal impairments must be tested, before simulations can be widely used to guide treatment decisions for patients. Some of the important challenges to be resolved in future studies are outlined below.

First, methods to accurately and efficiently characterize the musculoskeletal geometry and the joint kinematics of children with cerebral palsy need to be developed. This is imperative because the results of simulations are often sensitive to the accuracy with which the lengths and moment arms of muscles can be estimated with a model. To date, studies of muscle function during movement have typically relied on generic models of adult subjects with normal musculoskeletal geometry. We have modified generic models to simulate bone deformities (Arnold et al. 1997, 2001, Arnold and Delp 2001), osteotomies (Free and Delp 1996, Schmidt et al. 1999), and tendon transfer surgeries (Delp et al. 1994). However, more work is needed to understand how variations in musculoskeletal geometry due to size, age, deformity, or surgery might influence the predictions of a model, and to determine when, and under what conditions, simulations based on generic models are applicable to individual patients. One approach might be to develop patient specific models from magnetic resonance images or ultrasonography scans that can estimate muscle lengths, moment arms, and joint kinematics *in vivo* (Sheehan et al. 1998, Wilson et al. 1999, Ito et al. 2000, Maganaris 2000). However, using image data alone to determine the lengths and moment arms of muscles at the wide range of body positions assumed during walking would require extensive imaging protocols to capture the muscle and joint geometry in many limb configurations. We suggest that a hybrid approach, which combines medical images with generic musculoskeletal models, offers a promising, tractable way to construct representative models of patients. For instance, it may be possible to transform a generic model to represent a range of individuals with cerebral palsy using multidimensional scaling techniques, algorithms for deforming bones, and a few patient specific parameters derived from image data or experimental measurements (Chao et al. 1993, Arnold and Delp 2001). We have begun to develop and evaluate such models (Arnold et al. 2001, Arnold and Delp 2001), and we believe that additional efforts are warranted.

Second, the model of muscle-tendon mechanics that we have used in simulations must be further tested. While this model captures many features of muscle force generation in unimpaired subjects, it does not account for adaptations that can occur in persons with neuromuscular disorders. For example, the model does not account for complexities associated with activation of spastic muscle, such as potential alterations in recruitment or rate modulation (Tang and Rymer 1981). Although we have attempted to account for decreases in the muscle fiber lengths that may occur with contracture, our simulations have not considered the effects of muscle-tendon remodeling, such as alterations in the peak force of a muscle (Williams and Goldspink 1978) or changes in the elasticity of tendon (Woo et al. 1982). Muscle-tendon models that characterize the effects of pathology, surgery, and other treatment modalities on the muscle force generating characteristics are needed to verify the accuracy of existing simulations and to enhance the value of new ones.

Perhaps the most profound limitation of the models described in this chapter is their exclusion of central nervous system control. Our analysis of equinus gait did not consider how tendon surgery or postoperative physical therapy might affect muscle force production through its influence on motor control. The dynamic simulations of stiff knee gait were performed open loop; that is, the synthesized motions had no ability to modulate the muscle excitation patterns through reflexes, as occurs *in vivo*. Certainly, the incorporation of accurate representations of sensorimotor control into dynamic simulations of abnormal movements is one of the most critical challenges that must be overcome if models are to be developed that can predict the outcomes of treatments.

Before any model can be used to make treatment decisions, the model must be tested. Sensitivity studies should be performed to determine whether the conclusions one draws from analysis of a model are sensitive to variations in the model parameters. If possible, simulation results should be compared with experimental data to verify that a particular model is of sufficient complexity to answer the clinical question being posed. Ultimately, controlled clinical studies are required to determine if the insights gained from a model can indeed improve treatment outcomes.

We believe that computer models of the neuro-musculoskeletal system play an important role in the assessment and treatment of gait abnormalities in persons with cerebral palsy. Musculoskeletal simulations are necessary for explaining the biomechanical causes of movement abnormalities and the consequences of common interventions; this information is essential for developing improved treatment plans.

Acknowledgements

We would like to thank Stephen Piazza, Kim Statler, Bill Hess, Deanna Asakawa, Silvia Blemker, Saryn Goldberg, Peter Loan, Ken Smith, Carolyn Moore, Stephen Vankoski, Claudia Kelp-Lenane, Julie Witka, and Rob Novak for help in the anatomical experiments, computer modeling, and data analysis. We are also grateful to Eugene Bleck, Norris Carroll, Luciano Dias, James Gage, Sylvia Õunpuu, Jacquelin Perry, George Rab and Felix Zajac for their helpful comments related to movement deformities and musculoskeletal modeling. This work was supported by NIH RO1HD33929 and RO1HD37639.

REFERENCES

Anderson FC, Pandy MG. (2001) Dynamic optimization of human walking. *J Biomech Eng* **123:** 381–390.

Arnold AS, Delp SL. (2001) Rotational moment arms of the medial hamstrings and adductors vary with femoral geometry and limb position: implications for the treatment of internally rotated gait. *J Biomech* **34:** 437–447.

Arnold AS, Komattu AV, Delp SL. (1997) Internal rotation gait: a compensatory mechanism to restore abduction capacity decreased by bone deformity. *Dev Med Child Neurol* **39:** 40–44.

Arnold AS, Asakawa DJ, Delp SL. (2000) Do the hamstrings and adductors contribute to excessive internal rotation of the hip in persons with cerebral palsy? *Gait Posture* **11:** 181–190.

Arnold AS, Blemker SS, Delp SL. (2001) Evaluation of a deformable musculoskeletal model for estimating muscle-tendon lengths during crouch gait. *Ann Biomed Eng* **29:** 263–274.

Bleck EE. (1987) *Orthopaedic Management in Cerebral Palsy.* London: Mac Keith Press.

Chao EY, Lynch JD, Vanderploeg MJ. (1993) Simulation and animation of musculoskeletal joint system. *J Biomech Eng* **115:** 562–568.

Chong KC, Vojnic CD, Quanbury AO, Letts RM. (1978) The assessment of the internal rotation gait in cerebral palsy: an electromyographic gait analysis. *Clin Orthop* **132:** 145–150.

Delp SL, Zajac FE. (1992) Force- and moment-generating capacity of lower-extremity muscles before and after tendon lengthening. *Clin Orthop* **284:** 247–259.

Delp SL, Ringwelski DA, Carroll NC. (1994) Transfer of the rectus femoris: effects of transfer site on moment arms about the knee and hip. *J Biomech* **27:** 1201–1211.

Delp SL, Statler K, Carroll NC. (1995) Preserving plantar flexion strength after surgical treatment for contracture of the triceps surae: a computer simulation study. *J Orthop Res* **13:** 96–104.

Delp SL, Arnold AS, Speers RA, Moore CA. (1996) Hamstrings and psoas lengths during normal and crouch gait: implications for muscle-tendon surgery. *J Orthop Res* **14:** 144–151.

Delp SL, Hess WE, Hungerford DS, Jones LC. (1999) Variation of rotation moment arms with hip flexion. *J Biomech* **32:** 493–501.

Dul J, Shiavi R, Green NE. (1985) Simulation of tendon transfer surgery. *Eng Med* **14:** 31–38.

Free SA, Delp SL. (1996) Trochanteric transfer in total hip replacement: effects on the moment arms and force-generating capacities of the hip abductors. *J Orthop Res* **14:** 245–250.

Friederich JA, Brand RA. (1990) Muscle fiber architecture in the human lower limb. *J Biomech* **23:** 91–95.

Gage JR. (1991) *Gait Analysis in Cerebral Palsy.* London: Mac Keith Press.

Gage JR, Perry J, Hicks RR, Koop S, Werntz JR. (1987) Rectus femoris transfer to improve knee function of children with cerebral palsy. *Dev Med Child Neurol* **29:** 159–166.

Gerritsen KG, van den Bogert AJ, Hulliger M, Zernicke RF. (1998) Intrinsic muscle properties facilitate locomotor control—a computer simulation study. *Motor Control* **2:** 206–220.

Goldberg S, Piazza SJ, Delp SL. (2001) The importance of swing phase initial conditions in stiff-knee gait: a case study. *Gait and Posture* **13:** 246–247. (Abstract.)

Hoffer MM. (1986) Management of the hip in cerebral palsy. *J Bone Joint Surg Am* **68:** 629–631.

Hoffinger SA, Rab GT, Abou-Ghaida H. (1993) Hamstrings in cerebral palsy crouch gait. *J Pediatr Orthop* **13:** 722–726.

Hollerbach JM, Flash T. (1982) Dynamic interactions between limb segments during planar arm movement. *Biol Cybern* **44:** 67–77.

Ito M, Akima H, Fukunaga T. (2000) In vivo moment arm determination using B-mode ultrasonography. *J Biomech* **33:** 215–218.

Lee CL, Bleck EE. (1980) Surgical correction of equinus deformity in cerebral palsy. *Dev Med Child Neurol* **22:** 287–292.

Lieber RL, Friden J. (1997) Intraoperative measurement and biomechanical modeling of the flexor carpi ulnaris-to-extensor carpi radialis longus tendon transfer. *J Biomech Eng* **119:** 386–391.

Lundy DW, Ganey TM, Ogden JA, Guidera KJ. (1998) Pathologic morphology of the dislocated proximal femur in children with cerebral palsy. *J Pediatr Orthop* **18:** 528–534.

Maganaris CN. (2000) In vivo measurement-based estimations of the moment arm in the human tibialis anterior muscle-tendon unit. *J Biomech* **33:** 375–379.

Neptune RR, Kautz SA, Zajac FE. (2001) Contributions of the individual ankle plantar flexors to support, forward progression and swing initiation during walking. *J Biomech* **34:** 1387–1398.

Perry J. (1987) Distal rectus femoris transfer. *Dev Med Child Neurol* **29:** 153–158.

Perry J. (1992) *Gait Analysis: Normal and Pathological Function.* Thorofare, NJ: Slack.

Piazza SJ, Delp SL. (1996) The influence of muscles on knee flexion during the swing phase of gait. *J Biomech* **29:** 723–733.

Root L. (1987) Treatment of hip problems in cerebral palsy. *Instr Course Lect* **36:** 237–252.

Rose SA, DeLuca PA, Davis RB 3rd, Õunpuu S, Gage JR. (1993) Kinematic and kinetic evaluation of the ankle after lengthening of the gastrocnemius fascia in children with cerebral palsy. *J Pediatr Orthop* **13:** 727–732.

Rose J, Haskell WL, Gamble JG, Hamilton RL, Brown DA, Rinsky L. (1994) Muscle pathology and clinical measures of disability in children with cerebral palsy. *J Orthop Res* **12:** 758–768.

Saraph V, Zwick EB, Uitz C, Linhart W, Steinwender G. (2000) The Baumann procedure for fixed contracture of the gastrosoleus in cerebral palsy. Evaluation of function of the ankle after multilevel surgery. *J Bone Joint Surg Br* **82:** 535–540.

Schmidt DJ, Arnold AS, Carroll NC, Delp SL. (1999) Length changes of the hamstrings and adductors resulting from derotational osteotomies of the femur. *J Orthop Res* **17:** 279–285.

Schutte LM, Hayden SW, Gage JR. (1997) Lengths of hamstrings and psoas muscles during crouch gait: effects of femoral anteversion. *J Orthop Res* **15:** 615–621.

Segal LS, Thomas SE, Mazur JM, Mauterer M. (1989) Calcaneal gait in spastic diplegia after heel cord lengthening: a study with gait analysis. *J Pediatr Orthop* **9:** 697–701.

Sharrard WJ, Bernstein S. (1972) Equinus deformity in cerebral palsy. A comparison between elongation of the tendo calcaneus and gastrocnemius recession. *J Bone Joint Surg Br* **54:** 272–276.

Sheehan FT, Zajac FE, Drace JE. (1998) Using cine phase contrast magnetic resonance imaging to non-invasively study in vivo knee dynamics. *J Biomech* **31:** 21–26.

Sutherland DH, Cooper L. (1978) The pathomechanics of progressive crouch gait in spastic diplegia. *Orthop Clin North Am* **9:** 143–154.

Sutherland DH, Schottstaedt ER, Larsen LJ, Ashley RK, Callander JN, James PM. (1969) Clinical and electromyographic study of seven spastic children with internal rotation gait. *J Bone Joint Surg Am* **51:** 1070–1082.

Sutherland DH, Santi M, Abel MF. (1990) Treatment of stiff-knee gait in cerebral palsy: a comparison by gait analysis of distal rectus femoris transfer versus proximal rectus release. *J Pediatr Orthop* **10:** 433–441.

Tachdjian MO. (1990) *Pediatric Orthopaedics.* Philadelphia: W.B. Saunders.

Taga G. (1995) A model of the neuro-musculo-skeletal system for human locomotion. I. Emergence of basic gait. *Biol Cybern* **73:** 97–111.

Tang A, Rymer WZ. (1981) Abnormal force–EMG relations in paretic limbs of hemiparetic human subjects. *J Neurol Neurosurg Psychiatry* **44:** 690–698.

Tardieu G, Tardieu C. (1987) Cerebral palsy. Mechanical evaluation and conservative correction of limb joint contractures. *Clin Orthop* **219:** 63–69.

Thompson NS, Baker RJ, Cosgrove AP, Corry IS, Graham HK. (1998) Musculoskeletal modelling in determining the effect of botulinum toxin on the hamstrings of patients with crouch gait. *Dev Med Child Neurol* **40:** 622–625.

Wickiewicz TL, Roy RR, Powell PL, Edgerton VR. (1983) Muscle architecture of the human lower limb. *Clin Orthop* **179:** 275–283.

Williams PE, Goldspink G. (1978) Changes in sarcomere length and physiological properties in immobilized muscle. *J Anat* **127:** 459–468.

Wilson DL, Zhu Q, Duerk JL, Mansour JM, Kilgore K, Crago PE. (1999) Estimation of tendon moment arms from three-dimensional magnetic resonance images. *Ann Biomed Eng* **27:** 247–256.

Woo SSY, Gomez MA, Woo JK, Akeson WH. (1982) Mechanical properties of tendons and ligaments II. The relationships of immobilization and exercise on tissue remodeling. *Biorheology* **19:** 397–408.

Yamaguchi GT, Zajac FE. (1990) Restoring unassisted natural gait to paraplegics via functional neuromuscular stimulation: a computer simulation study. *IEEE Trans Biomed Eng* **37:** 886–902.

Zajac FE. (1989) Muscle and tendon: properties, models, scaling, and application to biomechanics and motor control. *Crit Rev Biomed Eng* **17:** 359–411.

Zajac FE, Gordon ME. (1989) Determining muscle's force and action in multi-articular movement. *Exerc Sport Sci Rev* **17:** 187–230.

Ziv I, Blackburn N, Rang M, Koreska J. (1984) Muscle growth in normal and spastic mice. *Dev Med Child Neurol* **26:** 94–99.

12
PATHOLOGICAL GAIT AND LEVER-ARM DYSFUNCTION

James R. Gage and Michael Schwartz

In the first section of this book we studied the brain, how it controls locomotion and the types of brain injuries that can occur in cerebral palsy. In the second section we discussed assessment of the patient via clinical examination, gait analysis and musculoskeletal modeling. Before we move on to treatment of gait disorders, we must now spend some time examining the pathology of gait itself.

First, it should be remembered that during normal locomotion the muscles and/or ground reaction force supply the necessary power for movement; the skeleton makes available the rigid lever arms these forces need to produce movement, and the joints provide the action points at which the movements occur. Normal locomotion, then, depends upon an appropriate and adequate force acting via a rigid lever of appropriate length on a stable joint (Fig. 12.1, and Dynamic 12.1 on the CD-Rom). "Normal gait" has several attributes or prerequisites that include (1) stability in stance, (2) clearance in swing, (3) pre-position of the foot in terminal swing, (4) an adequate step length, and (5) conservation of energy. Because of the neuromuscular problems that occur in cerebral palsy, all of these attributes are lost in varying degrees.

When looking at pathological gait, it is important to remember that what we are seeing is a combination of cause and effect. For example, look at a typical brain injury, such as the one illustrated in Figure 2.4, which often results from periventricular leukomalacia secondary to preterm birth. This type of brain damage can interfere with gait in several specific ways: (1) through loss of selective control of muscles, particularly those in the distal part of the limb, (2) because of difficulties with balance, and (3) because of abnormal muscle tone (usually spasticity). We refer to these abnormalities of gait as the primary effects of the brain injury. "*Primary effects*" occur at the moment of brain injury and as a direct result of the injury. In general they are permanent, and to a large extent cannot be corrected.

However, it should also be remembered that the child is growing, and the everyday forces imposed upon the child's muscles and bones play a large part in governing normal growth. In simple terms, growing bones and muscles follow the *Star Wars* principle: "May the force be with you!" Because the primary effects of the brain injury impose abnormal forces on the skeleton, neither bone nor muscle grows normally. Yet these changes, which we refer to as the *secondary effects* of the brain injury, are not immediate. Since muscles and bones grow slowly over time, these skeletal deformities also emerge slowly over time, and in direct proportion to the rate of skeletal growth.

180

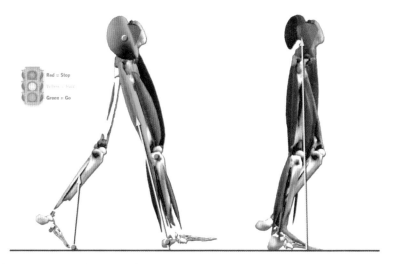

Fig. 12.1. See CD-Rom, Figure 12.1, for a dynamic illustration of muscle action and bone movements during normal gait. The muscles act on the skeletal levers to produce moments that make the joints move.

Finally, we find ourselves with a child who is trying to walk while burdened with dynamic and structural deformities, some of which are primary and some of which are secondary. It is not easy, and the child must learn to cope with his or her problems. For example, a child with hemiplegia and spasticity of the rectus femoris on the affected side may have great difficulty in getting the affected knee to bend and, as a result, would tend to drag his or her foot during the swing phase of gait. The child may cope with this problem in one of several ways: by vaulting on the sound side, by circumduction of the affected limb on the swing side, and/or by hyperflexion of the hip on the swing side. While one or all of these mechanisms may solve the problem, they are also abnormalities of gait and, in general, increase the energy cost of walking. We refer to these "coping mechanisms" as the *tertiary effects* of the brain injury.

Pathological gait, then, is a mixture of *primary*, *secondary* and *tertiary* abnormalities. It is important to discriminate between these different types of abnormalities, for as we said earlier the primary abnormalities of gait usually are permanent, the secondary abnormalities can frequently be corrected, and the tertiary abnormalities (coping responses) will disappear spontaneously once they are no longer required. This fact provides us with the foundation of our treatment program for gait problems in cerebral palsy, which was perhaps expressed best by Reinhold Niebuhr (Simpson 1988):

> *God, give us grace to accept with serenity the things that cannot be changed, courage to change the things which should be changed and the wisdom to distinguish the one from the other.*

Our task then is to sort out the primary, secondary and tertiary abnormalities of gait, to determine which ones can and should be corrected, and to exercise the wisdom to leave the rest of the pathology alone. The remainder of this book will be dedicated to the successful execution of that task. For the present, however, we must look at the primary, secondary and tertiary gait abnormalities in more detail.

Gait abnormalities
THE PRIMARY ABNORMALITIES OF GAIT

Before reading this section, it would be well for the reader to go back and review the first three chapters dealing with control of locomotion, cerebral injury patterns in cerebral palsy, and the genesis of spasticity. Injuries to specific brain centers will generate fairly specific types of functional loss. For example, injury to the cerebellum will produce a specific abnormality of gait that we refer to as ataxia. Consequently, although injury to different brain control centers may generate different types of functional loss, they all contribute in different ways to the three primary abnormalities of gait: (1) loss of selective motor control, (2) impaired balance, and (3) abnormal tone. As discussed in Chapter 2, in children with spastic diplegia secondary to preterm birth the most common type of neurological injury is called *periventricular leukomalacia*. This neurological injury is typically (but not necessarily symmetrical) bilateral and occurs most frequently in the white matter adjacent to the frontal horns of the lateral ventricles, as well as toward the posterior aspects of the ventricles in the peritrigonal white matter. Since the axons conducting input to the lower extremities course through the frontal regions, injury in this location produces the typical clinical picture of spastic diplegia, in which the most prominent feature is motor impairment in the legs (see Fig. 2.4).

It should be remembered that the degree of loss of selective motor control is directly related to the degree of central nervous system injury. In a child with the classic injury of periventricular leukomalacia secondary to preterm birth, the abnormal tone present is spasticity, with loss of selective motor control mainly in the distal portion of the limb, lesser involvement of the knee and relative sparing of the hip. By definition, in children with mixed tone there is injury to the basal ganglia. As was pointed out in Chapter 1, the basal ganglia contain "motor memories" of previous similar movement patterns. Consequently, *injury to the basal ganglia usually results in severe loss of selective motor control*. Because of this, to our mind, the term "mixed diplegia" is a non sequitur. We believe that children with mixed tone, unlike children with purely spastic tone, have a more severe loss of selective motor control which affects all four extremities to some degree, and for this reason should be considered to have quadriplegic involvement.

Selective motor control
Since the pyramidal tract is distributed mainly to the distal end of the extremity, loss of selective motor control is more severe in the distal portion of the limb than the proximal. For example, just as the child with spastic hemiplegia often has good control of the shoulder, limited control of the elbow, and poor control of the wrist and hand, the child with spastic diplegia will usually demonstrate fairly good selective motor control at the hip, limited control of the knee, and poor control of the ankle and foot. In addition, from a control standpoint, biarticular muscles (which span two joints) are more severely involved than those that are monoarticular. The specific reason why this is true is not clear, but one can speculate as to

why this might be true. First, biarticular muscles tend to be made up of non-pennated, fast-twitch fibers. Therefore the muscle spindles would be oriented along the longitudinal axis of the muscle, and for that reason, might be more directly affected by stretch and secondarily affected by spasticity, since spasticity itself is velocity dependent. Secondly, the pyramidal tracts are distributed primarily to the distal ends of the limbs and these tracts are directly affected by the lesion of *periventricular leukomalacia* (see Chapter 2 for a review as to why this is true). Thirdly, biarticular muscles are made up largely of fast-twitch fibers and have a more complex task to perform. Thus the speed and precision of action of a biarticular muscle is greater than that of a monoarticular muscle. Consequently, an axiom to remember in treating cerebral palsy is that *the distal, biarticular muscles are involved primarily and more severely than those that are monoarticular and/or proximal*. The classification system that we developed for hemiplegia is based on this premise (Winters et al. 1987). This maxim also has a lot of implications in the treatment of cerebral palsy. Look, for example, at the triceps surae. It is made up of a monoarticular muscle (the soleus) and a biarticular muscle (the gastrocnemius). The axiom above predicts that the biarticular gastrocnemius should be more severely involved than the monoarticular soleus, and in fact this has been shown to be true (Rose et al. 1993, Delp et al. 1995). Yet tendo-Achilles lengthening (TAL/ETA), the procedure most commonly done to correct contracture of this muscle, lengthens both equally—often to the great detriment of the patient. A similar situation exists with the iliopsoas at the hip. The psoas is biarticular, and the iliacus monoarticular. In the past a recession of the iliopsoas tendon from the lesser trochanter to the capsule was often done to correct contracture of this muscle (Bleck 1971). However, this is analogous to tendo-Achilles lengthening at the ankle because the iliacus, which usually is not contracted, is lengthened along with the contracted psoas. For that reason, we feel that intramuscular lengthening of the psoas alone is a better procedure (Novacheck et al. 2002).

Balance
Dysequilibrium is another of the primary problems of cerebral palsy. Hagberg and colleagues (1972) have likened the falling of a child with abnormal equilibrium reactions to a "felled pine-tree". All children with quadriplegia have significant balance problems and most require aides such as walkers or crutches for ambulation. The walking aide stabilizes the balance problem, but significantly increases the energy cost of walking (see Chapter 10). However, even children who have spastic diplegia with fairly minimal involvement have deficient equilibrium reactions to some degree. These usually become apparent when balance is stressed, for example, when avoiding an object and/or rapidly changing direction.

Although sophisticated force platforms for testing balance now exist, Bleck (1987) pointed out that equilibrium reactions can easily be tested clinically by gently pushing the child from side to side and anteriorly and posteriorly. Able-bodied children will easily maintain their balance and if necessary make a stepping response to regain their equilibrium, whereas the child with deficient equilibrium reactions will topple over (Fig. 12.2). Hopping or standing on one foot is also a strong indication of good balance. A child with relatively normal balance should be able to stand unsupported on one foot for at least 10 seconds. Dr Bleck states that children with spastic diplegia, who can walk without aides, often fail this

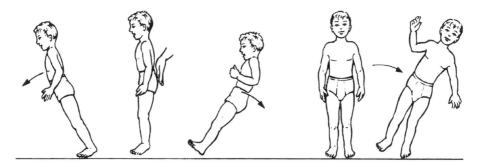

Fig. 12.2. Standing equilibrium reactions. Lack of normal equilibrium is easily demonstrated by pushing forward, backward, and/or from side to side. The child will fall down as opposed to demonstrating a normal stepping response. (Reproduced from Bleck 1987, fig. 2.15, p 32, by permission.)

test on one or both sides. Because of these deficiencies in lateral equilibrium reactions, to maintain balance these children are forced to shift their trunk over the stance side. Since this same coping response is also necessary in the face of weak hip-abductors, balance problems may well be misinterpreted as hip-abductor weakness. Bleck feels that if a child has adequate side to side but poor fore and aft equilibrium reactions, crutches will be required for support. If lateral equilibrium reactions are also deficient, a walker will be required. However, he contends that even children with spastic diplegia who walk without aids generally have poor posterior equilibrium reactions and so may fall backwards with very little provocation (Bleck 1987).

There is an argument in the literature over whether or not deficient equilibrium reactions can be improved by training and/or therapy (Liao et al. 1997). Following surgery in which the limbs have been realigned and stance-phase stability restored, it is certainly common to see a child discard crutches or aides as s/he becomes accustomed to the new positions of her/his limbs in space. However, this does not necessarily mean that the child's underlying balance mechanisms have improved. Providing the child with a better base of support is one thing that has been shown to be helpful in improving balance. In this regard orthotics are very helpful (Butler et al. 1992, Burtner et al. 1999). Bleck (1987) states: "Of all the motor problems in cerebral palsy, deficient equilibrium reactions interfere the most with functional walking." Although we certainly agree with his statement, we must confess to our shame that we have not instituted a formal balance-testing program at our hospital. It needs to be done.

Abnormal tone
Abnormal tone is a universal finding in cerebral palsy. Minear (1956) proposed the present classification of cerebral palsy. He classified abnormal tone as spastic, athetoid or mixed. Although this is a workable classification, it is not ideal. In fact, now that we have a better understanding of the function of the central nervous system, we would suggest that a better classification is needed. In the first place, athetosis describes only one type of abnormal

tone emanating from injury to the basal ganglia. Dystonia, chorea, and/or rigidity are also abnormal muscle tones that may arise as a result of basal ganglia injury. Furthermore, primary injury to the cerebellum, in addition to producing ataxia, can also produce hypotonia. To better understand the mechanism by which these abnormal tones arise, the reader should read or review the first three chapters in this book, by Warwick Peacock and Adré du Plessis. It is fairly clear now that spastic muscle tone arises as a result of injury to the cortical connections to the vestibular and/or reticular brainstem nuclei, the nuclei themselves, and/or the tracts emanating from them. Injury to the motor cortex was once thought to produce spasticity. However, it has now been shown that damage to the motor cortex and/or corticospinal tract alone only produces loss of fine motor control in distal-limb muscles without spasticity (Hepp-Reymond et al. 1974, Kuypers 1981).

Of the abnormal muscle tones present in cerebral palsy, spasticity is the most common. As stated in Chapter 3, spasticity arises as a result of loss of central nervous system inhibition. Its hallmark feature is that it is velocity dependent. That is, the higher the angular velocity of joint movement, the more resistance to movement that is encountered. There are several ways in which spasticity interferes with function in cerebral palsy: (1) it acts like a brake on the system and this drag on movement increases energy consumption; (2) it inhibits voluntary control of movement; (3) it interferes with the stretch on muscles that normally occurs during activity and so inhibits growth; and (4) it contributes to bony deformity of the growing skeleton by inducing excessive torques on long bones during gait.

Although it is sometimes argued that spasticity can be thought of as a compensation for weakness, the increased muscle tone induces abnormal movement patterns and frequently leads to deformities such as muscle contractures and joint dislocations. At the present time, spasticity is the only type of abnormal tone—indeed, it is the only primary abnormality—which we can address surgically (see Chapter 18). However, Albright (1996) and his colleagues (1996, 2001) have claimed some success in the treatment of dystonia with the intrathecal baclofen pump. The ability to reduce spastic tone has represented a major advance in the treatment of cerebral palsy. In fact Dr Albright believes it is the most significant treatment advance that he has seen in his 30 years of practice.

Abnormalities of tone arising from injury to the basal ganglia (athetosis, dystonia, chorea and/or rigidity) are always associated with severe loss of selective motor control. As such it is difficult to determine whether abnormal muscle tone emanating from basal ganglia injury is a problem in itself or whether the abnormal tone merely represents a symptom of the problem, i.e. the underlying injury to the control system in the basal ganglia.

THE SECONDARY ABNORMALITIES OF GAIT

As stated earlier, the secondary abnormalities arise as a result of the abnormal forces imposed on the skeleton by the effects of the primary brain injury. By definition, therefore, the secondary abnormalities are anomalies of muscle and/or bone growth. As was pointed out earlier, these skeletal deformities emerge slowly over time, and in direct proportion to the rate of skeletal growth. There are two types of secondary abnormalities: (1) muscle contractures, and (2) abnormal bone growth, which can take a variety of forms. We refer to these latter types of growth anomalies as *lever-arm dysfunction*. Unlike the primary abnormalities of cerebral palsy, which are usually permanent, the secondary abnormalities are frequently amenable to correction. To understand why and how they arise, however, we first need to understand the normal growth process.

Muscle growth

In an able-bodied child, muscles and bone grow proportionally. Therefore a mechanism for muscle growth must exist to keep muscles growing in proportion to bone (Ziv et al. 1984) showed that muscle growth takes place at the musculotendinous junction, which they term the *muscle growth-plate* and that the stimulus to longitudinal growth of muscle is stretch. Since muscles grow in proportion to the bone to which they are attached, it means that a muscle must double its length during the first four years of life and double it again between the age of four and adulthood. In spastic mice, they found that the rate of growth was reduced by 45%, which resulted in contractures (Ziv et al. 1984).

If we accept that the stretch necessary for daily muscle growth is incurred during the play activities of an able-bodied child, it becomes apparent that muscle growth in a child with cerebral palsy will be abnormal for the following reasons. (1) The primary problems of cerebral palsy (loss of selective motor control, impaired balance, and abnormal tone) prevent normal play activities. (2) A spastic muscle will not allow stretch to the same degree as one with normal tone. As a result a muscle that initially has dynamic contracture secondary to the spasticity itself will eventually develop true contracture as muscle growth fails to keep pace with growth of the bone. (3) The distal biarticular muscles are more severely involved. The reasons for this are not precisely known.

Bone growth

Growth of the long bones occurs by means of epiphyseal plates or, in the case of cartilaginous bone, appositionally via the periosteum. However, it is the forces that act upon bone during growth that determine its ultimate shape. There are two laws of bone growth from the old German literature. The first is the Heutter-von Volkmann principle, which states that excessive pressure inhibits epiphyseal growth. The second is Wolff's law, which states that bone remodels in response to the stresses that act upon it (Zaleske et al. 1990). To these one could add the four postulates listed by Arkin and Katz (1956). (1) When a growing epiphysis is subjected to a stress, the rate or direction of the growth of that epiphysis or both are modified so as to yield to that stress. (2) Pressures applied in directions parallel to the direction of epiphyseal growth inhibit the rate of such growth. While considerable pressures are necessary to stop cartilaginous growth completely, slight or even intermittent pressures can slow or hinder it. (3) Pressures applied in directions perpendicular to the direction of epiphyseal growth deflect the direction of such growth, resulting in lateral or spiral (torsional) displacement of the newly laid-down bone. (4) The ease with which angular or torsional deformities may be produced in a growing bone varies inversely with its diameter. The narrower the bone, the greater is its "plasticity".

In simple terms, what they are saying is that if you put a twist on a growing bone, it takes the twist, which is why I stated earlier that growing bone follows the Star Wars principle, "May the force be with you!" For those with more literary tastes, the words of

Alexander Pope also apply: "Just as the twig is bent, the tree's inclined."[1]

The implications of this are that following the onset of cerebral palsy, future bone growth may be abnormal. However, it was some time before we realized that the errors of bone modeling imposed by the primary abnormalities of cerebral palsy work in two directions. That is, bones not only fail to mold or model normally as they grow; they also fail to remodel normally. The best example of this is femoral anteversion. Sommerville (1957) pointed out that in the 30th week of gestation anteversion of the femoral neck is about 60°. He then described how pressure of the femoral head and neck against the anterior iliofemoral (Bigalow's) ligament acts to reduce normal anteversion to about 10°–15° by adulthood, with most of the anteversion molding away in the first few years of life. The mechanism by which this occurs depends upon the fact that at about 10–12 months of age when a child starts pulling to stand and/or starts walking the upper ends of the femurs are still largely cartilaginous. With standing the hip is extended and Bigalow's ligament presses firmly against the cartilaginous, soft, moldable, rapidly growing femoral head and neck. Given the postulates of Arkin and Katz just discussed, one would expect that this mechanism would produce rapid remodeling of femoral neck anteversion, which in fact is what occurs. In a child with cerebral palsy, therefore, there are several reasons to explain the process by which femoral anteversion remodels fails. (1) The age of standing and/or walking is delayed and so by that time the child starts to walk, much of the proximal femur has ossified and so is much less malleable. (2) The rate of remodeling is directly proportional to the rate of growth, which is greatest in the first year of life and decreases steadily thereafter. Consequently, by the time a child starts to stand or walk, the rates of both growth and remodeling have slowed. (3) Remodeling of the proximal femur is dependent on the pressure of Bigalow's ligament against the femoral head and neck, which is greatest when the hip is in full extension. However, the child with cerebral palsy typically stands and walks with hips and knees in some flexion.

For the reasons listed above, children with cerebral palsy retain what Sommerville (1957) terms *persistent fetal alignment.*

Because of the abnormal forces imposed on the skeleton during walking, however, forward or future modeling of the long bones of the lower extremity is also abnormal. For example, it has been pointed out that internal rotation gait restores the strength of the hip abductors (Arnold et al. 1997, Arnold 1999), and Delp and colleagues (1999) have shown that in flexion the gluteus minimus is a strong internal rotator of the hip. Accordingly, in a child who walks with her/his hips in flexion, and/or internal rotation, the gluteus minimus exerts a strong internal rotation torque on the proximal femur, which with time and growth, would tend to increase anteversion.

Lever-arm dysfunction
In Chapter 4 we introduced the concept of levers, forces and moments. It was pointed out that joints are moved by moments. Forces acting on skeletal levers produce these moments.

---

[1] Alexander Pope (1688–1744), British satirical poet; Epistle to Cobham, l: 149–150.

Therefore, since the bones constitute the levers upon which muscles act, we have coined the term *lever-arm dysfunction* to describe the distortions of bone that regularly occur in a child with cerebral palsy. Lever-arm dysfunction refers to the alteration in the leverage relationships necessary for normal gait. In particular, lever-arm dysfunction describes a set of conditions in which internal and/or external lever arms become distorted because of bony or positional deformities. Lever-arm deformities are commonly associated with neuromuscular conditions, but can also occur in patients with non-neurological conditions, such as a mid-foot amputation.

In this chapter, we will concentrate on those deformities that are common in the lower extremities of children and adults with cerebral palsy. These include torsional deformities of long bones (femurs and/or tibias), hip subluxation or dislocation, foot deformities and positional anomalies (e.g. crouch gait).

Clinicians and engineers in the field of gait analysis have been slow to recognize the role and importance of lever-arm dysfunction. There is a tendency to think of muscles as force generators. However, modern research into the functional micro- and macro-anatomy of muscle tissue makes it clear that muscles are actually highly optimized generators of rotation (Zajac and Gordon 1989, Lieber 1997).

It is also common to think of the power-generating capacity of muscles as being directly related to muscle force. But again, since power is the product of force and motion, the force that a muscle produces cannot generate or absorb power without a concomitant joint motion. To fully understand the pathogenesis and treatment of the gait disorders common in cerebral palsy, it is necessary to think of muscles as generators of rotation. This thought process will naturally lead to the analysis of muscle moments, which in turn points directly at the issue of lever-arm dysfunction.

Although little can be done to increase the power generated by a muscle, correcting the lever-arm dysfunction that is present can increase the magnitude of the moment acting on a joint. Furthermore, lever-arm dysfunction, once recognized, can usually be corrected. For example, the flexible lever-arm dysfunction created by a severe pes valgus might be remediable with an appropriate foot orthosis and/or with appropriate surgery to stabilize the foot. Torsional deformities of long bones are easily corrected with derotational osteotomies. Once lever-arm dysfunction is recognized, therefore, correction of the problem is generally straightforward. However, to understand this concept, one first needs to understand the mechanics of levers.

LEVERS

The basic elements common to all levers are the fulcrum, load, effort, and the lever itself (Fig. 12.3). The fulcrum is the fixed point about which motion, in the form of rotation, occurs. The load and the effort are the forces acting on the lever. The lever itself is a rigid body on which the load and the effort act. In gait, bones form the levers; body segment weight, ground reaction forces, and inertial forces of motion create the load; active and passive muscle forces supply the effort; and the joints act as fulcrums.

There are three classes of levers aptly named first-, second- and third-class levers. The purpose of a lever is to produce either a mechanical advantage over the load or a rapid motion of the load. The mechanical advantage of a lever is the ratio of the load to the effort:

Mechanical advantage = Load/Effort

This ratio, in turn, can be expressed in terms of the relative lever arms (d) of the load and effort:

Mechanical advantage = ^{d}effort/^{d}load

There is an inherent compromise between goals of mechanical advantage and rapid motion. That is, to achieve a mechanical advantage inherently involves losing the capacity for rapid motion. In contrast, rapid motion of loads requires effort in excess of the load.

In first-class levers, the effort and the load are on opposite sides of the fulcrum (Fig. 12.3a). This type of lever is commonly exemplified by a teeter-totter (see-saw). In a balanced teeter-totter, the weight of one individual (load) multiplied by his/her distance from the fulcrum (lever arm) is equal to the weight of another individual (effort) times his/her distance from the fulcrum (lever arm). First-class levers can have a mechanical advantage either greater than or less than one. An example of a biomechanical first-class lever is the pelvis during single leg support. The body weight is the load; the hip-abductor force, primarily supplied by the gluteus medius, is the effort; and the hip joint acts as a fulcrum (Fig. 12.3 a). First-class levers are simple to conceptualize but are only one of three types of levers that occur in the body.

In second-class levers, the fulcrum is at one end, the load is in the middle, and the effort is at the other end of the lever (Fig. 12.3b). Second-class levers can be used to slowly move large loads (mechanical advantage >1.0). An everyday example of a second-class lever system is a *wheelbarrow*. A biomechanical example of a second-class lever is the foot at toe-off. In this case, the load is the body weight acting at the ankle, the triceps surae force is the effort, and the foot acts as the lever.

In a third-class lever, the fulcrum is at one end, the effort is adjacent to the fulcrum, and the load is at the other end of the lever (Fig. 12.3c). A *catapult* is an example of a third-class lever. In the body, an excellent example of a third-class lever can be found in the forearm. There, the action of the biceps brachii on the radius supports a weight carried in the hand with a fulcrum at the elbow. These types of levers can produce very rapid motions (such as a pitched baseball) at the cost of large effort demands. In general, the bones, joints, ligaments and muscles comprising the skeletal system represent combinations of all three types of levers.

Moments and motions

The study of motion alone is called kinematics (see Chapter 7). The study of the forces related to these motions is called kinetics (see Chapter 8). Together, the two areas comprise what is known as dynamics. Any motion can be broken down into a translational and a rotational component. Newton's second law of motion states that the force (F) acting on a particle is equal to the mass (m) of the particle times its acceleration (a),

$$F = ma.$$

Newton's second law of motion for a particle can be generalized to a system of particles,

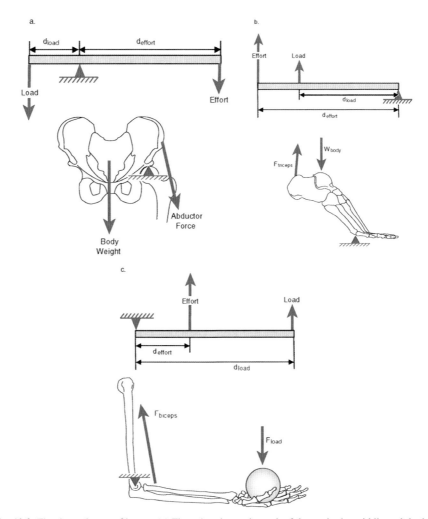

Fig. 12.3. The three classes of levers. (a) First-class levers have the fulcrum in the middle and the load an effort at opposite ends. The common example of a first-class lever is a teeter-totter (see-saw). A biomechanical example is the pelvis during single limb support. The load is the body weight, the effort is the hip abductor force, and the fulcrum is the hip joint. First-class levers can have a mechanical advantage either greater or less than one depending on the relative lengths of the two lever arms. (b) Second-class levers have the fulcrum at one end, the load in the middle, and the effort at the other end. A common example of a second-class lever is the wheelbarrow. The foot during push-off is a good biomechanical example. Here the fulcrum is the metatarsal heads, the load is the body weight acting through the ankle joint, and the effort is the force of the ankle plantarflexors. The advantage of a second-class lever system is that large loads can be supported with small efforts. (c) Third-class levers have the fulcrum at one end, the effort in the middle, and the load at the opposite end. Although now usually seen only in pictures, the medieval catapult is an excellent example. In the body, the best example would be the forearm when throwing a ball. In this case the ball is the load, the effort is the force of the elbow flexors, and the fulcrum is the elbow-joint. The advantage of third-class lever systems is speed. However, this speed comes at the expense of the need for a relatively large effort. (Reproduced from Gage and Schwartz 2002, fig. 22.1, p 762, by permission.)

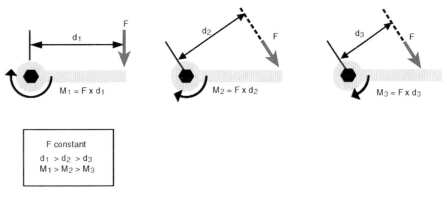

Fig. 12.4. Moments and lever arms. The magnitude of a moment is the product of force times the length of the lever arm. A lever arm is defined as the perpendicular distance between the force and the center of rotation. A change in either the position or the orientation of the applied force will cause a change in the magnitude of the moment. To create the largest moment, the force must be perpendicular to the lever. (Reproduced from Gage and Schwartz 2002, fig. 22.2, p 764, by permission.)

such as a rigid body like a bone. In this case, the net force on the body is equal to the body's mass times the acceleration of its center of mass. This governs the translation of the body.

To determine the rotational motion of a body, an additional set of rules needs to be satisfied. These rules can be summarized as stating that the net moment acting about a body's mass center is proportional to the rotational/angular acceleration of the body,

$$M = I\alpha.$$

The constant of proportionality (I) is called the moment of inertia, and is a measure of the distribution of mass within the body. The angular, or rotational, acceleration is denoted by (α). M is the net moment acting on the body. A moment is the rotary impetus occurring at a pivot point (fulcrum) generated by forces acting at a distance. The magnitude of a moment is the product of force (measured in Newtons) times the length of a lever arm (measured in meters). Consequently, the units of a moment are Newton meters.

The direction of a moment depends on the relative orientation of the force and the center of rotation about which the force acts. A simple analogy can be found in the tightening of a bolt with a wrench. One applies a force to the end of the wrench and rotation of the bolt occurs. The direction of rotation depends on the direction in which the force is applied. The magnitude of the moment depends on the magnitude of the force applied to the wrench, the length of the wrench handle, and the angle of application of the force (Fig. 12.4).

We can better understand the above equation by the example of a balanced teeter-totter (Fig. 12.5). It was stated that the product of weight (force) times the distance to the fulcrum (lever arm) of each occupant is equal. In mechanical terms, this statement can be summarized as "the net moment acting on the teeter-totter is zero". That the net moment acting about the fulcrum of the teeter-totter is zero means that the left-hand side of the above equation (M) is zero. This, in turn, means that there is no angular acceleration (a), and, hence, the teeter-totter does not rotate.

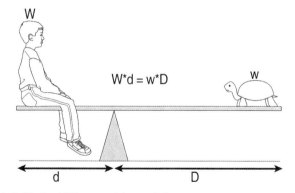

$$W*d = w*D$$

Fig. 12.5. Two individuals of different weights can balance a teeter-totter (see-saw) so long as the product of the weight of one individual times his/her distance from the pivot point is equal to the other individual times his/her distance from the pivot. The teeter-totter can be set in motion when one of the individuals pushes against the ground. When this occurs, the effective weight of that individual on the teeter-totter is decreased. Since the moment on the other side is unchanged, static equilibrium is no longer present and so the system becomes dynamic, i.e. the teeter-totter starts to move. Changing the length of the lever, for example if the turtle walks towards the fulcrum, will also set the teeter-totter in motion. (Reproduced from Gage and Schwartz 2002, fig. 22.3, p 764, by permission.)

Rotation of the teeter-totter can occur when one occupant pushes against the ground or changes his/her position on the teeter-totter. In the former case, the effective weight (load) of the restless occupant is decreased and therefore the moment about the fulcrum is decreased. Because the weight of the other occupant (effort) is unchanged, the moments no longer balance. At this point, the system transforms from static to dynamic. There is angular acceleration, which, when integrated over time, produces angular velocity and, hence, motion of the teeter-totter (see-saw). The magnitude of the angular acceleration is equal to the net unbalanced moment divided by the moment of inertia of the teeter-totter and its occupants. In the alternate case, in which one occupant moves, the load is unchanged, but the lever arm of the load is altered. Again, if the effort and its lever arm remain fixed, the moment about the fulcrum is unbalanced and the system again becomes dynamic. From this simple example, we can begin to gain an appreciation for both forces and lever arms in everything from teeter-totters to people.

The way in which the body produces motion is similar to the example just described. In a stationary posture, all accelerations (translational and rotational) are zero. The ground reaction force passes directly through the body's center of mass, and the net moments about each joint are zero. This means that the external moments due to the ground reaction force and body segment weight are exactly balanced by the internal moments produced by muscles, tendons and ligaments. Initiation of motion can be achieved by changing the level of muscle activation to produce an unbalanced moment. The unbalanced moment results in angular accelerations of various body segments, and the body begins to move.

Using modern motion capture systems, one can measure the rotational and translational motions of the body. The external ground reaction forces can be measured with force plates, and the segment mass distributions can be estimated with fair accuracy. The internal

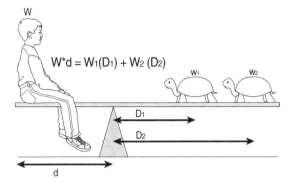

$$W*d = W_1(D_1) + W_2(D_2)$$

Fig. 12.6. A teeter-totter (see-saw) can be used to illustrate the problem of redundancy. If the child on the left side of the teeter-totter remained in place, but the turtle on the other side were replaced with two turtles, there would be an infinite variety of positions on the teeter-totter where the turtles could be placed to balance the child.

moments cannot be measured directly, but can be calculated by simultaneously solving the equations of motion for each body segment (inverse dynamics).

Redundancy

The action of individual muscles is of primary interest in lever-arm dysfunction. Much of the discussion to this point has referred to muscle forces and the levers on which they act. However, an estimation of the internal joint moments is not sufficient to determine the forces in individual muscles (Fig. 12.6). Numerous muscles and ligaments span each joint in our bodies. The number of unknown forces produced by these structures exceeds the number of mathematical equations produced by the governing laws of motion. This situation is known as redundancy. Redundancy in man-made structures is often used to add strength and stability. While this is advantageous from a functional point of view, it poses an analytical difficulty that complicates the analysis of lever-arm dysfunction. Namely, there are an infinite number of combinations of muscle forces that could produce the same net joint moment.

To calculate individual muscle forces, some way is needed to deduce the proportion of force that each muscle is contributing is needed. There is a significant body of current research aimed at this specific task (Pedotti et al. 1978, Davy and Audu 1987, Tsirakos et al. 1997, Anderson and Pandy 1999a, b). This work generally involves modeling muscle geometry and physiology and exploiting mathematical optimization schemes to estimate the individual muscle forces that occur during motions. To accomplish this, it is necessary to know the origin, insertion, and wrapping points of each muscle as well as its cross-sectional area, fiber type, pennation angle, and other anatomic and physiological parameters. In terms of skeletal information, accurate estimates of joint centers and the torsion of the various bones are also needed. Currently, the technology to achieve this is not perfected. However, promising results from this branch of research continue to be achieved (see Chapter 11).

Since the focus of this chapter is on clinical understanding of lever-arm dysfunction, and not mathematical modeling, a simplified version of the situation in the body will be adopted. The simple lever ideas described earlier will be used, and the actions of individual muscles or muscle groups will be considered independent of the exact value of the forces they can/do produce. When a net joint moment is present, we will discuss the muscle(s) likely to be causing that moment without concerning ourselves overly with some of the subtle issues of redundancy. Although this clearly is a simplification, it will allow us to look the clinical pathology of lever-arm dysfunction.

Normal function

In normal gait, internal moments produced by the action of muscle and ligamentous forces act in concert with external moments due to ground reaction and inertial forces. If the moments are equal, no accelerations are present and a steady state of motion continues. This steady state could be static posture or it could be dynamic equilibrium. If either the internal or external moments become dominant, the state of the system transforms. A simple conceptual example of this is the initiation of gait from a standstill. In reality, these transformations of dynamic state occur continuously throughout any motion and require an elegant and impenetrably complex motor control system. Normal motion depends on this control system. In addition to the gross and fine motor control (the software), skeletal motion also requires a mechanical structure (the hardware). This hardware consists of appropriate and adequate forces acting, via rigid levers of proper length and orientation, on a stable joint (see CD-Rom, Fig. 21.1, for a dynamic illustration). The breakdown of part or all of this mechanical system is the crux of lever-arm dysfunction.

MECHANICS OF THE ANKLE: FIRST ROCKER

To gain a better idea of how muscles and lever arms function during normal gait, consider the normal function of the ankle and foot. The action of the ankle in stance was described in terms of three rockers in Chapter 4 (see Fig. 4.15). Recall that during normal gait, first rocker uses the heel as a fulcrum and the foot as a lever. The load is the body's weight acting at the ankle, and the effort is the force of the pretibial muscles. Posterior protrusion of the heel creates a lever arm for the body's weight equal to 25% of the foot's total length. The immediate effect of the load (body weight) is to cause a moment about the heel (fulcrum) that rotates the toes toward the floor. Figure 12.3b shows that this is an example of a second-class lever.

MECHANICS OF THE ANKLE: SECOND ROCKER

Second rocker begins when the entire plantar surface of the foot is in contact with the floor. The fulcrum has moved from the heel to the ankle joint. The ground reaction force is the load acting through the lever arm of the forefoot and the soleus acting through the lever arm of the heel provides the effort. This is an example of a first-class lever (Fig. 12.3a).

MECHANICS OF THE ANKLE: THIRD ROCKER

During third rocker, the gastrocnemius and other plantarflexors have joined the soleus to arrest the forward progression of the tibia at the ankle. This forces the fulcrum of the foot lever forward to the metatarsal heads, and the heel rises off the ground. Consequently, the foot then acts again as a second-class lever (this time in the opposite direction) with the effort (triceps surae force) at the proximal end, the load (body weight) in the middle, and the fulcrum (metatarsal heads) at the distal end (Fig. 12.3b).

Pathological function

In a neuromuscular condition such as cerebral palsy, the muscle forces and ground reaction forces are neither appropriate nor adequate. This shortcoming arises as a result of muscle contractures, poor body segment balance and/or positioning, poor selective motor control, and abnormal bone lever arms. With respect to the lever arms themselves, five distinct types of deformity exist: (1) short lever arm, (2) flexible lever arm, (3) malrotated lever arm, (4) abnormal pivot or action point, and (5) positional lever-arm dysfunction. In addition to neuromuscular conditions, other causes, such as trauma, can also produce each of these deformities. Potential treatment of each type of lever-arm dysfunction is discussed briefly at the end of each section.

SHORT LEVER ARM

Examples of a short lever arm can include pathological abnormalities such as mid-foot amputation, fracture of a long bone that healed with significant shortening, coxa breva, and coxa valga. How does coxa valga create lever-arm dysfunction? The answer lies in the fact that a moment-arm is defined as the *perpendicular* distance from the center of rotation (hip-joint center) to the line of action of the muscle (Fig. 12.7b). Thus, even though the femoral neck is of appropriate length, the effective abduction lever is reduced due to the change in the line of action. Because the abduction moment is the abductor force multiplied by the lever arm, the effect of a shortened lever arm is to reduce the magnitude of the internal abduction moment (effort) in exact proportion to the shortening of the lever arm itself. If no postural compensation occurs, an increased hip-abductor force is required because the external moment of the body weight (load) is unchanged. Often, the abductors cannot meet this demand. Consequently, it is common to see postural adjustments, such as shifting the upper trunk over the stance limb, which has the effect of moving the body's center of mass closer to the fulcrum, thereby reducing the load (Fig. 12.8). If shifting the trunk cannot sufficiently compensate, pelvic drop (Trendelenburg sign) is seen with each single leg stance. This example indicates how an "effective" hip-abductor insufficiency can arise in a patient with normal muscle strength and control.

Treatment of short lever-arm dysfunction is often possible, particularly at the hip. Lever-arm dysfunction induced by coxa valga can be corrected with a varus osteotomy to restore the normal neck-shaft angle. However, an adverse effect of this is to move the insertion of the hip abductors closer to their origin (reduce the articular-trochanteric distance), thereby creating functional abductor insufficiency. In a young child, this may correct spontaneously with growth or a trochanteric epiphysiodesis can be performed (Gage and Cary 1980). The problem with varus osteotomy in an older child is that there is insufficient growth remaining to re-tension the abductor muscles. As such, abductor insufficiency is often permanent. Because of this, in an older child a distal transposition of the trochanter

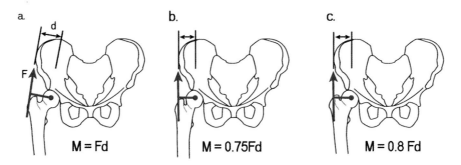

Fig. 12.7. Hip-abductor moments. (a) Abduction moment acting on a normal hip. Lever arm "d" is the perpendicular distance from the hip-joint center to the abductor muscle. The moment generated about the hip is equal to the muscle force times the length of the lever. A moment of Fd is generated in this case. (b) Hip joint with excessive valgus. In this example, the lever arm is shortened by 25% because the gluteus medius insertion has been drawn closer to the hip joint center by the effect of the valgus. The result is that, even though the muscle force is unchanged, the magnitude of the moment has been reduced by 25%. (c) Effect of a coxa breva that can occur following a fracture in an adult or avascular necrosis of the capital femoral epiphysis in a growing child. Again, the effect of the femoral neck shortening is to draw the gluteus medius closer to the center of the hip joint (by 20% in this example). As a result the magnitude of the moment has been reduced to 80% of normal despite normal muscle strength. (Reproduced from Gage and Schwartz 2002, fig. 22.5, p 767, by permission.)

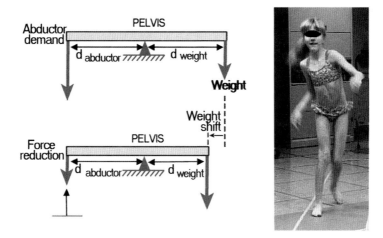

Fig. 12.8. Gait compensation for a short hip abduction lever. (a) If the location of the body weight (load) is unchanged a higher force will be demanded of the hip abductors. If this effort cannot be supplied, a compensatory posture will be found that reduces the lever arm of the external force, thereby reducing the demand on the hip abductors. Trendelenburg gait is an example of this sort of compensation. (b) The girl in the photograph has an upper body shift and a pelvic drop (Trendelenburg sign) during single limb stance. (Reproduced from Gage and Schwartz 2002, fig. 22.6, p 768, by permission.)

is usually necessary to restore the gluteal muscles to their functional length. The technique used for trochanteric transfer will vary depending on what one wishes to accomplish. If the goal were to re-tension the hip abductors, the osteotomy of the trochanter would need to

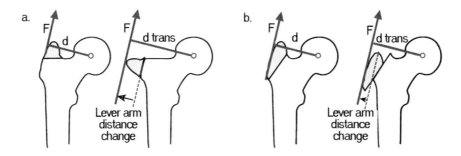

Fig. 12.9. (a) An illustration of a trochanteric transfer in which the trochanter is cut off horizontally and then transferred to the lateral aspect of the femoral shaft. This has the effect of lengthening the lever arm of the hip abductors. Assuming that muscle strength was unchanged, the abduction moment would be increased by the percentage by which the abductor lever arm was lengthened. This would be the preferred method of trochanteric transfer to correct coxa breva. (b) If the trochanter is cut off at an angle, the transposition of the trochanter is more distal than lateral. The abductor muscle is tightened, but the percentage of increase in the lever arm length is much less than in example (a). Since the increase in the magnitude of the abduction moment is directly proportional to the increase in the lever-arm length, the amount of improvement of the abduction moment would be much less as well. This would be the preferred way of transferring the trochanter following varus osteotomy of the hip in an older child, since the goal here would be to tighten the hip-abductor muscle rather than to lengthen the lever arm. (Reproduced from Gage and Schwartz 2002, fig. 22.8, p 769, by permission.)

be done in a more vertical direction (Fig. 12.9b). On the other hand, in a condition such as coxa breva, where the goal is to lengthen the abductor lever-arm, it is important to make the osteotomy more horizontal such that the abductor insertion is carried laterally rather than distally (Fig. 12.9a).

FLEXIBLE LEVER ARM
The problems associated with a flexible lever-arm dysfunction can be likened to attempting to pry up a rock with a rubber crowbar. In a child with spastic diplegia the classic example of this is flexible pes valgus (Fig. 12.10). Since these children have a "midfoot break" with forefoot abduction, dorsiflexion and abduction deformation of the forefoot reduces both the magnitude and the direction of the moment. The reason for this is that the lever is not rigid enough to transmit the force and, as a result, bends as the force increases. This, in turn, shortens and maldirects the lever arm. The effect of a moment on a non-rigid body, then, is to produce deformation rather than rotation. In spastic diplegia flexible pes valgus is one of the principal causes of crouch gait because it results in substantial loss of the normal plantarflexion/knee-extension (PF/KE) couple that provides about half of the support necessary for upright posture. The PF/KE couple and its effects were described in Chapter 4 and will be discussed in more detail when we come to crouch gait.

Treatment of this type of lever-arm dysfunction is usually possible. In the case of flexible pes valgus, lengthening of the lateral column of the foot in conjunction with reefing of the talonavicular joint capsule are usually sufficient (Mosca 1995, 1998). However, because of the muscle imbalance that exists in children with cerebral palsy, these procedures

197

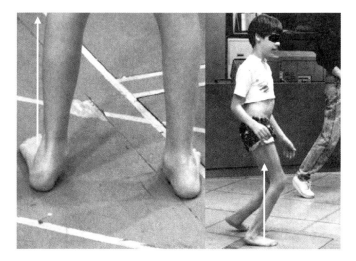

Fig. 12.10. Flexible lever-arm dysfunction. (a) During terminal stance the heel normally moves into relative varus and the arch lifts as the plantar fascia is winched around the metatarsal heads. These actions render the foot rigid so that it is an excellent lever for push-off. In pes valgus, the hindfoot remains in valgus and the forefoot in abduction and supination throughout stance. As such the foot is externally rotated to the knee axis and there is excessive motion in the midfoot. This means that the lever arm is not only maldirected (it is not in the plane of progression): it is also flexible, like a crowbar made of rubber. (b) Boy with spastic diplegia and severe pes valgus. It is apparent that no PF/KE couple can be generated since the GRF is always behind the knee axis. This means that the entire task of sustaining lower-extremity extension falls to the hip- and knee-extensors. Unfortunately in an adult there is not enough power in these two muscle groups to assume this burden and so crouch gait invariably occurs. (Reproduced from Gage and Schwartz 2002, fig. 22.9, p 770, by permission.)

need to be supplemented with an appropriate foot orthosis and/or subtalar arthrodesis.

MALROTATED LEVER ARM

The most common examples of malrotated levers in the body are torsional deformities of the long bones of the lower extremities. In the case of cerebral palsy, this occurs because of failure to remodel fetal anteversion, with resultant femoral torsion usually in conjunction with further plastic deformation of bone during growth. In spastic diplegia this often leads to both femoral anteversion and external tibial torsion, a combination often referred to as the *malignant malalignment syndrome* (Fig. 12.11). To understand this type of lever-arm dysfunction, it is necessary to visualize its effects in the transverse plane.

Figure 12.12b depicts the effect of external tibial torsion. In the sagittal plane, it can be seen that the relative length of the knee-extension lever arm of the ground reaction force has been reduced. In the transverse plane, the malrotation of the foot can be seen. From this perspective, it can be noted that valgus and external rotation moments about the ankle/knee have been introduced as well. Hence, malrotated levers produce two effects: (1) reduction of the magnitude of the primary or intended moment, and (2) introduction of secondary moments. It is important to remember, however, that both the external and

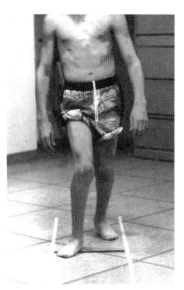

Fig. 12.11. An illustration of a young man with "malignant malalignment syndrome". This condition features the combination of internal femoral torsion (femoral anteversion), in conjunction with external tibial torsion and/or pes valgus. The result is that the foot and knee are not aligned to the plane of progression and the normal PF/KE couple cannot occur.

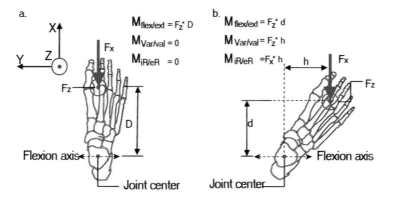

a.

$$M_{flex/ext} = F_z^* D$$
$$M_{Var/val} = 0$$
$$M_{iR/eR} = 0$$

b.

$$M_{flex/ext} = F_z^* d$$
$$M_{Var/val} = F_z^* h$$
$$M_{iR/eR} = F_x^* h$$

Flexion axis

Joint center

Joint center

Flexion axis

Fig. 12.12. Malrotated lever-arm dysfunction, external tibial torsion. (a) Malrotated lever arms most commonly occur in the long bones of the lower extremity (femoral anteversion, tibial torsion). (a) Normal anatomy and alignment. Note the relative length of the extension moment Fz * D and that the varus/valgus and rotational moments are zero. (b) External tibial torsion causes the GRF to move posterior and lateral to its normal position. This has the effect of shortening the extension moment lever arm, which means that the knee-extension moment is reduced. In addition, valgus and external rotation moments are introduced that will generate valgus and external rotation forces at the foot, shank and knee. In a growing child these abnormal forces acting over time will produce pes plano-valgus, further external tibial torsion and genu valgum. (Reproduced from Gage and Schwartz 2002, fig. 22.10, p 771, by permission.)

internal moments can be affected. With femoral anteversion, the specific effect would depend on the relative positions of the hip and knee during gait. For example, if an individual with 45° of excessive anteversion were to walk with the knee directed anteriorly, the insertion point of the gluteus minimus referable to the hip joint center would have to be

199

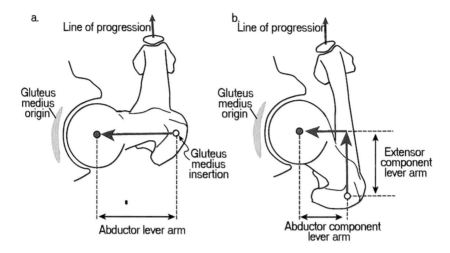

Fig. 12.13. Malrotated lever arm, femoral anteversion. (a) Just as tibial torsion generates lever-arm dysfunction at the foot, so femoral anteversion will generate lever-arm dysfunction at the hip. This figure depicts a transverse view of normal anatomy at the hip. The gluteus medius insertion point is directly lateral to the hip and as such the moment produced by this muscle would be only abduction. The product of the extension and external rotation moments would be zero. (b) Severe femoral anteversion. By internal rotation of the entire limb, the individual is able to neutralize some of the anteversion. However, the portion that is not neutralized with internal rotation of the limb has the effect of carrying the gluteus medius insertion point posteriorly. The abduction moment of the gluteus medius would thus be reduced in magnitude, and hip-extension and internal-rotation moments that are not normally present would be introduced. (Reproduced from Gage and Schwartz 2002, fig. 22.11, p 772, by permission.)

rotated externally by the same 45°. This would reduce the abduction moment on the hip by an amount proportional to the reduction of length of the abduction lever arm. In addition, it would introduce a hip-extension moment of approximately equal magnitude (Fig. 12.13).

It is important to recognize that the introduction of secondary moments and the reduction of primary moments can occur without any change in the *magnitude* of the muscle forces. Hence, a lever of proper length can cause pathological abnormality solely as a result of its improper orientation. From our earlier discussions on the mechanism of bone growth, it should be remembered that growing bone is plastic and remodels in accordance with the stresses that are imposed on it. Therefore the long-term effect of malrotated lever-arm dysfunction in a growing child is to generate further deformity of the long bones and feet.

The treatment of a malrotated lever arm is straightforward. The malrotation must be surgically corrected, either acutely via osteotomy and internal fixation of the affected bone or slowly via a derotation component in an Ilizarov frame.

UNSTABLE FULCRUM

A good example of an unstable fulcrum is hip subluxation or dislocation (Fig. 12.14). In this case, even in the presence of an adequate force and lever, an effective moment cannot be generated. Because the hip is subluxated, there is no stable fulcrum. As a result, a normal

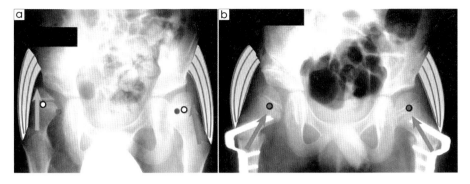

Fig. 12.14. (a) Unstable fulcrum, hip subluxation. Hip subluxation or dislocation provides an excellent example of the effect of an unstable fulcrum. The right hip joint is severely subluxated and unstable. Consequently, contraction of the hip abductors will not produce abduction, but rather upward translation of the femoral head and neck. On the opposite side the femoral head is stable in the acetabulum, but the severe coxa valga has the effect of shortening the abduction lever arm (short lever-arm dysfunction). (b) After bilateral varus-derotational femoral osteotomy and a right acetabuloplasty both hips are stable and normal hip-abduction lever arms have been restored. (Reproduced from Gage and Schwartz 2002, fig. 22.12, p 773, by permission.)

hip abductor muscle would not produce abduction, but rather upward subluxation of the femoral head. There is an element of similarity between the effect of a flexible lever and that of an unstable fulcrum, but the underlying causes are substantially different.

Treatment would depend on the integrity of the joint and the length of time the condition had been present. For example, a hip subluxation or dislocation in a child with cerebral palsy can usually be corrected with open reduction plus appropriate femoral and acetabular osteotomies. However in an adult with cerebral palsy and concurrent degenerative joint disease, a total hip replacement might be required to remedy this situation.

POSITIONAL ABNORMALITIES
Positional lever-arm dysfunction is a bit more difficult to understand. One of the best examples of it is seen in the effect of a crouch gait. As was discussed in Chapter 4, despite the fact that hamstrings are biarticular muscles, in normal gait they function as hip-extensors during the first half of stance phase (Fig. 12.15a). Despite the fact that the hamstrings are biarticular muscles, this is possible because the distal joint (the knee) is locked (initially by the action of the vasti and later by the effect of the PF/KE couple). In addition, with erect posture, the lever arm of the hamstrings at the knee, as compared to its lever arm at the hip, is relatively short. Because of this, concentric action of the hamstrings is able to augment hip extension without flexing the knee. Almost 30 years ago Dr Jacquelin Perry, one of the pioneers of gait analysis, demonstrated the effectiveness of the hamstrings as hip-extensors (Waters et al. 1974); and over a decade ago, she pointed out their function in cerebral palsy (Perry and Newsam 1992). Much of this knowledge has still not been assimilated by the orthopaedic community at large. Now, however, there is further evidence from the modeling community showing that the hamstrings act as knee extensors during

201

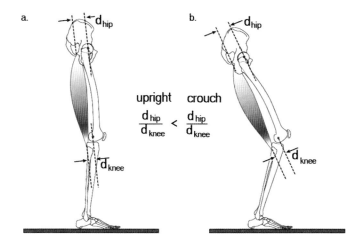

Fig. 12.15. (a) In erect posture, the hip-extension lever arm of the hamstrings significantly exceeds that of the knee-flexion lever arm. (b) As one begins to crouch, the ratio of hip-flexion lever to knee-flexion lever decreases, making the hamstrings relatively stronger knee-flexors. The rectus femoris is recruited to help extend the knee. Unfortunately this muscle is also a powerful hip-flexor and thus places a higher demand on the hamstrings to extend the hip. This in turn produces further flexion at the knee. This vicious cycle frequently leads to a downward spiral into further crouch. As higher knee-extension forces are required the combination of knee pain (secondary to patellar stress-fracture or patellar–femoral arthritis) and/or increased energy consumption often lead to loss of ambulation. (Reproduced from Gage and Schwartz 2002, fig. 22.13, p 774, by permission.)

stance (Arnold 1999). This is a result of induced accelerations arising from a coupled, closed, kinematic chain.

During crouch gait, however, the situation changes dramatically (Fig. 12.15b). Because the ground reaction force now lies well behind the knee, the PF/KE couple is no longer operative. In fact, because the ground reaction force is now posterior to the knee, it acts to generate a strong external flexion moment that must be resisted by the quadriceps. Furthermore, since the ground reaction force now passes in front of the hip, it also generates an external hip-flexion moment. The hip-flexion moment must be resisted by the hip extensors, including the hamstrings. However, the flexed posture of the hip and knee has now changed the relative length of the proximal and distal lever arms of the hamstrings (the lever-arm length at the knee has increased relative to that of the hip). Furthermore, the knee is now unlocked. Put these effects together and the hamstrings now become highly effective knee-flexors.

The secondary results of the large flexion moments at the hip and knee are twofold: (1) the patellar–femoral pressures increase, and (2) the rectus femoris and hamstrings are called on for more assistance to resist the moments. However, biarticular muscles act at two joints. Therefore, in addition to being a knee-extensor, the biarticular rectus femoris is also a strong hip-flexor. And the hamstrings, in addition to their action as hip-extensors, are strong knee-flexors. Thus with rectus femoris and hamstring activity, even larger extension moments are required at the hip and knee to resist their collapse into flexion. If

202

hamstring and rectus femoris activity result in an increase in knee and/or hip flexion, the ground reaction force will move even further from the hip and knee, thereby increasing the external lever arm and the magnitude of the flexion moment at each joint. The result is a vicious cycle in which the hip- and knee-flexion moments get progressively larger and the extension moments become progressively more inadequate. Eventually, the increased energy requirements and knee pain from increased patellar–femoral pressure or patellar stress fracture make walking impossible (see dynamic CD-Rom, Fig 21.2d).

Since the problem can arise from a variety of causes, the treatment of positional lever-arm dysfunction is complex. For example, in a neuromuscular condition such as cerebral palsy, the problem can be secondary to problems relating to balance, loss of selective motor control, abnormal muscle tone, muscle weakness, an increase in body mass, and/or other types of lever-arm dysfunction discussed earlier in this chapter. In paralytic conditions such as myelomeningocele or polio, the problem often emanates from distal weakness of the triceps surae, which in turn produces an inadequate PF/KE couple during mid-stance.

However, primary lever-arm dysfunction such as severe pes valgus or external tibial torsion can also produce a reduction in the external ground reaction moment such that the PF/KE couple is not sufficient to sustain knee extension in mid-stance. Consequently, success of treatment depends on a correct understanding of the source(s) of the pathological abnormality. It is important to remember that this particular type of lever-arm dysfunction often arises as a consequence of the presence of some of the other types of lever-arm dysfunction that were discussed earlier. Since the treatment of positional lever-arm dysfunction is complex and relates directly to the treatment of crouch gait, we will discuss it more completely when we come to crouch gait in the treatment section of this book.

REFERENCES

Albright AL. (1996) Intrathecal baclofen in cerebral palsy movement disorders. *J Child Neurol* **11** (Suppl. 1): S29–35.

Albright AL, Barry MJ, Fasick P, Barron W, Shultz B. (1996) Continuous intrathecal baclofen infusion for symptomatic generalized dystonia. *Neurosurgery* **38:** 934–939.

Albright AL, Barry MJ, Shafton DH, Ferson SS. (2001) Intrathecal baclofen for generalized dystonia. *Dev Med Child Neurol* **43:** 652–657.

Anderson FC, Pandy MG. (1999a) A dynamic optimization solution for vertical jumping in three dimensions. *Comput Methods Biomech Biomed Engin* **2:** 201–231.

Anderson FC, Pandy MG. (1999b) *Static and dynamic optimization solutions for gait are practically equivalent.* Paper presented at the 23rd annual meeting of the American Society of Biomechanics, Pittsburgh.

Arkin AM, Katz JF. (1956) The effects of pressure on epiphyseal growth. *J Bone Joint Surg* **38A:** 1056–1076.

Arnold AS. (1999) Quantitative descriptions of musculoskeletal geometry in persons with cerebral palsy: Guidelines for the evaluation and treatment of crouch gait. *Doctor of Philosophy Dissertation in the Department of Biomedical Engineering. Northwestern University, Evanston, Illinois.*

Arnold AS, Komattu AV, Delp SL. (1997) Internal rotation gait: a compensatory mechanism to restore abduction capacity decreased by bone deformity. *Dev Med Child Neurol* **39:** 40–44.

Bleck EE. (1971) Postural and gait abnormalities caused by hip-flexion deformity in spastic cerebral palsy. Treatment by iliopsoas recession. *J Bone Joint Surg Am* **53:** 1468–1488.

Bleck EE. (1987) *Orthopaedic Management in Cerebral Palsy.* London: Mac Keith Press.

Burtner PA, Woollacott MH, Qualls C. (1999) Stance balance control with orthoses in a group of children with spastic cerebral palsy. *Dev Med Child Neurol* **41:** 748–757.

Butler PB, Thompson N, Major RE. (1992) Improvement in walking performance of children with cerebral palsy: preliminary results. *Dev Med Child Neurol* **34:** 567–576.

Davy DT, Audu ML. (1987) A dynamic optimization technique for predicting muscle forces in the swing phase of gait. *J Biomech* **20:** 187–201.

Delp SL, Statler K, Carroll NC. (1995) Preserving plantar flexion strength after surgical treatment for contracture of the triceps surae: a computer simulation study. *J Orthop Res* **13:** 96–104.

Delp SL, Hess WE, Hungerford DS, Jones LC. (1999) Variation of rotation moment arms with hip flexion. *J Biomech* **32:** 493–501.

Gage JR, Cary JM. (1980) The effects of trochanteric epiphyseodesis on growth of the proximal end of the femur following necrosis of the capital femoral epiphysis. *J Bone Joint Surg* **62A:** 785–794.

Gage JR, Schwartz MH. (2002) Dynamic deformities and lever-arm considerations. In: Paley D, editor. *Principles of Deformity Correction.* Berlin: Springer. p 761–775.

Hagberg B, Sanner G, Steen M. (1972) The dysequilibrium syndrome in cerebral palsy. Clinical aspects and treatment. *Acta Paediatr Scand* **226:** 1–63.

Hepp-Reymond M, Trouche E, Wiesendanger M. (1974) Effects of unilateral and bilateral pyramidotomy on a conditioned rapid precision grip in monkeys (*Macaca fascicularis*). *Exp Brain Res* **21:** 519–527.

Kuypers H. (1981) *Anatomy of the Descending Pathways,* vol. 2. Bethesda, Maryland.

Liao HF, Jeng SF, Lai JS, Cheng CK, Hu MH. (1997) The relation between standing balance and walking function in children with spastic diplegic cerebral palsy. *Dev Med Child Neurol* **39:** 106–112.

Lieber RL. (1997) Muscle fiber length and moment arm coordination during dorsi- and plantarflexion in the mouse hindlimb. *Acta Anat (Basel)* **159:** 84–89.

Minear WL. (1956) A classification of cerebral palsy. *Pediatrics* **18:** 841–856.

Mosca VS. (1995) Calcaneal lengthening for valgus deformity of the hindfoot. Results in children who had severe, symptomatic flatfoot and skewfoot. *J Bone Joint Surg Am* **77:** 500–512.

Mosca VS. (1998) The child's foot: principles of management. *J Pediatr Orthop* **18:** 281–282.

Novacheck T, Trost J, Schwartz M. (2002) Intramuscular psoas lengthening improves dynamic hip function in children with cerebral palsy. *J Pediatr Orthop* **22:** 158–164.

Pedotti A, Krishnan VV, Stark L. (1978) Optimization of muscle-force sequencing in human locomotion. *Math Biosci* **38:** 57–76.

Perry J, Newsam C. (1992) Function of the hamstrings in cerebral palsy. In: Sussman M, editor. *The Diplegic Child: Evaluation and Management.* Rosemont, IL: American Academy of Orthopaedic Surgeons. p 299–307.

Rose SA, DeLuca PA, Davis RB 3rd, Õunpuu S, Gage JR. (1993) Kinematic and kinetic evaluation of the ankle after lengthening of the gastrocnemius fascia in children with cerebral palsy. *J Pediatr Orthop* **13:** 727–732.

Simpson JB. (1988) *Simpson's Contemporary Quotations.* Boston: Houghton Mifflin.

Sommerville EW. (1957) Persistent foetal alignment of the hip. *J Bone Joint Surg Br* **39:** 106.

Tsirakos D, Baltzopoulos V, Bartlett R. (1997) Inverse optimization: functional and physiological considerations related to the force-sharing problem. *Crit Rev Biomed Eng* **25:** 371–407.

Waters RL, Perry J, McDaniels JM, House K. (1974) The relative strength of the hamstrings during hip extension. *J Bone Joint Surg Am* **56:** 1592–1597.

Winters TF Jr, Gage JR, Hicks R. (1987) Gait patterns in spastic hemiplegia in children and young adults. *J Bone Joint Surg Am* **69:** 437–441.

Zajac FE, Gordon ME. (1989) Determining muscle's force and action in multi-articular movement. *Exerc Sport Sci Rev* **17:** 187–230.

Zaleske DJ, Doppelt SH, Mankin HJ. (1990) Metabolic and endocrine abnormalities of the immature skeleton. In: Morrissy RT, editor. *Lovell and Winter's Pediatric Orthopaedics,* vol. 1. Philadelphia: J.B. Lippincott. p 205.

Ziv I, Blackburn N, Rang M, Koreska J. (1984) Muscle growth in normal and spastic mice. *Dev Med Child Neurol* **26:** 94–99.

13
SPECIFIC PROBLEMS OF THE HIPS, KNEES AND ANKLES

James R. Gage

Now that we have discussed the overall mechanisms by which gait pathology arises in cerebral palsy, we are ready to discuss in more detail the specific problems that arise at each of the lower-extremity joints. Based on what was discussed in Chapter 12, it should now be evident that a cascade of events occur, beginning with the neurological injury. If we take the case of a boy with spastic diplegia (such as the one shown in Fig. 13.1), that neurological lesion would most likely be periventricular leukomalacia, which is typically a bilateral lesion in the white matter adjacent to the frontal horns of the lateral ventricles. Since the axons conducting input to this boy's lower extremities course through the frontal regions, injury in this location produced the typical clinical picture in which the most prominent features are motor impairments in his lower extremities (distal > proximal), impaired balance and spasticity. This complex of neurological injury is what we referred to in the last chapter as the primary effect of the brain injury. However, the consequences of the primary effect to this boy were such that normal play activities such as running and jumping, which promote muscle-stretching, were not possible. The spasticity in his rectus femoris muscles made it difficult for him to flex his knees adequately during the swing phase of gait, so he tended to drag his feet. As each foot dragged across the floor/ground, it tended to rotate into external rotation. The spasticity and foot-drag greatly increased the energy cost of his walking. In addition, his spasticity, which tended to be the worst in the distal biarticular muscles, impeded stretch of these particular muscle-groups even more. Furthermore, the child was now forced to spend much more of his time sitting, and the sitting posture itself tended to favor hip- and knee-flexion contractures. As a consequence of the spasticity, inadequate muscle-stretch during growth and the sitting postures, over time he developed contractures of his psoas, hamstrings and gastrocnemius bilaterally.

He started walking late, at about 3 years of age, and because of his balance problems and hip- and knee-flexion contractures, he never stood completely erect. In addition, by the time he started walking his rate of growth had slowed and his proximal femora had ossified. Consequently the upper ends of his femora were no longer as malleable as they had been during the first few years of his life when they were still cartilaginous. As a result he was left with persistent fetal alignment of his femurs because his femoral anteversion, which we all have at the time of birth, did not remodel.

With time and growth, the under- or overactivity of certain muscle groups, and the torsional effects of the walking pattern imposed upon him by the neurological injury, abnormal

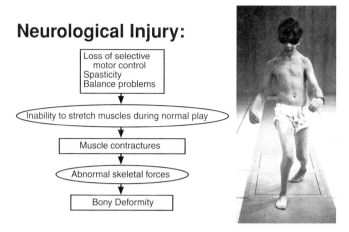

Neurological Injury:

Loss of selective motor control
Spasticity
Balance problems

↓

Inability to stretch muscles during normal play

↓

Muscle contractures

↓

Abnormal skeletal forces

↓

Bony Deformity

Fig. 13.1. Typical boy with spastic diplegia whose gait demonstrates bilateral femoral and tibial torsion. The sequence of events that led to the deformities is shown at left.

forces were generated on his growing bones. His anteversion worsened and other secondary bony problems developed, which included pes valgus and external tibial torsion. As a consequence, we now find ourselves confronted with a typical child of about 8 years of age with spastic diplegia, who in addition to having the primary abnormalities of cerebral palsy that have been with him since birth, has additional bilateral secondary abnormalities which include (1) femoral anteversion, (2) external tibial torsion, and (3) contractures of his psoas, hamstrings, and gastrocnemius. Now that we can visualize the scenario by which he arrived at this state of development, we should look more closely at the functional and structural abnormalities that might be present in each of the major joints of his lower extremities.

The foot and ankle

MAJOR FUNCTIONS IN NORMAL GAIT

Quadrupeds have paws or hooves, and bipeds have feet. With four paws a dog, cat or cougar has no need for feet. However, we do, because as bipeds we must spend time with only one foot on the ground. The foot is the platform upon which we stand and balance, and for that matter, upon which we push off from the ground to walk, run or jump. For the foot and ankle to function normally the knee and foot have to be appropriately aligned to the plane of progression, the foot is required to function as a stable platform, the ankle needs to have an adequate range of motion, and the power generations/absorptions of the muscles that serve the ankle and foot must be appropriate. Since we are about to talk about ankle and foot pathology, perhaps this may be a good time to go back to Chapter 4, to review the foot-rockers, their purpose, and the prerequisites/attributes of normal gait, i.e. (1) stability in stance, (2) clearance in swing, (3) pre-position of the foot at initial contact, (4) an adequate step length, and (5) energy conservation. Recall also from Chapter 4 that our Creator has ingeniously crafted our foot so that at impact and during loading response the foot is in

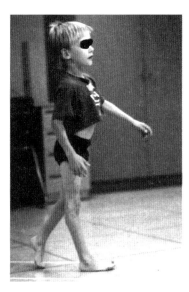

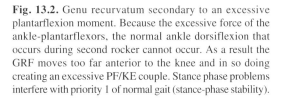

Fig. 13.2. Genu recurvatum secondary to an excessive plantarflexion moment. Because the excessive force of the ankle-plantarflexors, the normal ankle dorsiflexion that occurs during second rocker cannot occur. As a result the GRF moves too far anterior to the knee and in so doing creating an excessive PF/KE couple. Stance phase problems interfere with priority 1 of normal gait (stance-phase stability).

relative valgus, and so functions as an ideal shock absorber. Whereas in terminal stance, the rotations of the ankle and hindfoot, plus the winching of the plantar fascia around the heads of the metatarsals, act to bring our foot into relative varus and render it rigid so that it can serve as an ideal lever arm for the ankle plantarflexors at push-off (Inman et al. 1994). In fact during normal walking about 50% of the total power required comes from this source, with most of the remaining 50% coming from muscles acting around the hip (Õunpuu et al. 1991, 1996, Winter 1991, Õunpuu 1994).

Pathology of the ankle and foot
STANCE PHASE

Loss of priority one (stability in stance) is the principal problem encountered here. Stability in stance may be lost as a result of malrotation (e.g. tibial torsion), varus or valgus deformities, and/or abnormal muscle moments that leads to equinus or calcaneus deformity. I have deliberately used the term "abnormal muscle moment" in this discussion, because by this point in the book I am hoping that the reader is thinking in terms of moments (force times lever arm) rather than muscles. In the untreated patient with cerebral palsy, the abnormal moment is almost always excessive equinus as a result of relative dominance of the triceps surae over the ankle-dorsiflexors (Fig. 13.2). Calcaneus is the norm in myelomeningocele, but in cerebral palsy it is nearly always iatrogenic as a secondary effect of tendo-Achilles lengthening, particularly in a child with mixed tone.

    Spasticity/contracture of all or part of the triceps surae is common in all types of spastic cerebral palsy. In hemiplegia the foot usually is stuck in the rigid posture of terminal stance (push-off). Spasticity/contracture of the tibialis posterior tends to dominate that of the peroneals and contracture is common in both the gastrocnemius and soleus components of the triceps surae. However, even if both muscles are contracted, they are not contracted to the same degree (Delp et al. 1995). Consequently, tendo-Achilles lengthening is probably not the best option. We will discuss this further when we come to treatment. As a result of the relative overactivity of the triceps surae and the dominance of the tibialis anterior and posterior over the peroneals and long toe-extensors, the typical foot posture is one of equinovarus, and because the soleus, which is a powerful plantarflexor, is involved, the deformity is often quite rigid. Initially the deformity is dynamic, but with time contracture of the plantar fascia, as well as bony deformity of the forefoot and/or hindfoot, may develop. In addition, depending on the patient's walking pattern, internal or external tibial torsion may occur, although external tibial torsion in conjunction with forefoot adduction and pronation (forefoot valgus) is more common.

With diplegia and quadriplegia, on the other hand, the foot is stuck in the posture of loading response (shock absorption). The tibialis posterior is relatively underactive and so the peroneus brevis tends to dominate pulling the forefoot into abduction. The gastrocnemius is overactive and usually contracted, but in diplegia the soleus is almost always relatively uninvolved and usually of normal length, although in quadriplegia it may become contracted to a minor degree. Because the gastrocnemius is overactive and the tibialis posterior is not strong enough to maintain the arch, the hindfoot commonly collapses into valgus, that is, the calcaneus rotates into valgus. This means that the sustentaculum tali is no longer a horizontal platform to support the talus. As a consequence the talus rotates medially and drops into equinus. The GRF then pushes the forefoot into supination (forefoot varus) and abduction such that the talonavicular joint is severely subluxated. The result is that the hindfoot is in relative equinus whereas the forefoot is dorsiflexed and abducted relative to the hindfoot. As such the midfoot is extremely mobile, a condition which is frequently referred to as a "midfoot break". Correction of this deformity is usually best accomplished by lengthening the lateral column, tightening the medial column, and, if necessary correcting the malrotation of the forefoot (Mosca, 1995, 1996, 1998). Once that is done, the gastrocnemius contracture becomes much more apparent and needs to be corrected as well.

SWING PHASE

Just as stability (priority 1) was the issue in stance, so clearance (priority 2) and position of the foot at initial contact (priority 3) are the issues during swing phase. Dynamic or static mal-position of the foot (varus, valgus and/or equinus) and/or abnormal muscle moments will account for virtually all of the deformities that are commonly seen. Varus or valgus mal-position of the foot generates problems with priority 3 (pre-position at initial contact) whereas equinus can cause difficulties with either priority 2 or 3 (clearance in swing and/or pre-position at initial contact) (Fig 13.3). We have already discussed static varus and valgus deformities. However, because of poor distal selective motor control that is present in nearly all of these patients, dynamic varus, valgus, and/or equinus deformities are common. In hemiplegia, the peroneal muscles and extensor digitorum longus are under active. In addition, the force of the plantarflexors, particularly the triceps surae, frequently overwhelms the dorsiflexors. As such dorsiflexion in swing, if it occurs at all, is usually accomplished with the tibialis anterior and flexor hallucis longus. If this is the case, the

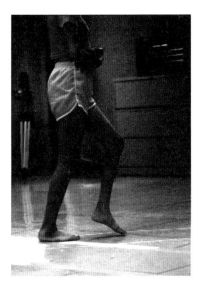

Fig. 13.3. A young man with a severe drop foot in swing. Swing-phase problems interfere with clearance (priority 2) or appropriate foot position at initial contact (priority 3 of normal gait).

forefoot will supinate and the feet will dorsiflex in a varus posture. In diplegia and quadriplegia, although the dorsiflexors are still often overwhelmed by the plantarflexors, they are better balanced. Consequently, if dorsiflexion occurs, the foot often comes up in a relatively neutral position. In diplegia, in fact, foot position relative to the tibia is usually normal and the individual lands in a foot-flat or forefoot initial contact position because of abnormal knee flexion. With slow-motion video, idiopathic toe-walking and diplegia can frequently be differentiated in this way since children with idiopathic toe-walking commonly have true ankle equinus and full knee extension at initial contact, whereas children with mild diplegia, with whom idiopathic toe-walkers are confused, usually have a flexed-knee posture with normal foot position relative to the shank at initial contact (Hicks et al. 1988). Dynamic equinus, in addition to causing clearance problems in swing, will also produce abnormal pre-position at initial contact. As such, first rocker will never occur. At best, the individual will land in a foot-flat position, but more commonly toe to heel (reverse first-rocker). The child may use a variety of "coping responses" to circumvent this problem, including hyperflexion of the hip, circumduction of the limb, and/or, in the case of hemiplegia, vaulting on the opposite side. Children with spastic diplegia and/or quadriplegia do not have enough selective motor control to vault, although diplegic children will often have what I refer to as "serendipitous spasticity". In this case the abnormal landing position and/or gastrocnemius spasticity on the opposite side induces premature activity of the gastrocnemius in early mid-stance. Since the upper body is directly over the foot at this time, it has the same effect as a vault. In my opinion, when sorting out deformities of the foot and ankle during swing and stance, slow-motion video is often more useful than gait analysis, although both are required. When evaluating foot and ankle pathology, in addition to kinematics and kinetics, I depend heavily on close-up standing videos of the foot including the Root test (see Chapter 5) plus slow-motion close-up videos of the lower extremities from the side, front and rear.

The knee

Again, if the reader is unclear as to the functions of the knee in normal gait, it would be useful to briefly review that portion of Chapter 4. The reader should recall that in stance the knee functions as a shock-absorber during loading response, and by helping to reduce the vertical excursion of the center of mass, it participates in the conservation of energy throughout stance phase. In addition, energy is conserved by maintaining knee stability via the plantarflexion/knee-extension (PF/KE) couple rather than the quadriceps during the latter two-thirds of stance phase. In swing the knee functions to provide foot clearance (priority 2). Since we can vary our speed, however, a mechanism is also required to allow us to vary our cadence.

PATHOLOGY OF THE KNEE IN STANCE

Except in the mildest cases of spastic diplegia, normal knee function typically is severely compromised in children with cerebral palsy. To begin with, the knee is frequently not aligned to the plane of progression. "Lever-arm dysfunction" is common in diplegia and quadriplegia as well as in the more severe cases of spastic hemiplegia. Consequently the "malignant malalignment syndrome" is often seen, which is the combination of internal femoral and external tibial torsion plus/minus pes valgus (Fig. 12.11). Since the knee is the pivot point upon which the shank rotates to clear the foot during swing phase, it should be readily apparent that if the hinge is 20° or more out of plane, as is often the case, normal function can not occur.

Normal loading response does not occur because the knee, instead of being extended, is usually flexed about 45° at initial contact. Consequently, heel strike and first rocker cannot take place. Instead the foot lands in a toe-down or foot-flat position. From the moment of initial contact, therefore, the knee begins to extend and the ankle dorsiflex. This means that the gastrocnemius, which normally does not come under tension until mid-stance, feels stretch from the instant of initial contact. This premature muscular tension, together with the muscle's innate spasticity, causes the gastrocnemius to fire early (usually at about 20% of the gait cycle). Since the origin of the gastrocnemius is proximal to the knee and the upper body is directly above the foot at this time, the effect of the premature action of the gastrocnemius is to drive the body upward and at the same time to produce a strong flexion moment at both the knee and hip. Consequently extra effort must then be expended by the quadriceps and the hip-extensors to maintain stability of these joints. The end result is a "bounce gait" in which the upper body rises and falls with each step. Because of the excessive vertical excursion of the body's center of mass and the additional muscular effort to stabilize the hip and knee, energy is wasted instead of being conserved.

A second period of "energy wasting" may occur during midstance. Recall that midstance is the period of second rocker during which the GRF passes through the forefoot creating a knee-extension moment (the PF/KE couple). As such the knee is stable and quadriceps action is not required. However if, as in crouch gait, the individual walks with excessive knee flexion during this period, the GRF will move behind the knee to create a flexion moment that must then be resisted by the quadriceps. Rotational lever-arm dysfunction as seen in the "malignant malalignment syndrome" compounds the problem for the reasons discussed in the previous chapter. Since hip flexion and knee flexion typically occur concomitantly, this usually means that the external flexion moment on the hip also increases as well, so that additional muscular effort also will be required to maintain stability in that joint.

PATHOLOGY OF THE KNEE IN SWING

Except in the mildest cases of diplegia and hemiplegia, in which the rectus femoris and hamstrings are relatively spared, knee pathology in swing phase is almost the norm. In order to fully understand why this is so, the reader may need to return to Chapter 4 to review the mechanism by which we vary our cadence during swing phase. Recall that the power that drives the knee into flexion during swing phase comes from the ankle plantarflexors during terminal stance and the hip flexors during pre-swing and initial swing. More speed requires more power, but since the lower extremity is a compound pendulum, the biarticular muscles (rectus femoris and hamstrings) must act to retard and dampen the excessive knee flexion that would otherwise occur. Given this information, plus the pathology of cerebral palsy (poor distal selective motor control and spasticity of the biarticular muscles) discussed in the previous chapter, the specific pathology that occurs at the knee can be anticipated. Recall that 50% of the power for walking comes from the ankle plantarflexors during terminal stance. However, because of the poor distal motor control, the magnitude of that power is greatly diminished and the timing of its delivery is frequently abnormal as well. Furthermore, because of the effects of the spasticity and loss of selective motor control on the biarticular muscles (gastrocnemii, hamstrings, and rectus femoris), their function is abnormal, too. Dr Perry (1988) has pointed out that because selective motor control is better proximally than distally, the *biarticular muscles join the proximal synergy*, that is, they act as though they belong to the proximal joint. Consequently the rectus femoris and hamstrings, instead of acting like springs or isometric straps to dampen knee flexion and extension respectively, act instead like prime movers of the hip. Moreover, because of their spasticity, even if their timing were normal, they would act excessively. Because of the poor distal selective motor control, push-off power from the triceps surae is greatly reduced. Consequently the power needed at push-off to launch the limb into the air and flex the knee is greatly diminished. This in turn results in inadequate knee-flexion forces. Because the rectus femoris has joined the proximal synergy of the hip, it acts as with the other hip-flexors during pre-swing and initial swing, but since it is also an extensor of the knee, its action there only serves to dampen knee flexion further. Furthermore, because of its spasticity, rectus femoris activity is greatly prolonged. Meanwhile the spastic hamstrings fire early, often before mid-swing, and act primarily as hip-extensors. The result is that both rectus femoris and hamstrings usually are acting throughout mid-swing (a time when both muscles are normally silent). The result is that the magnitude of peak knee flexion is greatly reduced and the timing of peak knee flexion is delayed from initial swing to mid-swing (Gage et al. 1987, Perry 1987, Sutherland et al. 1990) (Fig. 13.4). Finally, since the principal use of the rectus femoris and hamstrings in normal gait is to allow variation of cadence, given the pathology of these muscles, it should be apparent that in cerebral-palsied gait, the ability to vary cadence is largely lost as well.

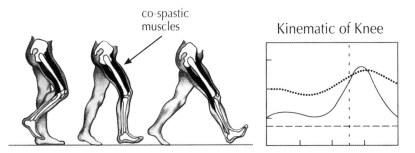

co-spastic
muscles

Kinematic of Knee

Fig. 13.4. Inadequate knee flexion in swing. Foot clearance in swing is dependent upon adequate hip and knee flexion and ankle dorsiflexion. Since the foot is still in equinus in initial swing, maximum knee flexion of approximately 60° is required at that point. Knee flexion in swing is dependent upon adequate acceleration forces at the ankle and hip and appropriate intensity and timing of action of the rectus femoris and hamstrings. Diagram on the left shows the common circumstance in cerebral-palsied gait in which the activity of both the hamstrings and rectus femoris is prolonged making the muscles "co-active" or "co-spastic" throughout the swing phase of gait. The result of this is shown in the kinematic graph of the knee (right) in which a typical knee curve of an individual with cerebral palsy (dotted line) is contrasted with that of a normal knee kinematic (solid line). Note that not only is the magnitude of knee flexion reduced, the timing of peak knee flexion is delayed as well.

The hip

MAJOR FUNCTIONS IN NORMAL GAIT

In Chapter 4 it was stated that the hip has three major functions. (1) It provides power for movement; during normal walking about half the necessary power comes from the hip with the other half coming from the ankle. (2) Balance of the hand and trunk segment is centralized at the hip. (3) Appropriate motion of the pelvis on the femur during gait allows conservation of energy because, as Inman and colleagues (1994) have pointed out, pelvic tilt and obliquity help to minimize the vertical excursion of the center of mass and pelvic rotation permits a longer step-length.

PATHOLOGY OF THE HIP IN CEREBRAL-PALSIED GAIT

If loss of selective motor control and spasticity extends to the hip, the situation is not unlike that of the ankle and knee, that is, all normal functions of the hip joint may be lost to some degree. Lever-arm dysfunction is extremely common at the hip. In fact, it is probably more common at the hip than the other major lower-extremity joints because, as we discussed in the previous chapter, these children almost invariably fail to remodel the femoral anteversion with which they are born: and so, in Sommerville's (1957) terms, they have persistent fetal alignment. This then produces the *malrotated* type of *lever-arm dysfunction* along with its attendant consequences (see Fig. 12.13). Other types of lever-arm dysfunction, such as coxa valga (*short lever-arm dysfunction*) and/or hip subluxation/dislocation (*unstable fulcrum*) are also very common, particularly in children who are minimal ambulators and/or have quadriplegic involvement. The coxa valga probably emanates from primary weakness of the hip-abductors, which in turn generates under growth of the trochanteric apophysis according to the laws of growth discussed in the previous chapter. For a more complete discussion of growth characteristics of the proximal femur, see Gage and Cary (1980). Coxa valga and anteversion by themselves may produce hip subluxation, but they are often aided and abetted by asymmetrical spasticity of the hip adductors, which in turn frequently leads to pelvic obliquity.

As we learned in the previous chapter, the general effect of lever-arm dysfunction is to reduce the magnitude of the primary moment and/or introduce secondary moments acting in other planes. Clinically this often manifests itself to the examiner as weakness. However, with both diplegia and quadriplegia primary muscle weakness, particularly of the hip-extensors and abductors, is also common. The individual is then forced to resort to tertiary abnormalities ("coping responses") to substitute for the deficient muscle function. Backward or lateral shifting of the upper trunk during stance phase is the common "coping response" use to substitute for weak hip-extensors or abductors, respectively. The previous chapter explained that selective motor control is better proximally and worse distally. Hence gait deviations are most common distally, whereas "coping responses" occur proximally, since one must be able to control the particular body part that is being used for the "coping response". One way to remember this is to think of the phrase, "proximal compensations for distal deviations". This is also true with respect to power for propulsion. Children who walk normally draw about half of the necessary power from their plantarflexors at push-off, and most of the remainder from their hips (Õunpuu et al. 1991, Winter 1991, Õunpuu 1994). However, this is not the case in cerebral palsy. Since selective motor control is poorest on the distal end of the limb, most children with cerebral palsy do not derive much walking power from their ankle-plantarflexors. As a result they must substitute by generating additional power from their hips and often from their knees as well (Gage 1994). The situation is not unlike walking in deep mud or snow. When doing so, one is forced to derive the power for mobility from "pull-up" from the hips and knees, as opposed to "push-off" from the foot and ankle.

Balance and equilibrium are abnormal in cerebral palsy, particularly in the anterior-posterior plane. Winter states that the body is an unstable pendulum, since two-thirds of the mass of the head, arms and trunk (HAT) is located at about two-thirds of the body's height above the ground. He then demonstrates that the hip is the center for balance control since the forces and/or postural compensations necessary to maintain the HAT segment balanced over the lower limbs are much smaller when applied at the hip than would be the case if they were applied more distally in the limb (Fig. 13.5) (Winter 1991). The situation, then, is not unlike that of a seal balancing a ball on its nose (Fig. 13.6), in which the ball represents the trunk, the seal the lower limbs and the seal's nose the hip joint. When we reflect on this a bit, we immediately realize that the task of the seal is quite complex, as is the task of maintaining balance while walking. An inebriated man, with alcohol-induced ataxia, can maintain balance and walks only with great difficulty, and I seriously doubt if an inebriated seal could balance a ball on his nose at all. The point of this is that if an individual is to maintain balance without the use of balance aides (such as crutches or a walker), good selective motor control and normally functioning muscles are mandatory. I suspect that this is also the case in cerebral palsy. We know that in the mildest cases of spastic diplegia (which are often confused with idiopathic toe-walking) only the distal biarticular muscles are

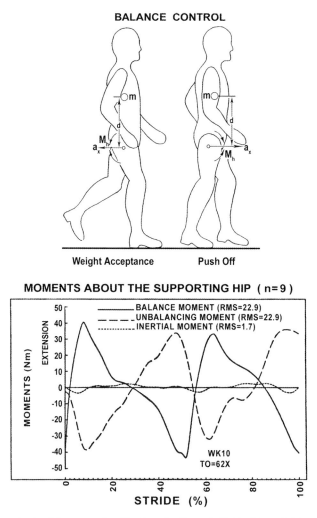

Fig. 13.5. Moments about the supporting hip. In order for an individual to maintain erect posture, the upper body (head, arms and trunk or HAT) must remain balanced over the lower extremities throughout the gait cycle. Winter (1991) has shown that an external (GRF and/or inertia) unbalancing moment is always counteracted by an internal balancing moment of equal magnitude. Thus the total inertial moment of HAT is always close to zero. (Reproduced from Winter 1991, fig. 6.12, p.79, by permission.)

involved (gastrocnemii). Furthermore, these children usually have excellent balance. We also know that as the severity of neurological involvement increases, so does the involvement of the proximal muscles. We have shown this to be true in hemiplegia (Winters et al. 1987), and I suspect that it is true in diplegia as well. From this I would infer that the child with diplegia who can walk without aides has reasonably normal muscle function and fairly good selective motor control around his/her hips, whereas the child who needs balance aides to walk probably does not.

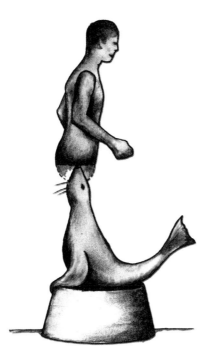

Fig. 13.6. A seal balancing the head and trunk (HAT) on its nose. If one equates the ball that a seal commonly balances on its nose with the HAT, the seal's nose with the hip joint, and the seal itself with the lower extremities, the feat is not unlike the one that we perform daily when we stand and/or walk.

REFERENCES

Delp SL, Statler K, Carroll NC. (1995) Preserving plantar flexion strength after surgical treatment for contracture of the triceps surae: a computer simulation study. *J Orthop Res* **13:** 96–104.

Gage JR. (1994) The clinical use of kinetics for evaluation of pathologic gait in cerebral palsy. *Instr Course Lect* **76A:** 622–631.

Gage JR, Cary JM. (1980) The effects of trochanteric epiphyseodesis on growth of the proximal end of the femur following necrosis of the capital femoral epiphysis. *J Bone Joint Surg Am* **62:** 785–794.

Gage JR, Perry J, Hicks RR, Koop S, Werntz JR. (1987) Rectus femoris transfer to improve knee function of children with cerebral palsy. *Dev Med Child Neurol* **29:** 159–166.

Hicks R, Durinick N, Gage JR. (1988) Differentiation of idiopathic toe-walking and cerebral palsy. *J Pediatr Orthop* **8:** 160–163.

Inman VT, Ralston HJ, Todd F. (1994) Human locomotion. In: Rose J, Gamble JG, editors. *Human Walking*. Baltimore: Williams and Wilkins. p 1–22.

Mosca VS (1995) Calcaneal lengthening for valgus deformity of the hindfoot. Results in children who had severe, symptomatic flatfoot and skewfoot. *J Bone Joint Surg Am* **77:** 500–512.

Mosca VS (1996) Flexible flatfoot and skewfoot. *Instr Course Lect* **45:** 347–354.

Mosca VS (1998) The child's foot: principles of management. *J Pediatr Orthop* **18:** 281–282.

Õunpuu S. (1994) The biomechanics of walking and running. *Clin Sports Med* **13:** 843–863.

Õunpuu S, Gage JR, Davis RB. (1991) Three-dimensional lower extremity joint kinetics in normal pediatric gait. *J Pediatr Orthop* **11:** 341–349.

Õunpuu S, Davis RB, DeLuca PA. (1996) Joint kinetics: methods, interpretation and treatment decision-making in children with cerebral palsy and myelomeningocele. *Gait Posture* **4:** 62–78.

Perry J. (1987) Distal rectus femoris transfer. *Dev Med Child Neurol* **29:** 153–158.

Perry J. (1988) *Normal muscle control sequence during walking.* Paper presented at the Instructional Course of Gait Analysis, Annual Meeting of the American Academy of Cerebral Palsy and Developmental Medicine, Toronto, Canada.

Sommerville EW. (1957) Persistent foetal alignment of the hip. *J Bone Joint Surg Br* **39:** 106.

Sutherland DH, Santi M, Abel MF. (1990) Treatment of stiff-knee gait in cerebral palsy: a comparison by gait analysis of distal rectus femoris transfer versus proximal rectus release. *J Pediatr Orthop* **10:** 433–441.

Winter DA. (1991) *The Biomechanics and Motor Control of Human Gait: Normal, Elderly, and Pathological,* 2nd edn. Waterloo, Ontario: University of Waterloo Press. p 35–52, 75–85.

Winters TF Jr, Gage JR, Hicks R. (1987) Gait patterns in spastic hemiplegia in children and young adults. *J Bone Joint Surg Am* **69:** 437–441.

14
PATTERNS OF GAIT PATHOLOGY

Sylvia Õunpuu

Over the past 20 years, clinicians have made great advances in the understanding of the pathomechanics of gait, using computerized gait analysis techniques (Davis and DeLuca 1996). Computerized gait-analysis techniques allow for the systematic review of kinematic and kinetic patterns both before and after treatment. The interpretation of kinematic and kinetic patterns requires considerable skill, and at least a cursory understanding of the methods used to obtain these data and the typical values associated with each parameter being examined (see Section 2 of this book). Also important is an understanding of the pathology being examined and the typical gait patterns expected in the pathology. Identifying typical gait patterns and using this terminology facilitates communication and ultimately understanding of atypical gait. As patterns represent a specific pathology and an associated set of possible causes, they can ultimately be connected with a specific treatment protocol.

There have been several attempts to identify patterns of movement in persons with cerebral palsy (CP), with the ultimate goal of associating a specific pattern with a specific set of treatments (Winters et al. 1987, Kadaba et al. 1991, Sutherland and Davids 1993). Due to the complexity of movement in all three planes of motion and of both lower extremities and the trunk, it may not be possible to categorize a person as a single pattern with a specific set of treatments. However, simplifying this approach to individual joints or combinations of joints is feasible and still useful. The purpose of this chapter is to illustrate typical gait patterns seen in persons with CP, initially at individual joints, followed by combinations of joint motion within a plane of motion, and finally across planes. Joint kinematic patterns will also be discussed in relation to their associated joint kinetic patterns as well.

Individual joint and segment kinematic patterns
The initial stage in interpreting gait analysis data is to identify abnormal joint and segment motion patterns versus a typical reference pattern. Due to the complexity of gait problems in persons with neuromuscular disorders, a gait deviation is seldom the result of pathology solely at the joint or segment of interest. Some of the exceptions will be discussed below.

DOUBLE-BUMP PELVIC PATTERN
This pattern is characterized by increasing anterior pelvic tilt that occurs twice during the gait cycle, once in stance and once in swing (Fig. 14.1). The peak anterior tilt always occurs in single-limb stance and the peak posterior tilt in double-limb stance. It is typically seen in persons with bilateral and symmetrical involvement. There is some debate about the causes of this motion pattern, but it seems clear that it involves the inability to dissociate pelvic from hip motion and thus involves both hip-flexors and extensors. That is, the pelvis is in

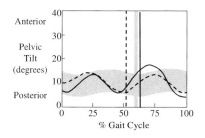

Fig. 14.1. Double-bump pelvic tilt pattern with increasing anterior pelvic tilt during stance and swing. Pelvic range of motion is increased in comparison with typical motion (solid band). *See CD-Rom, Figure 14.1, for a dynamic illustration.*

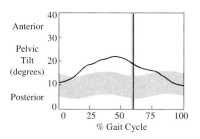

Fig. 14.2. Single-bump pelvic tilt pattern with increasing anterior pelvic tilt throughout the stance phase in comparison with the typical motion pattern (solid band). *See CD-Rom, Figure 14.2, for a dynamic illustration.*

its most anterior position in single stance when weak hip-extensors and/or spastic hip-flexors (the hip is extending in this phase) are allowing the pelvis to tip forward. In double stance, the pelvis is in the most posterior position when the maximum length is required of the hamstrings on one side, which pulls the pelvis into a more posterior position.

SINGLE-BUMP PELVIC PATTERN

This pattern is characterized by increasing anterior pelvic tilt through out the stance phase to a peak just before toe-off with a return to a baseline tilt through out the swing phase (Fig. 14.2). This pattern is typically seen in persons with hemiplegia. Like the double-bump pattern it is caused by an inability to dissociate pelvic from thigh motion, which happens on one side only. It is generally accepted that as the hip extends throughout stance, the pelvis is pulled anteriorly through pull of the spastic and/or tight hip-flexors. During swing, the pelvis returns to the baseline position as the stretch on the hip-flexors ends when the hip moves into flexion.

INTERNAL HIP ROTATION

This pattern is characterized by increased internal hip rotation through out the gait cycle (Fig. 14.3). There is typically a correlation between increased internal hip rotation and increased femoral anteversion as estimated on clinical examination (Ruwe et al. 1992). Spasticity of the medial rotators of the thigh may also result in internal hip rotation (Tylkowski 1982).

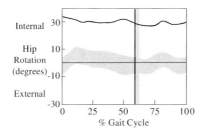

Fig. 14.3. Internal hip-rotation pattern throughout the gait cycle in comparison with the typical motion pattern (solid band). *See CD-Rom, Figure 14.3, for a dynamic illustration.*

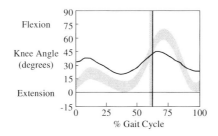

Fig. 14.4. Excessive knee-flexion pattern throughout the stance phase in comparison with the typical motion pattern (solid band). *See CD-Rom, Figure 14.4, for a dynamic illustration.*

EXCESSIVE KNEE FLEXION (CROUCH)

This pattern is characterized by greater than normal knee flexion throughout the stance phase (Fig. 14.4) and is very common in CP. Although there is some debate about the pathomechanics of crouch, there is general consensus that it is a result of any one of the following, or a combination of them, in terms of the knee: hamstring tightness, hamstring spasticity, hamstring weakness and severe knee-flexion contracture (Sutherland and Cooper 1978). Other causes not related to the knee include ankle-plantarflexor weakness and/or excessive length of the plantarflexors. Clinical examination results will help determine the cause(s).

EXCESSIVE KNEE HYPEREXTENSION

This pattern is characterized by greater than normal knee extension throughout the stance phase (Fig. 14.5). There may or may not be excessive flexion at initial contact, though there is typically a rapid knee extension during the loading response. Knee hyperextension is primarily a function of excessive plantarflexor tightness that does not allow the tibia to advance normally in second rocker, thus contributing to knee hyperextension. Over time, this leads to increasing knee hyperextension in stance and on clinical examination. This pattern is often present with an associated anterior tilt of the trunk.

DOUBLE-BUMP ANKLE PATTERN

This pattern is characterized by a double-bump shape of the ankle kinematic (Fig. 14.6).

219

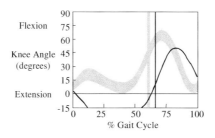

Fig. 14.5. Knee-hyperextension pattern during stance in comparison with the typical motion pattern (solid band). *See CD-Rom, Figure 14.5, for a dynamic illustration.*

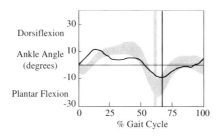

Fig. 14.6. Double-bump ankle pattern in stance with dorsiflexion followed by premature plantarflexion followed by a second dorsiflexion and plantarflexion motion. Typical motion is represented by the solid band. *See CD-Rom, Figure 14.6, for a dynamic illustration.*

Although ankle angle at initial contact may be normal, there is a toe- or foot-flat initial contact due to excessive knee flexion. After initial contact there is a rapid dorsiflexion followed by plantarflexion (possibly a response to the quick stretch on the plantarflexors). This pattern is repeated in the second half of stance. A full description of this pattern can be found in the section on joint kinetic patterns below.

INTERNAL FOOT PROGRESSION

This pattern is characterized by increased internal foot progression in comparison to the direction of progression (Fig. 14.7). This may be result of deformity at the foot and ankle, leading to adductus of the forefoot such as posterior tibialis over-pull. Foot progression, however, is the net result of all that takes place above, and abnormal patterns may have nothing to do with pathology at the foot (see example below).

Multiple joint-segment patterns within one plane

The following section deals with some of the possible combinations of joint motion within a plane. These examples in many cases build on the examples in the previous section. The reader will gain an appreciation of how motion at one joint is not isolated but may affect motion at adjacent joints as well.

220

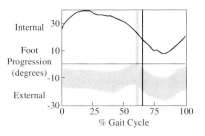

Fig. 14.7. Internal foot progression throughout the gait cycle. Typical motion is represented by the solid band. *See CD-Rom, Figure 14.7, for a dynamic illustration.*

RELATIONSHIP BETWEEN PELVIC AND ANKLE MOTION

A common abnormality in gait in persons with CP is an excessive plantarflexion/knee-extension (PF/KE) couple where the tibia does not advance normally over the plantargrade foot. As a result, it is harder for the person to move the center of gravity forward along the direction of progression. Another mechanism that can allow forward progression is a forward trunk and associated anterior pelvic tilt (Fig. 14.8a). Although this relationship between ankle and pelvic motion is not obvious at initial glance, examination of the same person with an ankle–foot orthosis (AFO) allows insight into the cause of the progressive anteriorly tilting pelvis in stance. With the AFO, the excessive PF/KE couple is eliminated as well as the need for the increasing anterior pelvic tilt (Fig. 14.8b).

SINGLE-BUMP PELVIS AND ASSOCIATED ASYMMETRY IN HIP MOTION

A single-bump pelvic tilt motion (as described above) is a unilateral problem with associated decrease in hip sagittal-plane motion as a result of the decreased disassociation between the pelvis and thigh segments. As a compensation for reduced hip motion, there is an increase in pelvic sagittal-plane motion to allow the thigh segment to rotate posteriorly during the stance phase. However, there is a secondary effect on the opposite side, which includes increased hip sagittal-plane motion (Fig. 14.9). The increase in contralateral hip range of motion during gait is a result of the increased pelvic range of motion and the timing of the peak anterior and posterior pelvic tilt. That is, when the contralateral hip is in the most extension the pelvis is in its most posterior position, and when the contralateral hip is in the most flexion the pelvis is in its most anterior position.

INTERNALLY ROTATED GAIT

A common gait abnormality seen in persons with CP is an internally rotated gait, which is usually characterized by internal foot progression (Tylkowski 1982). One might also observe bilateral in-pointing knees. There are lots of "levels" where abnormal transverse-plane motion can occur, e.g. internally rotated hips, internal tibial torsion, internal knee rotation and/or forefoot adductus. The best way to dissect an internally rotated gait pattern is to use a combination of clinical estimates of bony torsions and transverse-plane kinematics. With this combination of information, the cause of abnormal internal foot progression can be isolated in some circumstances to increased internal hip rotation alone (Fig. 14.10).

221

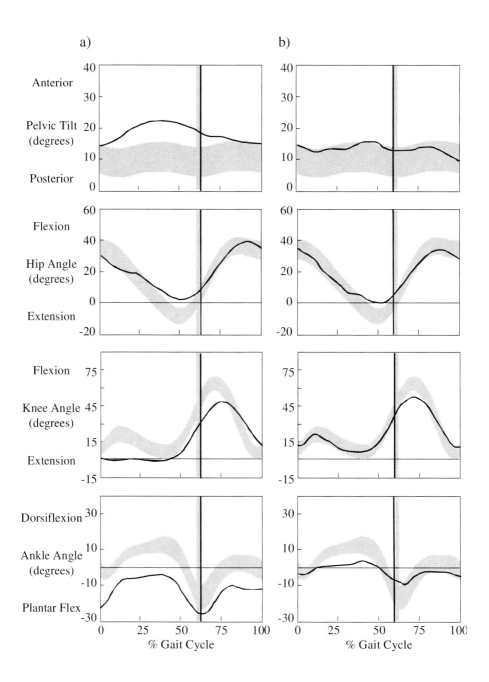

Fig. 14.8. Anterior pelvic tilt and excessive equinus. (a) An increase in anterior pelvic tilt is noted through out the stance phase secondary to progressive equinus in stance during barefoot walking. (b) With an AFO, the excessive equinus is resolved and the increasing anterior pelvic tilt is no longer necessary. *See CD-Rom, Figure 14.8, for a dynamic illustration.*

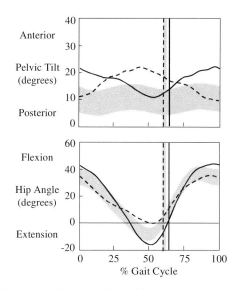

Fig. 14.9. Single-bump pelvic tilt pattern (dashed line) with associated bilateral asymmetric hip motion. With a single-bump pelvic tilt pattern, there is decreased hip range of motion on the ipsilateral side (dashed line) and secondary increased hip range of motion on the contralateral side (solid line). The typical motion pattern is represented by the solid band. *See CD-Rom, Figure 14.9, for a dynamic illustration.*

ASYMMETRICAL HIP ROTATIONS AND ASSOCIATED ASYMMETRICAL PELVIC ROTATION

Unilateral internal hip rotation is typically found in persons with hemiplegia (Õunpuu and DeLuca 2000). If left uncompensated, there would be an in-pointing knee during ambulation. The individual with hemiplegia, however, typically compensates to correct for an in-pointing knee with external rotation of the ipsilateral hemipelvis. As a result of this pelvic rotation, there is an associated internal rotation of the contralateral hemipelvis with compensatory external rotation of the contralateral knee. This complex series of secondary effects and compensations in the transverse plane is plotted in Figure 14.11. The net result of these asymmetries at the hips and pelvis is normal foot progression if no deformity is present below the femur.

Joint kinematic patterns across planes

The above discussions of typical gait patterns have been presented using a single-plane approach to develop our understanding of the primary causes of gait abnormalities at an individual joint, and the possible effect of a gait abnormality on adjacent joints and segments. To be complete, however, gait-analysis data interpretation must also include an understanding of the specific patterns of gait deviations that occur from one plane to another. This is facilitated with data presentation formats that include the coronal-, sagittal- and transverse-plane kinematic plots on one page, which encourages the understanding of the interaction of joint motion across planes, and ultimately other possible causes of certain gait abnormalities. The following examples illustrate combinations of motion relationships that occur from plane

223

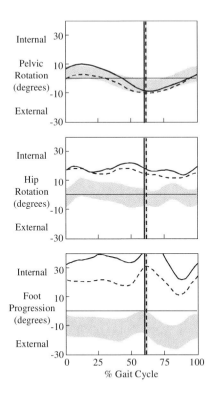

Fig. 14.10. Bilateral internally rotated gait. The transverse-plane kinematics show bilateral internal hip rotation with associated bilateral internal foot progression in comparison with the typical motion pattern (solid band). *See CD-Rom, Figure 14.10, for a dynamic illustration.*

to plane. Identifying these patterns will facilitate the interpretation of gait-analysis data and allow identification of primary versus secondary problems and/or voluntary compensations ("coping responses").

INCREASED PELVIC TRANSVERSE-PLANE MOTION/REDUCED SAGITTAL-PLANE MOTION

Increased pelvic transverse-plane motion is often secondary to reduced sagittal-plane motion. A primary problem of reduced sagittal-plane motion at the bilateral knee and hip joints, which limits step length, can be minimized by a compensatory increase in the transverse-plane motion of the pelvis to increase step length (Fig. 14.12).

INCREASED HIP ABDUCTION IN SWING/REDUCED SAGITTAL-PLANE MOTION

A primary problem of reduced sagittal-plane motion at the bilateral ankle, knee and hip joints may result in a typical compensation of increased hip abduction or circumduction in swing to improve clearance (Fig. 14.13).

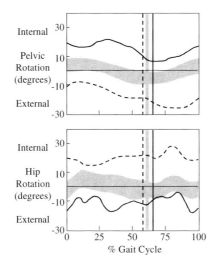

Fig. 14.11. Asymmetrical pelvic rotation compensation. Unilateral internal hip rotation (dashed line) results in a compensatory external rotation of the same side hemipelvis (dashed line). The associated internally rotated right hemipelvis (solid line) results in a secondary external rotation of the right hip (solid line). *See CD-Rom, Figure 14.11, for a dynamic illustration.*

INCREASED CORONAL-PLANE HIP MOTION/INCREASED TRANSVERSE-PLANE PELVIC MOTION

In persons with increased transverse-plane pelvic motion there will be a secondary deviation of increased coronal-plane hip motion (Fig. 14.14). For example, excessive internal rotation of the pelvis at initial contact will result in associated excessive hip abduction at initial contact. As the pelvis rotates through a large range of motion during loading response (from internal to external rotation), there is a simultaneous hip adduction.

INCREASED ASYMMETRIC CORONAL-PLANE HIP MOTION/TRANSVERSE-PLANE PELVIC ASYMMETRY

When there is asymmetry in the transverse-plane pelvic motion there is associated asymmetry of the coronal-plane hip motion (Fig. 14.15). For example, excessive internal rotation of the pelvis at initial contact will result in associated excessive hip abduction at initial contact. Conversely, excessive external rotation of the pelvis at initial contact will result in associated excessive hip adduction at initial contact. The degree of asymmetry at the pelvis is correlated with the degree of asymmetry at the hip. This pattern is typically seen in persons with hemiplegia.

PROGRESSIVE PELVIC EXTERNAL ROTATION/EXCESSIVE PLANTARFLEXION/KNEE-EXTENSION COUPLE

An excessive plantarflexion knee-extension couple characterized by delayed dorsiflexion in second rocker can drive the ipsilateral pelvis into external rotation towards toe-off as the

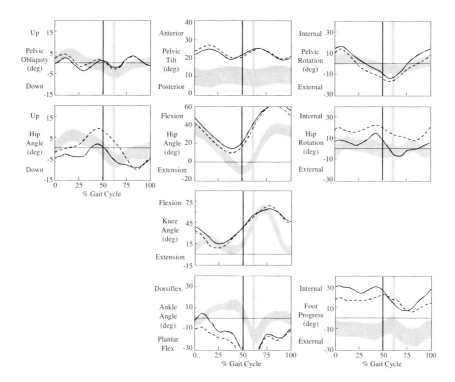

Fig. 14.12. Increased pelvic transverse-plane motion/reduced sagittal-plane motion. The increased transverse-plane pelvic motion (first plot right column) is a compensation for reduced sagittal-plane motion of the knee (third plot middle column) that allows for increased step lengths. Gait data are presented, with the first column representing the coronal, the second column the sagittal, and the third column the transverse planes for the pelvis, hip, knee and ankle. All the following figures are presented using this format. The typical reference data (solid band) were collected in the same gait laboratory. *See CD-Rom, Figure 14.12, for a dynamic illustration.*

rest of the body moves forward (Fig. 14.16). This pattern is typically seen in persons with hemiplegia.

Typical Joint-Kinetic Patterns

A joint kinetic pattern is a specific pattern of joint moment and sometimes power that reflects a specific kinematic presentation. Again, as in the discussion of kinematic patterns it serves as a terminology that facilitates communication in regards to pathological gait as well as understanding of the pathomechanics of pathological gait. A description of the various hills and valleys in these curves has also been described with respect to normal gait and where appropriate are also indicated in the examples below (Winter 1991). The joint kinetic patterns illustrated in this section are all formatted in a similar way, that is, the joint kinematic, followed by the joint moment, followed by the joint power. This allows examination of each parameter with regard to specific phases in the gait cycle. An understanding of the

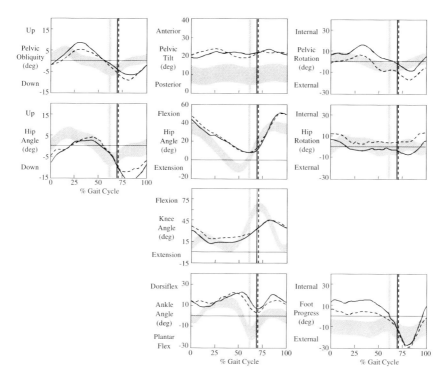

Fig. 14.13. Increased hip abduction in swing secondary to reduced sagittal-plane motion. The increased hip abduction in swing or circumduction (second plot, left column) is a compensation for reduced and delayed peak knee flexion in swing (third plot, middle column) to allow for clearance in swing. *See CD-Rom, Figure 14.13, for a dynamic illustration.*

joint kinetic patterns with associated kinematic and electromyographic data and related clinical information will improve our understanding of the impact of pathology and ultimately the mechanisms of pathological gait. Although the role of joint kinetic patterns in suggesting specific treatments may be limited at this time (Õunpuu et al. 1996), joint kinetic data can provide valuable information about the impact of treatment.

DOUBLE-BUMP ANKLE PATTERN
The double-bump ankle pattern is an extension of the double-bump ankle kinematic pattern, and is defined by a double bump shape not only in the ankle kinematic curve, but in the moment and power curves as well (Fig. 14.17). The use of this terminology, with a background understanding of its basis, reduces the detailed description needed to describe the various aspects of this curve with respect to the phases of the gait cycle. This pattern is found in persons who have spastic plantarflexors, clonus of the plantarflexors and a toe- or foot-flat initial contact during gait. This is the one kinetic pattern that has been connected to a particular treatment protocol (Rose et al. 1993). The specifics of the typically associated ankle joint kinematics and kinetics are described in Table 14.1.

227

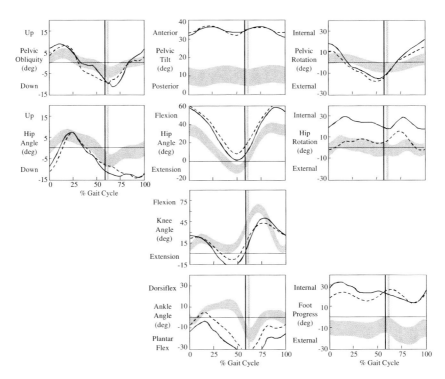

Fig. 14.14. Increased coronal-plane hip motion in loading response secondary to increased transverse-plane pelvic motion. The increased coronal-plane hip motion (second plot in left column) is secondary to the increased transverse-plane pelvic motion (first plot, right column). As the pelvis externally rotates and the hip extends, there is a simultaneous adduction of the hip. *See CD-Rom, Figure 14.14, for a dynamic illustration.*

TABLE 14.1

Specifics of the typically associated ankle-joint kinematics and kinetics: double-bump ankle pattern

Joint kinematic

Neutral or excessive plantarflexion at initial contact

Rapid dorsiflexion which results in a quick stretch of the spastic ankle plantarflexors, which respond by contracting and producing premature plantarflexion

Repeat dorsiflexion followed by plantarflexion in last half of stance (using a similar mechanism as above)

Less than typical dorsiflexion from mid-stance through toe-off

Joint moment

Development of a premature plantarflexor moment in early stance, followed by rapid decrease, increase and decrease in plantarflexor moment (double bump)

Plantarflexor moment 100% stance

Ankle plantarflexor dominance throughout stance

Joint power

Large power absorption in early stance (eccentric contraction of ankle plantarflexors)

Premature power-generation in mid-stance (concentric contraction of ankle plantarflexors)

Inappropriate power generation in mid-stance drives body up not forward

Second-power absorption and generation (A2)

Second-generation peak may be within normal limits

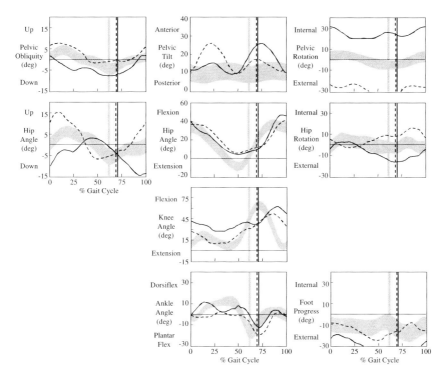

Fig. 14.15. Increased asymmetric coronal-plane hip motion secondary to transverse-plane pelvic asymmetry. At initial contact, when the hip is maximally flexed, there is increased adduction of the left hip (dashed line) and abduction of the right hip (solid line) (second plot, left column) secondary to asymmetry of the pelvis in the transverse plane (first plot, right column). *See CD-Rom, Figure 14.15, for a dynamic illustration.*

KNEE-FLEXOR MOMENT PATTERN

The knee-flexor moment pattern is an extension of the knee hyperextension pattern and is defined by full knee extension or hyperextension in stance, a knee-flexor moment in stance and typically excessive power absorption during loading response (Fig. 14.18). This pattern is found in those persons with full knee extension or knee hyperextension on passive range of motion, plantarflexor spasticity contributing to an excessive PF/KE couple and more often than not a forward trunk lean (see discussion of impact of trunk position below). This pattern is seen also in persons with quadriceps insufficiency such as found in polio (Õunpuu 2002), however, this pathology is not seen in persons with CP. The specifics of the typically associated knee-joint kinematics and kinetics are described in Table 14.2.

KNEE-EXTENSOR MOMENT PATTERN

The knee-extensor moment pattern is an extension of the crouch pattern and is defined by excessive knee flexion in stance, an associated knee-extensor moment in stance and an amodular power pattern (Fig. 14.19). This pattern is typically found in those persons with reduced hip-extensor and or ankle-plantarflexor strength leading to excessive knee flexion

229

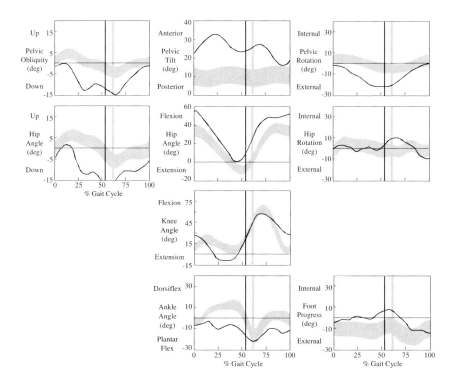

Fig. 14.16. Progressive pelvic external rotation in stance secondary to an excessive plantarflexion knee-extension couple. There is increasing external rotation of the pelvis during stance (first plot, right column) secondary to an excessive PF/KE couple and associated premature plantarflexion and knee hyperextension (third and fourth plots, middle column) which does not allow typical forward rotation of the tibia and "drives" the hemipelvis externally. *See CD-Rom, Figure 14.16 for a dynamic illustration.*

TABLE 14.2

Specifics of the typically associated knee-joint kinematics and kinetics: knee-flexion moment pattern

Joint kinematic
Typically greater than normal knee flexion at initial contact
Rapid knee extension after initial contact
Usually knee hyperextension in mid-stance (not required)
Prolonged knee extension in terminal stance

Joint moment
Rapid development of a knee-flexor moment during loading response
Excessive knee-flexor moment during the majority of stance
Knee-flexor dominance, which may be muscular or ligamentous (and can be confirmed using knee plots, clinical exam and EMG data)

Variable knee moment in pre-swing
Joint power
Increased power absorption during period of rapid knee extension in stance
Associated eccentric contraction of the knee-flexors and/or stretching of the soft-tissue structures

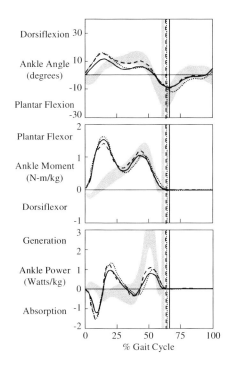

Fig. 14.17. Double-bump ankle pattern. The ankle kinematic, moment and power for three gait cycles for a patient with spastic diplegic cerebral palsy is plotted versus the typical reference band. The double-bump shape is reflected in the three plots during the stance phase. *See CD-Rom, Figure 14.17, for a dynamic illustration.*

or crouch (Õunpuu 2002). The knee-extensor moment pattern is characterized by continuous coactivity of the quadriceps and hamstrings. However, there is a net knee-extensor dominant moment required to prevent collapse. The specifics of the typically associated knee-joint kinematics and kinetics are described in Table 14.3.

HIP-EXTENSOR MOMENT PATTERN
The hip-extensor moment pattern is characterized by a shift towards increased hip flexion in stance, an associated increased hip-extensor moment and power generation in stance with delayed crossover to a flexor moment pattern or power-absorption pattern (Fig. 14.20a). The cause of the hip-extensor pattern varies and is not, in many cases, a result of pathology at the hip joint itself. A hip-extensor moment pattern may be secondary to excessive knee flexion and its associated causes and/or anterior pelvic (Fig. 14.20b) and forward trunk tilt and their respective causes. The specifics of the typically associated hip-joint kinematics and kinetics are described in Table 14.4.

HIP-ABDUCTOR AVOIDANCE MOMENT PATTERN
The hip-abductor avoidance (adductor) moment pattern is characterized by a minimal or

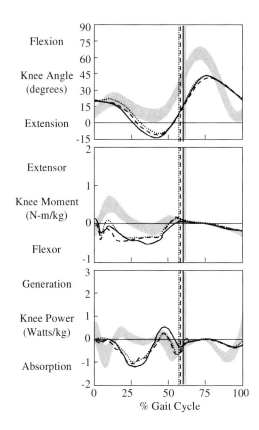

Fig. 14.18. Knee-flexor moment pattern. The knee kinematic, moment and power for three gait cycles for a patient with spastic diplegic cerebral palsy is plotted versus the typical reference band. There is knee hyperextension, a large knee-flexor moment and associated inappropriate power absorption. *See CD-Rom, Figure 14.18, for a dynamic illustration.*

TABLE 14.3

Specifics of the typically associated knee-joint kinematics and kinetics: knee-extensor moment pattern

Joint kinematic
Greater than normal knee flexion at initial contact
Continued excessive knee flexion during 100% stance
Minimal knee sagittal-plane range of motion in stance

Joint moment
Rapid development of extensor moment during loading response
Knee-extensor moment 100% stance phase
Associated with dominant and continuous activity of the quadriceps

Joint power
Varies depending on knee range of motion in stance
Typically no significant increase in power absorption/generation

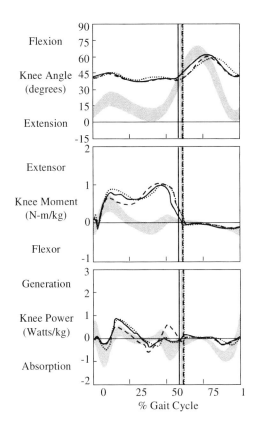

Fig. 14.19. Knee-extensor moment pattern. The knee kinematic, moment and power for three gait cycles for a patient with spastic quadriplegic cerebral palsy is plotted versus the typical reference band. There is knee flexion, a large knee-extensor moment throughout stance and an amodular power pattern. *See CD-Rom, Figure 14.19, for a dynamic illustration.*

TABLE 14.4
Specifics of the typically associated hip-joint kinematics and kinetics: hip-extensor moment patten

Joint kinematic
Shifting towards increased hip flexion throughout the gait cycle

Joint moment
Prolonged and greater than normal hip-extensor moment stance
Associated with increased hip-extensor activity
Reduced or minimal and delayed hip-flexor moment near toe-off

Joint power
Prolonged and greater than normal hip-power generation from initial contact through to terminal stance (concentric contraction of the hip-extensors)
Reduced and delayed power absorption in terminal stance

233

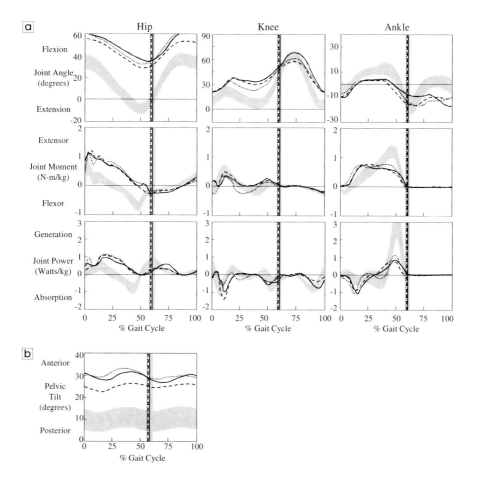

Fig. 14.20. Hip-extensor moment pattern. (a) The hip, knee and ankle kinematic, moment and power for three gait cycles for a patient with spastic quadriplegic cerebral palsy is plotted versus the typical reference band. The increased hip-extensor moment is required both to sustain the excessive knee flexion in stance to prevent collapse and to support the anterior pelvic tilt (b) and forward trunk lean (not shown). *See CD-Rom, Figure 14.20a, for a dynamic illustration.*

TABLE 14.5
Specifics of the typically associated hip-joint kinematics and kinetics: hip-abductor avoidance pattern

Joint kinematic
Lateral trunk lean during stance when there is the largest demand on the hip-abductors
Ipsilateral hemipelvic depression in stance with associated contralateral pelvic elevation in swing
Abnormal hip motion throughout the stance phase (similar modulation as pelvis)

Joint moment
Reduced hip-abductor moment throughout stance

Joint power
Minimal

234

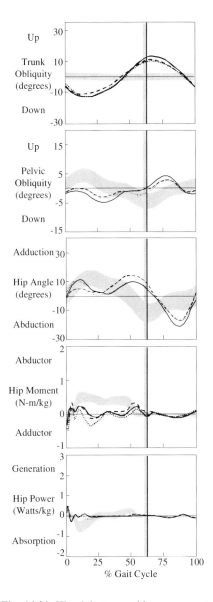

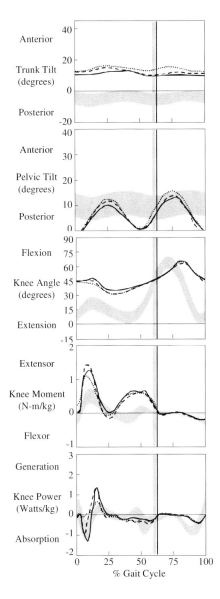

Fig. 14.21. Hip-abductor avoidance moment pattern. The shoulder and trunk kinematics and hip kinematic, moment and power in the coronal plane for three gait cycles for a patient with spastic diplegic cerebral palsy is plotted versus the typical reference band. The large lateral trunk lean shifts the centre of gravity laterally and results in a reduction of the hip-abductor moment. *See CD-Rom, Figure 14.21, for a dynamic illustration.*

Fig. 14.22. Knee-extensor moment pattern. The sagittal-plane kinematics for the shoulder, upper body and pelvis and kinematics and kinetics for the knee for three gait cycles for a patient with spastic diplegic cerebral palsy is plotted versus the typical reference band. The large forward trunk lean results in the reduction of the knee-extensor moment pattern from what it would have been given the knee flexion in stance alone. *See CD-Rom, Figure 14.22, for a dynamic illustration.*

no hip-abductor moment in stance (Fig. 14.21). This is typically seen in patients with hip-abductor insufficiency that does not allow a typical hip-abductor moment in stance. The patient will then compensate by shifting the body center of gravity laterally through a lateral trunk lean. This will minimize the strength demands on the hip-abductors as the resultant ground reaction force passes closer and closer to the hip center. The specifics of the typically associated hip-joint kinematics and kinetics are described in Table 14.5.

ROLE OF UPPER-BODY (TRUNK) POSITION AND MOTION ON KINETIC PATTERNS
A discussion of joint kinetic patterns is not complete without some discussion of the role of trunk position and motion on the lower-extremity joint kinetics. As discussed in Chapter 8, knowledge of trunk motion during gait will aid in the understanding of the lower-extremity kinetics, which in many cases is related to muscle-strength issues. Adaptations in trunk motion can result in reduction of specific muscle demands by reducing the external moments (Õunpuu et al. 1996). This is seen commonly in persons with CP who have hip-abductor insufficiency as seen in the above example. To minimize the requirements of the hip-abductors and therefore reduce the hip-abductor moment, the body center for gravity may be shifted laterally.

An atypical trunk position as a result of other causes, such as a forward trunk-tilt due to severe anterior pelvic tilt, will also affect the lower-extremity kinetics by shifting the body center of gravity forward. This can lead to unexpected moments in the lower extremity. For example, it would be predicted that a person with severe knee flexion in stance would have a net internal knee-extensor moment pattern. However, a forward trunk-lean will reduce the magnitude of the moment even with the relatively severe knee flexion in stance (Fig.14.22). In this example, appreciating trunk position allows the clinician to better interpret the knee moments.

Conclusions
The above examples in no way provide a complete list of all the gait patterns and relationships that occur in persons with CP, but they illustrate a framework for the interpretation of gait data. It is through this systematic approach in the interpretation of gait analysis data from the individual joint, followed by multiple joints in one plane to examining the relationships across planes that a comprehensive understanding of gait pathology is possible. The addition of the kinetics patterns allows us to appreciate the mechanics of these atypical gait patterns and provides us with a better understanding of the role of trunk position in pathological gait. Typically, a specific joint kinematic or kinetic pattern is associated with a specific list of possible causes. This provides us with a framework with which to identify the problems and possible causes of gait pathology and allows a more systematic approach for making treatment decisions. The specific treatment approach related to a particular gait pattern, however, is dependent on the philosophy of the treating physician and not dictated by the gait pattern itself. The gait analysis data provides information with which to make more informed treatment decisions. Ultimately with this approach there will be better outcomes. Although the patterns discussed in this chapter are typical for patients with CP, the concepts apply to gait analysis data interpretation in any gait pathology.

REFERENCES

Davis R, DeLuca P. (1996) Clinical gait analysis: current methods and future directions. In: Harris GE, editor. *Human Motion Analysis: Current Applications and Future Directions*. Piscataway, NJ: IEEE Press. p 17–42.

Kadaba MP, Ramakrishnan HK, Wootten ME, Cochran GV. (1991) Gait pattern recognition in spastic diplegia. *Dev Med Child Neurol* **33:** 28. (Abstract.)

Õunpuu S. (2002) Gait analysis in orthopaedics. In: Fitzgerald R, Kaufer H, Malkani A, editors. *Orthopaedics*. St Louis: C.V. Mosby. p 86–107.

Õunpuu S, DeLuca PA. (2000) Gait analysis. In: Neville B, Goodman R, editors. *Congenital Hemiplegia*. London: Mac Keith Press. p 81–97.

Õunpuu S, Davis RB, DeLuca PA. (1996) Joint kinetics: methods, interpretation and treatment decision-making in children with cerebral palsy and myelomeningocele. *Gait Posture* **4:** 62–78.

Rose SA, DeLuca PA, Davis RB 3rd, Ounpuu S, Gage JR. (1993) Kinematic and kinetic evaluation of the ankle after lengthening of the gastrocnemius fascia in children with cerebral palsy. *J Pediatr Orthop* **13:** 727–732.

Ruwe PA, Gage JR, Ozonoff MB, DeLuca PA. (1992) Clinical determination of femoral anteversion. A comparison with established techniques. *J Bone Joint Surg Am* **74:** 820–830.

Sutherland DH, Cooper L. (1978) The pathomechanics of progressive crouch gait in spastic diplegia. *Orthop Clin North Am* **9:** 143–154.

Sutherland DH, Davids JR. (1993) Common gait abnormalities of the knee in cerebral palsy. *Clin Orthop* **288:** 139–147.

Tylkowski CM. (1982) Internal rotation gait in spastic cerebral palsy. In: Nelson JP, editor. *The Hip: Proceedings of the 10th Open Scientific Meeting of the Hip Society*. St Louis: C.V. Mosby. p 89–125.

Winter DA. (1991) *The Biomechanics and Motor Control of Human Gait: Normal, Elderly and Pathological*. Waterloo, Ontario: University of Waterloo Press.

Winters TF Jr, Gage JR, Hicks R. (1987) Gait patterns in spastic hemiplegia in children and young adults. *J Bone Joint Surg Am* **69:** 437–441.

15
AN OVERVIEW OF TREATMENT

James R. Gage

The previous chapters have provided us with a background on which to build a program of treatment for pathologic gait in cerebral palsy. We now know something about how the brain controls locomotion, and the typical patterns of cerebral injury in cerebral palsy. We have studied normal gait and how it can be measured. We have learned about the static and dynamic assessment of the involved child, including physical examination, observation of gait, gait analysis and energy assessment. Finally, we have considered the mechanisms by which pathologic gait arises and which elements of that pathology are amenable to correction. As such we can now start to consider a logical approach to treatment that is based on that pathology.

Recall that in a child with cerebral palsy, the sequence of events starts with the primary abnormalities (balance difficulties, loss of selective motor control and abnormal tone), and that these occur as a direct result of the neurologic injury. These primary abnormalities then disturb normal growth processes and, by so doing, generate the secondary abnormalities that are related to growth (muscle contractures and lever-arm dysfunction). Consequently, if we wish to maximize function and minimize deformity, we must try to minimize the primary problems produced by the neurological injury and prevent, to the greatest degree possible, the secondary abnormalities of growth. Obviously this is easier said than done, but with a rational approach to treatment of each child we encounter, we can achieve it to varying degrees. In any discussion of treatment principles, however, we must go back to the first principle of medical treatment that was put forward by Hippocrates, i.e. do the sick no harm. Although the ability to walk is very important to all of us, it is not the most important objective for the adult patient with cerebral palsy.

Goal-setting

Bleck (1987) reported that when adults were questioned about their goals, they reported the following priorities: (1) communication, (2) activities of daily living, (3) mobility, and (4) walking.

Parents in particular tend to fixate on walking as the most important goal for their children. I have encountered many cases where parents and/or physicians have had such unrealistic expectations about a child's ability to walk that it has resulted in the loss of both independent mobility and activities of daily living (Fig. 15.1). Realistic goal-setting must therefore be the first priority. For example, although many children with spastic quadriplegia have some ability to walk, Root states that only about 22% of quadriplegic cerebral palsy patients are ambulatory as adults (Bleck et al. 1977). As such, for most quadriplegic patients wheelchair mobility with independent transfer may be a more realistic goal than independent

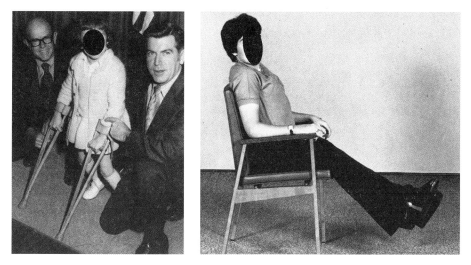

Fig. 15.1. Unrealistic expectations combined with iatrogenic injury. A montage of a patient preoperatively as a child and 12 years later as an adult. In the interim she had six major bilateral lower-extremity surgeries which included subtalar arthrodeses, tendo-Achilles lengthenings, distal hamstring releases, adductor tenotomies with anterior branch neurectomies, and bilateral varus derotational femoral osteotomies with iliopsoas recessions. Not only has she lost her ability to walk, but with her stiff extended knees she has lost her ability to transfer. The iatrogenic problems created by an unrealistic effort to improve her ambulation have resulted in a loss of independent mobility and activities of daily living. As physicians we must be very careful not to add iatrogenic problems to children who already bear a heavy disability

ambulation. Therefore it is important to set specific treatment objectives that are realistic for each individual. In this we have received invaluable guidance from a personal communication by Dr James Cary, who until his retirement was the Director of Education at Newington Children's Hospital. During the first week of each new orthopaedic residency rotation, he would give a lecture to the incoming residents in which he put forth these orthopaedic treatment principles for a child with a neuromuscular disability. (1) Define the end-product in terms of long-range treatment objectives. (2) Identify the patient's problems, both immediate and future, with precision. (3) Analyze the effects of growth on the problems, with and without the proposed treatment. (4) Consider valid treatment alternatives, including non-treatment. (5) Treat the whole child, not just his motor-skeletal parts.

This, then, is our task when faced with a child with cerebral palsy. We must do a thorough history and clinical examination, identify and categorize the problems, and then formulate valid treatment objectives in each of the areas in which the child is involved. Since many body systems are involved and we wish to optimize the outcome in each of the areas of involvement, evaluation is best done with a team of specialists.

The needs of a particular patient relate directly to the type of cerebral palsy and the degree of involvement. For example, because of their poor selective motor control, the major needs of children with athetosis (one of the abnormal tone patterns that can arise from injury to the basal ganglia) are usually communication and activities of daily living. Independent mobility may also be a goal, but this is usually accomplished with a power-chair (often with a custom-built control system that has been specifically adapted for the child by the orthotist). Seizures and mental retardation are uncommon in these children. From an orthopaedic standpoint, fixed contractures are uncommon and, in general, surgery designed to improve ambulation is unpredictable and fraught with hazard. For example, if the hip-adductors are lengthened, these children will often develop a fixed abduction deformity, something that is much less likely to occur in a child with pure spasticity. In addition to poor selective motor control, children with injury to the basal ganglia also have severe difficulties with balance and use of the upper extremities. Thus walking is rarely an achievable goal in this group of patients, and so the developmental pediatrician, therapists and orthotists are much more likely to be the primary-caregivers than the orthopaedic surgeon.

Children who are involved in all four limbs (quadriplegia) have a more extensive brain lesion than those with diplegia. Consequently they have more proprioception problems, poor selective motor control (only about 22% of them are able to ambulate as adults), and a higher incidence of mental retardation and seizures. From an orthopaedic standpoint, in children with total body involvement, ambulation is often not practical and/or possible (Bleck et al. 1977). The goal is frequently independent or assisted transfers, with some limited household ambulation (if possible). The major orthopaedic problems of these children center on scoliosis, hip subluxation/dislocation and/or severe foot deformities: so the goal of the orthopaedist for these children is to prevent spinal deformity, maintain the hips located and mobile, prevent knee contractures, and keep the feet plantargrade and shoeable. The specifics of the orthopaedic management of these problems have been adequately discussed in other orthopaedic texts and will not be reiterated here (Bleck 1987, Rang 1990). Residential care will eventually be necessary in about 82% of these individuals (Bleck et al. 1977).

Children with spastic diplegia and/or hemiplegia nearly always walk. In general, however, previous orthopaedic treatment has not been based on the pathophysiology of the condition. Because of this, plus the fact that surgical evaluation was usually based entirely on the physical examination and visual observation of gait without the benefit of gait analysis, I feel that the majority of our previous orthopaedic interventions were poorly conceived and often harmful. The initial surgery usually consisted of muscle-tendon lengthening (typically tendo-Achilles and/or hamstring lengthening). Bony deformities were generally ignored, unless there was hip subluxation and/or severe foot deformities. Following surgery, the child was immobilized in plaster for prolonged periods while the muscles healed. Then s/he underwent an extended period of therapy after each procedure. The usual end-result was excessive morbidity and permanent weakness. Furthermore, since the pathology was never addressed in a comprehensive manner, surgery was generally repeated multiple times during the course of the patient's childhood. Consequently, the individual spent most of her/his childhood either having or recovering from surgery. Mercer Rang referred to this as the "diving or birthday syndrome" (Rang 1990) (Fig. 15.2). That is, "the child had an operation every birthday and physical therapy all year long".

Team treatment
Appropriate treatment of this complex condition not only demands a team: the team must

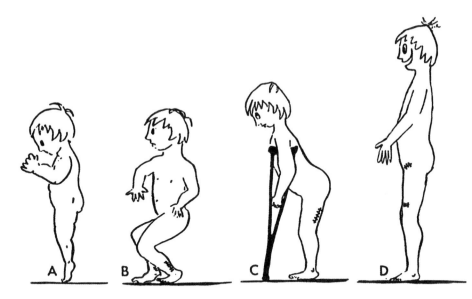

Fig. 15.2. Staging of orthopaedic surgery. The typical dilemma of the child with staged surgery. The child on the left has equinus contractures, but has increased tone in his hip flexors and hamstrings as well. Following tendo-Achilles lengthening a crouch gait develops. The hamstrings are lengthened next, but since the hip-flexors are still contracted, the child must now stand with hip flexion and so can not balance his body mass over his base of support without crutches. Following a fourth surgical procedure to lengthen the hip-flexors, the child can finally stand erect. Mercer Rang refers to this sequence of surgeries as the "diving or birthday syndrome", i.e. an operation each birthday and physical therapy all year long. (Drawing used by permission of the artist, Mercer Rang MD, Toronto.)

be one in which the members communicate with each other. The team approach has become the cornerstone of our treatment program. This does not mean that the child needs to see each member of the team at each visit. For that matter, s/he may never need to see some members of the team at all. Rather it means that each member of the team is familiar with all of the elements of the cerebral palsy problem and is also aware of the specific contributions that each of the other members might offer to the solution of the problem. As such, each member of the team must be willing to refer the patient to the appropriate member of the team for treatment when s/he encounters a problem that is outside her or his expertise. Because of the diverse nature of these children's problems, the team needs to be diverse as well. At our center, the cerebral palsy team embraces the following disciplines: developmental pediatrics, orthopaedic surgery, neurosurgery, ophthalmology, physical and occupational therapy, speech and hearing therapy, orthotics, psychology and social work. It is difficult to treat these children well without access to a specialized center that contains these many disciplines. At the end of the clinic visit at our center, a clinical nurse reviews the problems with the patient and family to ensure that all of the needs have been met.

In our program, the physician who first sees the child is generally a pediatric neurologist, a developmental pediatrician or a pediatric physiatrist. Each of these specialists is qualified to make the diagnosis of cerebral palsy, but the pediatric physiatrist usually does the initial

241

treatment and follow-up. S/he supervises the child's physical/occupational therapy programs, requests appropriate orthotics, and monitors not only the development of specific structures such as the hips and feet, but also global development as a whole. In addition, the physiatrist has the training and expertise to apply stretching casts, administer oral drugs to control tone and/or use injectable drugs such as botulinum toxin and/or phenol to prevent the development of contractures. My personal feeling is that a pediatric orthopaedist should also see the child at about 1 year of age and then at appropriate intervals of a year or more, depending upon the relationship between the physiatrist and orthopaedist and the physiatrist's comfort with orthopaedic problems.

Treatment protocols

The development of treatment protocols is also an integral part of team treatment. These are needed to ensure that the diagnosis is correct, and that associated deformities are not missed. If this is not done, disasters are sure to arise. As an example, a 5-year-old child with the diagnosis of spastic diplegia was once referred to me by a qualified pediatric neurologist. Unfortunately the correct diagnosis of medulloblastoma of the cerebellum was not made until after we had started to notice progression of neurological involvement into her upper extremities and had ordered an magnetic resonance imaging study of her brain. The lesson is that the diagnosis should never be presumed until one is sure that the specific, necessary, diagnostic studies have been done to rule out other treatable conditions. Even when the diagnosis of cerebral palsy is established, apparent neurological progression should trigger a referral back to the pediatric neurologist or neurosurgeon, as this may be indicative of a correctible problem (for example, hydrocephalus secondary to shunt obstruction). I have also had children referred to me on several occasions with dislocation or severe subluxation of the hip simply because the physician did not suspect the condition and take a routine anteroposterior roentgenogram of the pelvis. We have found that without the benefit of treatment protocols that are worked out and agreed upon by all members of the team, it is difficult to avoid such errors.

The treatment plan

At the appropriate stage in the child's development, his or her tone should be assessed and a decision made as to whether or not surgical reduction of tone is warranted. For most children, the optimal window of time to consider spasticity reduction is between about 5 and 8 years of age. By this age the neurological and social development of the child is usually adequate to go through both the surgery and the rehabilitation that follows. In addition, if a baclofen pump is being considered, the child is usually not large enough to allow its implantation until at least age 5. At our center we have put together a "spasticity evaluation team" to do this evaluation. This team consists of a pediatric orthopaedist, a physiatrist and a neurosurgeon. Ideally it would be nice to have the luxury to refer most of the children in our clinic to the spasticity evaluation team, but their number is too large to allow that. Instead we rely on the expertise of the child's principal physician (physiatrist or orthopaedist) to determine whether or not referral to the spasticity evaluation team is warranted. If a child is referred for spasticity evaluation, gait analysis will usually be done prior to that

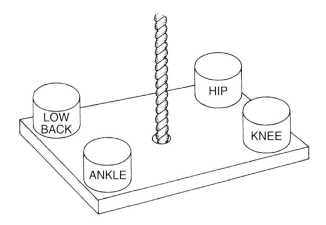

Fig. 15.3. Balance between joints. A board suspended from a rope with a weight at each corner illustrates the concept of balance between the lower-extremity joints and lumbar spine. For example, if surgery such as a tendo-Achilles lengthening is done in isolation, it will upset the balance between the ankle below and the knee and hip above. The usual result is a reduction in the plantarflexion/knee-extension couple such that the hip- and knee-flexors become dominant and contractures develop at those joints. The gastrocsoleus is no longer strong enough to restrain the tibia in the face of the contractures above, and the knee passes through the plane of the ground reaction force so that it now generates an external flexion moment. The result is a crouch gait which is progressive over time.

referral, provided that the child walks well enough to allow it. In that way, the results will be available to the spasticity evaluation team at the time of the child's initial visit. Based on the evaluation by the spasticity evaluation team, one of four decisions is usually made: (1) tone reduction is not indicated at this time; (2) oral medications should be tried to control the abnormal tone; (3) the child is a good candidate for selective dorsal rhizotomy; or (4) the child is a good candidate for the intrathecal baclofen pump.

If tone reduction is elected, the pediatric physiatrist monitors the postoperative rehabilitation.

Finally, once the child's gait has matured and is stable and issues relating to abnormal muscle tone have been addressed, consideration should be given to single-stage correction of his/her remaining growth deformities (muscle contractures and/or lever-arm dysfunction). Based on the pathophysiology of cerebral palsy, which we have discussed in previous chapters, we should now be well aware of the concept of *balance between joints*. Many of the muscles in the lower extremities are biarticular so that if a surgeon performs a procedure at the ankle, it will also have an effect on the knee. Similarly, an isolated procedure at the knee will affect the ankle and the hip as well (Fig. 15.3). We want to avoid Rang's "diving or birthday syndrome".

In our center, therefore, all of the child's orthopaedic deformities are corrected as part of a single surgical procedure. We refer to this as multiple lower-extremity procedures (MLEP). In the case of hemiplegia, one surgeon can do all the corrections. In children with diplegia, however, two teams of surgeons are used (one team operating on each side), in order to allow correction of all of the bony and soft tissue deformities within a reasonable period of time. The specifics of how this is accomplished will be discussed in more detail when we come to the chapters dealing with the treatment of hemiplegia and diplegia.

With this background in mind, we are now ready to discuss the various types of treatment that are available for cerebral palsy. We will begin with non-operative treatment. Following that we will discuss the surgical treatment of spasticity, and then go on to the correction of growth deformities (lever-arm dysfunction and muscle contractures).

REFERENCES

Bleck EE. (1987) *Orthopaedic Management in Cerebral Palsy*. London: Mac Keith Press. p 17–64, 142–143, 392–480.
Bleck EE, Root L, Silver CM. (1977) Orthopaedic surgery in cerebral palsy: hemiplegia, diplegia, and quadriplegia. *AAOS Instructional Course Lecture*.
Rang M. (1990) Cerebral palsy. In: Morrissy R, editor. *Pediatric Orthopaedics*. Philadelphia: J.B. Lippincott. p 465–506.

16
NON-OPERATIVE TREATMENT

Mark E. Gormley, Linda E. Krach and Sue Murr

Physical therapy

Although no definitive evidence exists to support the positive or negative effects of physical therapy (PT) on the movement dysfunction associated with cerebral palsy (CP) (Campbell et al. 1990, Anderson et al. 1992), children diagnosed with CP are often referred to PT as one of the first interventions of choice. This seems to indicate that clinical practices and beliefs continue to be based more on experience and empirical evidence than clinical research. Campbell and colleagues (1990) surveyed a sample of 200 physician members of the American Academy of Pediatrics and the American Academy of Cerebral Palsy and Developmental Medicine, to obtain their opinions of the efficacy of PT for children with cerebral palsy. These physicians were asked to rate both positive and negative potential outcomes, grouped into five categories: (1) physical and motor outcomes, (2) neurologic, (3) cognitive, (4) social and family, and (5) functional outcomes. The results indicated that more than 50% believed that PT for children with CP is likely to result in the prevention of contractures and deformities, improved functional abilities, independence through the use of assistive technology, and endurance and ability to profit from education, and that it can maintain functional motor performance. More than 75% of physicians also believe that therapists enhance parental abilities to manage their children and cope with the consequences of disability. About 30% believe that PT leads to excessive costs and time demands on the family.

Physical therapists who treat these children need to evaluate the evidence available concerning the variety of treatment techniques and develop examination and intervention strategies that are logical and assist the family in their goals. Many physical therapists may help families in long-term management of their child with cerebral palsy, assisting with referrals to appropriate providers, communication among health-care professionals and community providers, and providing direct episodes of therapy dependent upon the child's age or timing of other interventions.

There are many challenges in determining the effectiveness of interventions chosen (Barry 1996) and defining optimal treatment with respect to treatment techniques, and frequency and duration of therapy. Interventions are chosen with the goal of addressing the areas of impairment, functional limitations or disability, three of the dimensions listed in the National Center for Medical Rehabilitation and Research's model for classifying the dimensions of disability. *Impairment* includes the loss or abnormality of physiological, psychological or anatomical structure or function. *Functional limitation* involves the restriction of the ability to perform a physical action, activity or task in an efficient, typically expected or competent manner. *Disability* refers to the inability to engage in age-specific, gender-related or sex-specific roles in a particular social context and physical environment (Butler and Darrah 2001). Previous outcomes research has focused primarily on impairment, with little known about the impacts of PT interventions on functional limitations and disability (Barry 1996). Information is needed to connect changes in impairment with improved function and diminished disability across a person's lifespan, and may require the use of multiple outcomes measures to determine.

The confounding factors in the efforts to study the efficacy of treatment interventions include the lack of consistency in descriptive terminology and the heterogeneity of patients with CP and the challenge to categorize them similarly by various medical professionals. The Gross Motor Function Classification System may help here. Palisano and colleagues (1997) have developed a 5-level classification system with clinically meaningful distinctions in motor function among levels. Level 1, the highest level, represents one end of this continuum of children with mild motor impairments; level 5, at the other end of the continuum, represents children who lack the most basic antigravity postural control.

Another deterrent to randomized controlled studies is the ethical concern of leaving a control group untreated, and the willingness of parents to include their child in a study which may lead to non-treatment for a period of time (Barry 1996).

Therapists working in clinical settings must make decisions about the interventions used and recommended for children and adults across their lifetime. All clinicians have assumptions about motor development and motor control that influence their examination and treatment of patients. These assumptions may not always be well articulated. The Guide to Physical Therapy Practice has established a framework to enable physical therapists, clinicians and researchers to analyze their patients and pose questions and hypotheses for interventions (Howle 1999). The five elements of patient management include examination, evaluation, diagnosis, prognosis and intervention, all of which are designed to maximize outcomes. Interventions are chosen according to the information gathered, and are synthesized during the examination, evaluation and development of a diagnosis and prognosis. The remainder of this chapter presents several of the more common interventions chosen for patients with CP, giving consideration to the concept of evidence-based practice.

NEURODEVELOPMENTAL TREATMENT

Neurodevelopmental treatment (NDT) is one of the most common approaches used by pediatric physical therapists treating children with cerebral palsy and movement disorders (Barry 1996, 2001). Karel and Berta Bobath began to develop neurodevelopmental treatment in the 1940s. Karel was a neuropsychiatrist who used his understanding of the neuroscience theories to explain the clinical observations of his wife Berta, a physical therapist. The Bobaths considered the treatment a "living concept", indicating the evolution of the treatment as their understanding of neuroscience and their clinical observations increased and evolved. The traditional tenets of NDT are to inhibit abnormal tone and persistent primitive reflexes and to facilitate normal movement (Bobath and Bobath 1984). In their efforts to give children with CP the experience and sensation of normal movement, they utilized reflex-inhibiting postures and focused on the normal developmental sequence. This practice has given way to an emphasis on functional goals and a lessening of the overemphasis of the inhibition of the primitive reflexes. Since functional carry-over did not necessarily occur as a result of the normal movement experience, the specific handling techniques learned by students in the 8-week training-course, once considered to be the essence of NDT, have been replaced by emphasis on achieving functional goals. Goals such as transitions from sit to stand, with emphasis on weightbearing and weight-shifts, are included in the discussion of improved quality of movement (Bly 1991).

Many researchers have studied the efficacy of NDT. The challenges to these studies include a lack of standardized treatments, variable state of practice in the field (with therapists practicing according to the tenets of NDT as taught at their course and not updated), and the skill level of the therapist (Butler and Darrah 2001).

STRETCHING

Another common treatment intervention initiated early for children with CP is stretching, both passive and active. The goals of stretching include maintaining or regaining range of motion in order to prevent or reduce contracture and maximize function (Cherry 1980). Tightness occurs in the muscles of children with cerebral palsy because of the overexcitation associated with hypertonicity and the co-contraction of muscles in abnormal patterns. This is especially true of the two joint muscles, such as the hamstrings, the rectus femoris and the gastrocnemius muscles in the lower extremity. When impaired selective motor control causes these children and adults to move with restricted movement patterns, full range of motion is not achieved and appropriate growth of the agonist and antagonist muscles does not occur.

Passive stretching can assist with lengthening the elastic portion of the muscle and improve passive range of motion. However, unless it is accompanied by active use of the muscles or passive positioning support such as orthoses, night splints, casting or the use of adaptive equipment such as standers, the benefits of stretching cannot be maintained. Tardieu and colleagues (1988) studied the optimal length of time a muscle, specifically the soleus muscle, must be stretched each day to prevent contracture. Their aim was not to evaluate different kinds of treatment, but to study the threshold time necessary to prevent contracture, regardless of the method of stretching. Their results indicate that to prevent contracture, the soleus muscle must be stretched for 6 hours in each 24-hour period.

STRENGTHENING

Many physical therapists were taught that strengthening a child with hypertonicity would lead to increased hypertonicity. The Bobaths supported this concern even though Dr Winthrop Phelps, a contemporary of theirs in the 1940s, was developing a program for patients with cerebral palsy that included resistive exercise (Barry 1996). Proponents of NDT still may have difficulty advocating strengthening exercises because of the concern that spasticity and associated reactions will increase and also because of a conviction that weakness is not a primary problem for patients with CP. This notion has been disputed by Wiley and Damiano (1998), in a study comparing lower-extremity strength in children with diplegia, children with hemiplegia and their age-matched peers without cerebral palsy. They found that children with CP do have weakness, especially in their distal musculature (Wiley and Damiano 1998, Damiano et al. 2001b).

It has been suggested that emphasis on strengthening weak muscles, combined with motor-learning principles, are of greater benefit than focusing on hypertonicity and its reduction (Guiliani 1991). Damiano and colleagues are advocates of strength training for children with cerebral palsy (Guiliani 1991, Damiano et al. 1995a, 1995b, 1999, 2000, 2001a, 2001b, 2002, Damiano and Abel 1998). They describe training protocols using at least 65% of the maximum voluntary contraction, four sets of five repetitions, with a training frequency of three times per week for six weeks. The results of a study using this protocol indicate that all 14 subjects with CP gained strength in the quadriceps femoris muscle and a reduction in crouch and increase in stride length per gait analysis. An additional study completed by this group demonstrated improved muscle strength as well as improvements in gait velocity and gross motor skills (Damiano and Abel 1998). MacPhail and Kramer (1995) found that an eight-week strengthening program for mildly affected adolescents yielded strength gains of 12%–30% in knee-extensors and flexors without an increase in spasticity.

There also seem to be additional benefits of a strengthening and fitness program when projected across a lifetime. Benefits are reported in the areas of quality of life in terms of interacting with peers, improving self-esteem, and taking responsibility for one's own health and fitness (Barry 2001). These outcomes need to be researched more fully, as do the functional changes attributed to strengthening. Modalities for strengthening provide patients with cerebral palsy choices for fitness much like their peers. These include the use of fitness centers rather than direct physical therapy, and other activities such as aquatics, cycling, and horse-riding. With adaptations to commercially available equipment, or the availability of specially designed adaptive equipment, many children and adults with CP can participate in active lifestyles with their families and friends.

ELECTROTHERAPY

Electrical stimulation is another treatment intervention used for patients with cerebral palsy. Included in the variety of goals for the use of electrical stimulation are: maintaining or improving range of motion, facilitating voluntary muscle control and increasing force production, improving functional activities such as gait, and reducing spasticity (Barry 1996). Pape and colleagues (1993) studied the use of low-intensity electrical stimulation, with no apparent muscle contraction, during sleep to produce muscle growth. They found increased muscle bulk as early as 6–12 weeks after the initiation of the stimulation. Hazelwood and colleagues have documented increase in range of motion, for example increased dorsiflexion when the tibialis anterior was stimulated, but with no significant improvements in gait (Hazlewood et al. 1994, Barry 1996).

Neuromuscular electrical stimulation has been used to stimulate a muscle to the level of contraction and has been used on both agonist and antagonist muscles. This can be especially helpful after other surgical interventions such as a selective dorsal rhizotomy or muscle transfer (Carmick 1993). Overall, the evidence for the efficacy of electrical stimulation is inconclusive (Barry 1996). Hence, more study of the efficacy of this treatment modality is needed.

Biofeedback and the use of surface electromyography (EMG) can help in the treatment of school-aged and adolescent children who have developed abstract thinking and sufficient cognitive ability to understand and use the information provided (Olney and Wright 2000). Positive results have been reported, but with limited carry-over to functional, real-life situations.

PATTERNING

Patterning, or the Doman–Delacato method, continues to be offered and implemented despite a lack of research support (Barry 1996). Proponents believe that the repetitious patterning promotes normal development in undamaged areas of the brain and externally imposes patterns of movement into the damaged areas of the brain (Barry 1996). The patterning involves movement in a prescribed manner: with the child in a prone position, the head is turned side to side while the extremities are moved through flexion and extension. This prescribed movement is to be repeated for 5 minutes, four times every day. In 1960, Doman and colleagues published a study of 76 children with brain injuries of vast diversity resulting in mild to severe motor impairments. These children received patterning over a 6- to 20-month period (Barry 1996). Improved mobility was reported, but the measure was a scale developed exclusively for the study, with no validity or reliability data available. Both the American Academy of Pediatrics and the American Physical Therapy Association have issued policy statements regarding this method of intervention, stating concerns about its lack of effectiveness and about the promotional methods used by the Institutes for the Achievement of Human Potential. (Barry 1996).

Oral medications and neurolytic blocks

Many neuromuscular and musculoskeletal problems interfere with the function, comfort, positioning, or the care of the child with cerebral palsy. In Chapter 12 we discussed the primary and secondary functional abnormalities produced by cerebral palsy. The primary problems include abnormal tone, problems with balance, and loss of selective motor control. The secondary (growth) problems include muscle contractures and abnormal bone growth (long bone torsion, hip subluxation/dislocation and/or foot deformities). Although current treatment cannot eliminate all of these problems, treatments do exist to minimize the impact that many of these problems, especially spasticity, can have on a child's function and quality of life (Table 16.1).

This portion of the chapter will focus on the treatment of spasticity and control of deformity through the use of neurolytic blocks and oral medications. Surgical methods of spasticity reduction such as selective dorsal rhizotomy and the intrathecal baclofen pump will be addressed in Chapter 18.

Over the last 10–15 years, significant advances have been made in the treatment of spasticity in children with cerebral palsy. Historically, spasticity in children was treated with oral medications such as valium, baclofen and dantrolene, phenol neurolytic blocks, range of motion exercises, bracing (Little and Merritt 1988) and orthopaedic surgery (Chambers 1997). With the relatively recent additions of selective dorsal rhizotomy, intrathecal baclofen pump, botulinum toxin injections and tizanidine, we now have many

TABLE 16.1
Treatment options for cerebral palsy: indications, advantages/disadvantages, and relative cost

	Type of tone problem	Age	Advantage	Disadvantage	Cost
PT/OT	All types	Any	Improves development	Expensive	$$$
Oral Meds	Diffuse	> 1 year	Works systemically	Sedating	$
Bracing/Casts	All types	Any	Improves joint position and range of motion	Fails to reduce deformity	$
Orthopaedic surgery	All types	5 years to adolescent	Corrects alignment	Temporarily reduces deformity	$$$
Neurolytic blocks	Focal	Any	Reduces spasticity	Temporary	$$
SDR	Diplegia	4–8 years	Eliminates spasticity	Irreversible	$$$$
ITB	Lower extremity	> 34 pounds	Adjustable tone reduction	20 % adverse effects	$$$$

more options to treat spasticity and its impact on a child's function.

When treating a child with spasticity the goal is to improve some area of function and/or quality of life. These goals should be clearly outlined before treatment. Spasticity should not be treated because of its mere presence, but only if it adversely affects some area of function or quality of life. Because of the complexity of treating a child with CP, in order to determine the best treatment modalities and optimize outcomes, these treatments should utilize a team approach with a variety of medical professionals.

Several factors influence the treatment modality chosen. The patient's age, size, functional status, risk of future musculoskeletal deformities, developmental potential and cognition all have an impact on the decision-making process. For example, selective dorsal rhizotomy is used in a specific age-range in children with CP, while implantation of an intrathecal baclofen pump is contraindicated until a child reaches a minimal size (see Chapter 18). If a child's spasticity is likely to lead to various musculoskeletal deformities, such as hip-dislocation contractures or torsional deformities, treatment may be warranted even if spasticity reduction would not improve other areas of a child's functional status.

Although children with cerebral palsy will have altered development because of their neurologic abnormality, they will still make developmental gains due to brain maturation. For example, without any specific medical intervention, a child with spastic diplegic cerebral palsy may still learn to walk. Medical interventions to reduce spasticity are intended to minimize the neurologic impairments and promote functional gains. Consequently, it is often difficult to discern whether the functional improvements that follow these interventions are due to brain maturation or to the interventions themselves. Although maturation may improve a child's developmental growth, it may also affect it adversely. For example, contractures often worsen in children during a growth spurt (O'Dwyer et al. 1989). Adolescents are particular susceptible to these changes during pubescent growth and functional deterioration is common at that time. Sometimes the skills lost are never regained (Johnson et al. 1997, Bell et al. 2002). Because of these various developmental factors, a child's function evolves continuously during maturation. Therefore development not only

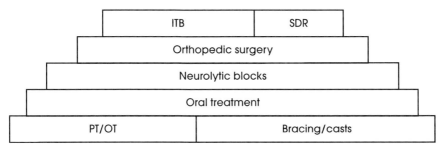

Fig. 16.1. Illustration of a traditional "pyramid" approach to the treatment of cerebral palsy. Modern treatment integrates many of these methods into a comprehensive approach designed to maximize the treatment outcome.

affects treatment of these children but also may complicate measurement of treatment outcomes.

Most children with spasticity do not have just one specific treatment modality for their spasticity, but rather benefit from a variety of treatments. Traditionally, treatment adopted a "ladder" or "pyramid" approach in which the most conservative measures were initiated first and more aggressive measures used when the more conservative treatment failed. More recently, treatment has used an integrated approach in which various different treatment options are utilized simultaneously. This might include a combination of bracing, stretching exercises, oral medications, neurolytic blocks, and/or surgery. To determine the most effective treatment options, each child should be assessed carefully and individually (Fig. 16.1).

Even the youngest child should be treated if a significant functional impairment is present. The brain is most plastic at an early age and that plasticity diminishes as adolescence is approached. For example, in a child with strabismus, if the non-dominant eye does not receive appropriate input at an early age, vision in that eye may be lost permanently even if the strabismus is corrected at a later age (Traboulsi and Maumenee 1990). Thus early intervention is important because appropriate and timely stimulation of the central nervous system promotes development of appropriate brain architecture and motor engrams (Mahajan and Desiraju 1988; "engram" is a term that Kottke coined in 1980 to describe memories of previous motor activities that have been learned through multiple repetitions of the activity). For this reason, even in a child under 1 year of age, if spasticity interferes with functional development it should be appropriately treated.

Spasticity is defined as velocity-dependent resistance to movement associated with increased deep tendon reflexes characteristic of upper motor-neuron impairment. It is associated with involvement of the pyramidal system (Young and Delwaide 1981, Davidoff 1985, Katz 1988, Alonso and Mancall 1991, Parziale et al. 1993, Young 1994, Dimitrijevic 1995). Many use the term spasticity to indicate all types of hypertonicity, but they are not equivalent. Rigidity is an increased resistance to passive stretch of muscles that is not velocity-dependent, and dystonia involves a variation in muscle tone often associated with increased extremity tone and decreased truncal tone that is associated with the tendency to assume postures. Rigidity and dystonia are considered extrapyramidal disorders (Young 1994). Some medications may be beneficial in the treatment of any of these disorders, but medications that affect muscle tone normally work on spasticity or dystonia, but not both.

Increased muscle tone may be exacerbated by medical problems, as any source of irritation can increase tone. It is therefore important to assure that potentially treatable causes of increased tone be eliminated before considering other interventions to reduce tone. Possible causes of increased tone include infection, ischemic ulcer, malnutrition, pain and sleep disturbance (Parziale et al. 1993, Young 1994, Bakheit 1996b). Sometimes even contractures themselves appear to play a role in perpetuating increased tone (Merritt 1981).

When evaluating an individual for the consideration of intervention to reduce muscle tone, one must carefully assess whether or not the increased tone is interfering with activity or care, or if the individual might actually be benefiting from it. This determination assists in the establishment of goals for tone reduction. Goals for improving function should be identified. These might include improved mobility, self-care and/or communication. For those who are dependent on others for care, goals could include increasing the ease of caregiving, improving positioning and/or decreasing discomfort (Whyte and Robinson 1990, Mayer 1991, Gracies et al. 1997). Tone reduction may also be considered if the individual is experiencing recurrent deformity secondary to the increased tone.

In some circumstances increased tone may be beneficial. For example, some individuals may learn to make use of their increased tone for weightbearing activities such as transfers or limited ambulation (Young 1994, 1997, Bakheit 1996b). Spasticity also may aid in the maintenance of muscle bulk and decrease the likelihood of ischemic ulcers. Finally, in those who have very limited mobility, it may assist in the prevention of deep venous thrombosis. Some of the more conservative medical treatment modalities include oral medications and neurolytic blocks. These will now be discussed in more detail.

ORAL MEDICATIONS

Consideration should be given to the use of oral medications when muscle tone is increased diffusely and interfering with function or the provision of care. In general, any of the oral medications used to treat increased tone has potential side-effects (Bakheit 1996a). The most common of these is sedation. Hence it is important to evaluate the response to the intervention carefully to decide whether the benefits noted are sufficient to merit continuing it.

BENZODIAZEPINES

Diazepam is the most commonly used oral medication for the treatment of spasticity. Despite not being labeled for this indication, it also has been used for this application for the longest period of time (Young 1997). Diazepam's mechanism of action is believed to relate to activation of gamma amino butyric acid-$_A$ (GABA$_A$) receptors by increasing the affinity of GABA to bind to the sites. This increases pre- and postsynaptic inhibition in the spinal cord and postsynaptic inhibition at supraspinal levels. It results in a reduction of mono- and polysynaptic reflexes (Davidoff 1985, Katz 1988, Whyte and Robinson 1990, Alonso and Mancall 1991, Parziale et al. 1993, Dimitrijevic 1995, Gracies et al. 1997).

Diazepam is well absorbed after oral administration. It is 98% protein-bound and has a half-life of 20–80 hours. Protein binding is important in that individuals with low serum proteins may have increased susceptibility to side-effects. It is metabolized in the liver and metabolites are excreted in the urine and feces (Young and Delwaide 1981, Gracies et al. 1997).

Diazepam's most frequent adverse effect is sedation. True physiologic dependence can also occur. After long-term use, therefore, it is necessary to taper the medication gradually. Since the half-life is long, symptoms of withdrawal may not occur until 2–4 days after it is acutely discontinued. In addition, diazepam may cause weakness, ataxia, depression and memory impairment (Young and Delwaide 1981, Katz 1988, Whyte and Robinson 1990, Alonso and Mancall 1991, Gracies et al. 1997, Young 1997). An advantage of diazepam in small children is that it is available in a liquid as well as tablet form. It is also well absorbed rectally and commercially available in a rectal form, if oral administration is not possible due to illness. It is available in an intravenous formulation as well. Typically dosing ranges from 0.12 to 0.8 mg/kg/day in divided doses (Gracies et al. 1997).

Effects of diazepam on children with cerebral palsy have been studied using a placebo-controlled double-blind study with doses from 3.75 to 20 mg/day. Using a subjective clinical evaluation, 12 of 16 children were noted to improve. Behavioral improvement was noted more than improvement in spasticity. Improvement was mild. Another study of children with CP showed greater improvement in children with athetoid rather than spastic CP. It was concluded that this was due to the general relaxation caused by diazepam (Whyte and Robinson 1990).

Other benzodiazepines may be helpful in the treatment of spasticity, but are less frequently used. Clorazepate is a benzodiazepine that undergoes metabolism to the same active metabolite as diazepam and therefore, may have similar effects on hypertonicity. Clonazepam is commonly used for seizures, but some have advocated its use for nighttime spasms and spasticity as well as dystonia. Sedation and fatigue limit its effectiveness for spasticity (Gracies et al. 1997).

Baclofen

Baclofen's chemical structure is similar to GABA and acts by binding at $GABA_B$ receptors. Binding occurs pre- and postsynaptically and results in inhibition of mono- and polysynaptic reflexes. Its effect on muscle tone appears to result from its activity in the spinal cord (Sachais et al. 1977, Young and Delwaide 1981, Davidoff 1985, Katz 1988, Whyte and Robinson 1990, Alonso and Mancall 1991, Gracies et al. 1997). Baclofen has also been reported to decrease the response to pain in experimental animals and, anecdotally, in people with spasticity (Davidoff 1985, Bakheit 1996b). Baclofen is used in its racemic form. l-baclofen appears to be responsible for the therapeutic effects and r-baclofen for most of the adverse effects (Davidoff 1985, Katz 1988, Herman and D'Luzansky 1991).

Baclofen is rapidly absorbed after oral administration. However, it is not available in an intravenous form and is not absorbed rectally (Kriel et al. 1997). Its half-life is about 3.5 hours. It is largely excreted through the kidneys, but the liver metabolizes about 15%. It is also available in an intrathecal formulation that will be discussed in Chapter 18 (Sachais et al. 1977, Terrence and Fromm 1981, Gracies et al. 1997, Young 1997). Due to its short half-life, frequent dosing is required to maintain a steady blood level (Herman and D'Luzansky 1991).

Sedation is also a common side-effect of baclofen, although it is noted to cause less sedation than diazepam. It can also cause dizziness, nausea, memory impairment and weakness. Individuals develop a physical tolerance to baclofen and experience withdrawal if it is discontinued acutely. Symptoms of withdrawal include seizures, hallucinations, increased tone, spasms, hyperthermia and confusion. Since it is not available in parenteral form and is not absorbed rectally, withdrawal symptoms can be seen if the drug is not tapered and discontinued prior to surgical procedures that result in an ileus and the inability to take oral medications (Terrence and Fromm 1981, Young and Delwaide 1981, Katz 1988, Whyte and Robinson 1990, Alonso and Mancall 1991, Mandac et al. 1993, Parziale et al. 1993, Gracies et al. 1997). The effect on seizure frequency during administration has been controversial, with some reporting increased seizure frequency, some reporting a decrease, and others no change (Terrence et al. 1983, Alonso and Mancall 1991).

The use of baclofen in the treatment of children with cerebral palsy has been studied. A double-blind placebo-controlled crossover trial in 20 children with CP demonstrated that baclofen was superior to placebo in decreasing Ashworth scores and allowing passive range of motion to be performed. Doses started at 5–10 mg/day in three doses for children aged 2–7 years, and gradually increased (Milla and Jackson 1977). Another double-blind study also demonstrated reduced tone in children with CP, with dosages of up to 30 mg/day in children up to age 6, and up to 70 mg/day in those who were older (Schwartzman et al. 1976).

Dantrolene sodium

Dantrolene sodium is unique among the medications commonly used to treat spasticity in that its effect is at the level of the skeletal muscle rather than the CNS. Some have suggested that this mechanism of action results in dantrolene being the preferred drug for the treatment of spasticity of cerebral origin (Katz 1988, Mayer 1991). Dantrolene interferes with the release of calcium from the sarcoplasmic reticulum of the muscle cell, which results in the uncoupling of the excitation/contraction. The effects are greatest during low frequencies of repetitive stimulation, on fast-contracting muscle and shorter muscle lengths (Pinder et al. 1977, Merritt 1981, Young and Delwaide 1981, Davidoff 1985, Katz 1988, Whyte and Robinson 1990, Gracies et al. 1997, Young 1997).

Dantrolene sodium is incompletely absorbed and is metabolized by the liver. The half-life is reported to be 7–8 hours. It is excreted in the urine and bile. It is available in both oral and intravenous forms. The intravenous form is generally used in the treatment of malignant hyperthermia. The initial dosage in children is about 0.5–1 mg/kg once or twice a day. Depending on clinical response, the dose can be increased every 4–7 days (generally to a maximum of 3 mg/kg four times a day or less than 100 mg four times a day) (Pinder et al. 1977, Young and Delwaide 1981, Katz 1988, Gracies et al. 1997). The most common side-effects noted are nausea and diarrhea. In addition, it can cause drowsiness, dizziness, weakness and fatigue. In ambulatory individuals, its mechanism of action and potential for causing weakness may limit its usefulness. The most serious potential side-effect is hepatotoxicity. Liver enzyme elevation has been reported in 1%–10% of patients and fatal hepatitis in 0.1%–0.3%. Consequently, hepatic function should be evaluated prior to the initiation of treatment with dantrolene sodium and periodically thereafter. Serum bilirubin was generally higher in fatal cases than non-fatal cases of hepatotoxicity. Toxicity was generally reported after at least 60 days of treatment. It was seen more frequently in women. It is believed that there is a dose-response relationship for the severity of hepatic injury. It is also appropriate to be cautious in using dantrolene with other medications know to potentially cause hepatotoxicity (Pinder et al. 1977, Merritt 1981, Young and Delwaide 1981, Katz 1988, Chan 1990, Gracies et al. 1997, Young 1997).

A few studies have also been done evaluating the effect of dantrolene sodium on spasticity associated with CP. One double-blind study of 26 children treated with dantrolene 1–3 mg/kg four times a day demonstrated reduction of spasticity and improved self-help skills. Another study of 18 children and adults with athetoid CP who received 5–100 mg of dantrolene or placebo four times a day showed a subjective improvement in athetoid movements and spasms in more than half of the subjects. In a third double blind study, however, in which children received 4 mg/kg/day increasing to a maximum of 12 mg/kg/day of dantrolene, almost half of the subjects did not demonstrate a difference between the placebo and active treatment periods. It was also noted that there was poor interrater reliability (Pinder et al. 1977, Whyte and Robinson 1990). A more recent open-label study of dantrolene reported that children aged 28–48 months receiving dantrolene were able to achieve better than predicted locomotor development, and an older group aged 5–13 years showed improved ease of movement (Badell 1991).

Alpha$_2$ adrenergic agonists
Two other medications that act on the CNS are used for the treatments of spasticity. These are clonidine and tizanidine.

Clonidine appears to have effects at the brain and spinal cord, decreasing the sympathetic outflow. It is thought to hyperpolarize motor neurons (Weingarden and Belen 1992). It may also inhibit afferent input to the reflex arc. It is available in oral, transdermal and intrathecal formulations. The transdermal formulation is believed to provide a more consistent delivery of the drug resulting in fewer peaks and troughs and therefore decreasing adverse effects (Weingarden and Belen 1992). The use of intrathecal clonidine has been reported in adults with spinal-cord injuries (Middleton et al. 1996, Remy-Neris et al. 1999). Clonidine is well absorbed orally and has a peak plasma level 3–5 hours after administration. Half is metabolized in the liver and the other half excreted in the urine. The half-life is 5–19 hours. In individuals with impaired renal function the half-life can increase to 40 hours. In adults, doses generally start at 0.1 mg/day (Gracies et al. 1997).

Adverse events include hypotension, particularly orthostatic hypotension, bradycardia and depression. Dry mouth, drowsiness, dizziness and constipation have also been noted (Gracies et al. 1997).

Clonidine has typically been used in spasticity due to spinal cord injury. One case report appeared in the literature of its use in a 17-year-old patient with CP who was no longer benefitting from diazepam and for whom baclofen produced no clinical effect. Transdermal clonidine 0.1 mg was used and subjectively tone was noted to improve enough that the patient's mother requested continuation of the drug (Dall et al. 1996).

Tizanidine has been more recently approved for use in spasticity, but again has generally been studied in adults with spasticity of spinal lesion origin. Postulated mechanisms of action are similar to clonidine. It is noted to have an anti-nociceptive effect as well (Kaplan 1997, Nance 1997, Young 1997). Tizanidine is well absorbed orally. It is metabolized in the liver and eliminated by both kidneys and gut. Half-life of tizanidine is 4–8 hours. The initial adult dose is generally 2–4 mg at bedtime. Gradual increase of dose is recommended to prevent sedation (Gracies et al. 1997, Kaplan 1997, Nance 1997).

Tizanidine's side-effects include sedation, dry mouth and dizziness. Fewer difficulties with hypotension have been reported with tizanidine than with clonidine. Rapid increase of dose may result in nausea and vomiting. Elevation of liver enzymes has been noted, so it is important to monitor liver enzymes prior to initiation and during treatment (Kaplan 1997, Nance 1997).

Tizanidine's efficacy has been reported in individuals with multiple sclerosis and spinal-cord injury. It has not been evaluated in spasticity of cerebral origin (Young 1997).

Gabapentin
Gabapentin is primarily prescribed as an anticonvulsant and for the treatment of neuropathic pain. It was developed as a GABA agonist that could cross the blood-brain barrier, but it has now been shown not to effect GABA receptors so its mechanism of action is unknown. It is well absorbed after oral administration, does not appear to have any drug interactions, is not protein-bound, and is excreted in the urine without having been metabolized. Side-effects can include sedation, dizziness and ataxia (Dunevsky and Perel 1998). Gabapentin's half-life is approximately 6 hours (Mueller et al. 1997). Reports have indicated that it can reduce muscle tone with no significant side effects in individuals with multiple sclerosis and spinal cord injury (Gruenthal et al. 1997, Mueller et al. 1997, Priebe et al. 1997, Cutter et al. 2000). Its efficacy in CP has not been reported.

SUMMARY OF ORAL AGENTS
The decision to recommend oral medication for the treatment of spasticity, as well as which medication to recommend, is not an easy one. The studies of these medications in individuals with CP are limited. Many of the studies that have been done use subjective measures, and do not examine changes in function. Oral medications have a systemic effect. They may reduce strength of muscles that are essential for head and trunk control. They frequently produce sedation. As such, in an attempt to minimize doses and reduce side-effects, it might be helpful to keep a particular drug's mechanisms of action in mind and consider using combinations of medications with different actions. Table 16.2 lists the mechanism of action and common side-effects of these drugs. Again, careful evaluation and goal-setting prior to the institution of any treatment is essential. Also, periodic assessment of the effectiveness of the intervention is imperative to assist in determining whether continuation of the medication is warranted.

TABLE 16.2
Drugs, mechanisms of action and side-effects

Drug	Mechanism of action	Common side-effects
Diazepam	Increase GABA affinity for GABA$_A$ receptors	Sedation, memory impairment, weakness, physical dependence
Baclofen	GABA$_B$ receptor agonist	Sedation, dizziness, weakness, physical dependence
Dantrolene sodium	Prevents release of calcium from the sarcoplasmic reticulum	Nausea, weakness, fatigue, potential hepatotoxicity
Clonidine	Alpha$_2$ agonist	Hypotension, dizziness, bradycardia, fatigue, depression
Tizanidine	Alpha$_2$ agonist	Fatigue, nausea, dry mouth potential hepatotoxicity
Gabapentin	Unknown	Sedation, dizziness, ataxia

NEUROLYTIC BLOCKS

Unlike oral medications, which are used to treat generalized spasticity, and selective dorsal rhizotomy or the intrathecal baclofen pump, which are considered to be regional treatments, neurolytic blocks are used for focal spasticity treatments. They cannot be used to treat generalized spasticity. However, if reducing spastic tone in only a few muscles improves their function, focal management of spasticity can still help a child with generalized spasticity. The most common neurolytic blocks used to treat spasticity in children are botulinum toxin type A and phenol blocks (Gormley 1999) (Table 16.3). Neurolytic blocks have an advantage over selective dorsal rhizotomy and the intrathecal baclofen pump in that they can be used in children of any age. As they become older and larger, however, children who respond to neurolytic blocks may be more appropriately treated with selective dorsal rhizotomy or an intrathecal baclofen pump (see Chapter 18).

Phenol neurolysis

Phenol or carbolic acid can denature protein and cause tissue necrosis in concentrations greater than 5% (Glenn 1990). When phenol is injected on to a motor neuron, a chemical neurolysis occurs, thus denervating that particular muscle. This can lead to a reduction in both the efferent and afferent impulses input to a muscle from the muscle spindle, both of which can reduce spasticity (Fig. 16.2). Phenol has been used for many decades to treat spasticity in children (Easton et al. 1984). Because it does not diffuse readily in tissue, phenol must be injected within a few millimeters of a motor neuron. This requires electrical stimulation to adequately localize the target nerve. Phenol can be injected into motor points, which are motor neurons within a muscle, or motor nerves before they innervate a muscle. Localization of the motor neuron needs to very precise and the child needs to be fully cooperative and move minimally during the procedure. Phenol neurolysis can take 10–60 minutes, depending on which and how many nerves are injected. Electrical stimulation can be uncomfortable and the phenol itself can be painful when injected. For these reasons phenol neurolysis in a child typically requires general anesthesia. The lethal dose of injected phenol

TABLE 16.3
Comparison of botulinum toxin A with phenol

Blocking agent	Administered	Effectiveness	Advantages	Drawbacks	Complications
Botulinum type A toxin	Injected into the muscle	Lasts 12–30 weeks	Easy to administer Diffuses readily into the muscle Painless Can be administered without anesthesia	Effects are always transient Lasts only 12–30 weeks Limited approval	No significant complications reported
Phenol block	Injected into the motor points of the involved muscle	Lasts 4–12 months	Use is widely approved Lasts longer than botulinum toxin Cummulative effects often occur	Can be painful May require general anesthesia during admini-stration Takes more skill to administer	Transient dysesthesias and numbness Hematomas may occur, which negate the effects of the treatment If a large intravascular injection occurs, phenol can cause systemic effects such as muscle tremors and convulsions, as well as depressed cardiac activity, blood pressure and respiration

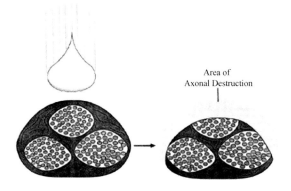

Area of
Axonal Destruction

Fig. 16.2. Distribution of axonal destruction created by dripping phenol onto a peripheral nerve (Glenn 1990).

is approximately 8.5 g in adults (Wood 1978). The recommended maximum dose is less than 1 g for one treatment session (Glenn 1990). Dosage guidelines have not been well established in children, but doses of less than 30 mg/per kg of body weight are considered safe (Morrison et al. 1991). This dosing guideline usually will allow treatment of two to four major muscle groups in a given session. For example simultaneous injection of bilateral adductors and hamstrings can be performed using several cubic centimetres of 5%–7% phenol in each muscle group.

The most common side-effect of phenol neurolysis is dysesthesias. It typically occurs

258

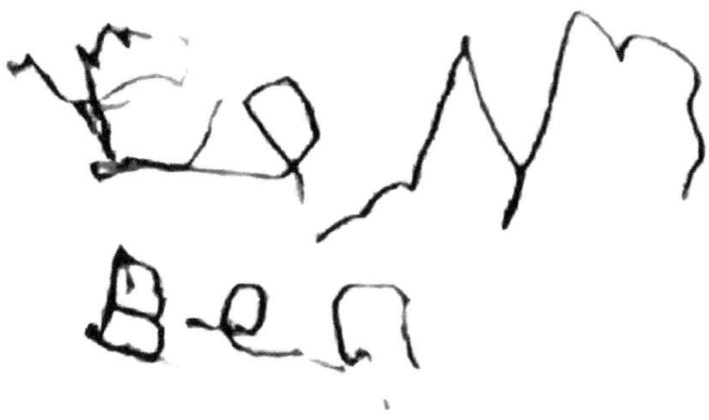

Fig. 16.3. Ben's signature. A 14-year-old boy's signature before (top) and after (bottom) phenol injections into forearm muscles.

if phenol is injected into a sensory nerve. This can result in a burning sensation and/or a hypersensitivity to touch that can last several weeks. Injections into the distal portion of the upper and lower extremities have the highest risk for dysesthesias, since motor and sensory neurons are in close proximity there. For that reason, it is probably best to confine phenol injections to muscles such as the hip-adductors, which are innervated nerves made up almost entirely of motor fibres, as opposed to muscles that are innervated by nerves that also carry a lot of sensory neurons. If dysesthesias occur, they can be treated with ibuprofen, gabapentin or carbamazepine. The incidence of dysesthesias in children is typically less than 5%, which is significantly less than the reported incidence of 15% in adults (Glenn 1990). The lower reported incidence of pain in children may just reflect the fact that children tend to complain less about pain than adults.

Phenol blocks are temporary and generally last 3–12 months (Spira 1971). Some cumulative effect can occur with repeat injections and the duration of the effect may be longer than 1 year. This increased duration of effect typically occurs in muscles with more easily accessible nerves. For example, the obturator nerve (hip-adductors) and the musculocutaneous nerve (biceps) are typically easy to locate, whereas motor points within the medial hamstrings and distal upper-extremity muscles are more difficult to find. However, even though the distal upper-extremity motor points may be more difficult to locate, phenol neurolysis in this area can still lead to significant improvement in function (Fig. 16.3).

Botulinum toxin type A, chemodenervation
Within the past 10 years botulinum toxin type A has been used to treat focal spasticity in children (Koman et al. 1993, Cosgrove et al. 1994, Sutherland et al. 1996). Botulinum toxin, when injected intramuscularly, blocks the release of acetylcholine at the neuromuscular junction (Kao et al. 1976). This essentially denervates the muscle and thus decreases tone. In addition to blocking neurotransmission of the alpha motor neurons, botulinum toxin also blocks the transmission of gamma motor neurons to the muscle spindle (Rosales et al. 1996). This has the effect of reducing spasticity directly by decreasing the tension of the intrafusal fibers in the muscle spindle, which in turn decreases the activity of the afferent nerve fibers of the reflex arc. For example, botulinum toxin injections into the gastrocnemius

259

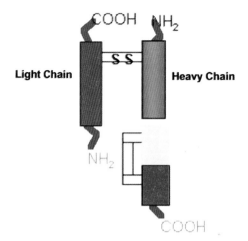

Fig. 16.4. Composition of botulinum toxin. Botulinum toxins have a heavy chain and a light connected by a disulfide bond.

soleus complex can decrease ankle clonus, which probably reflects its effect on the muscle spindle.

Botulinum toxin is an exotoxin secreted by the bacterium clostridium botulinum. There are seven neurotoxin serotypes: A, B, C1, D, E, F and G (Schantz and Johnson 1992, Aoki 2001). Botulinum toxin is a large molecule of approximately 150,000 daltons (Fig. 16.4) composed of a heavy chain and a light chain connected by a disulfide bond. Because of the molecule's large size it must be actively endocytized into the distal axon to have its toxic effect. The heavy chain has a great affinity for the distal axon and, when attached to a receptor on the distal axon, the toxin is endocytosed. The light chain is subsequently released and blocks the release of acetylcholine by lysing fusion proteins which are necessary for synaptic vesicles containing acetylcholine to dock to the distal axon basement membrane (Rosales et al. 1996) (Fig. 16.5).

The effect of botulinum toxin A on the distal axon is to cleave the fusion protein, Snap-25, and by so doing interfere with the release of acetylcholine from the neuromuscular endplate. Other botulinum toxins have different sites of action (Fig 16.6). The effect is temporary, lasting approximately 12–16 weeks. This neural recovery requires repeat injections for continued effect. Recent studies have revealed that initial neural recovery comes about as the affected distal axon sprouts new nerve-endings. In later stages of neural recovery the original neuromuscular junction begins to function normally again and the terminal sprouts regress (Fig. 16.5d) (Aoki 2001, Aoki and Guyer 2001).

Botulinum toxin was initially used as a therapeutic agent in the 1960s by Alan B. Scott, an ophthalmologist in San Francisco, while testing a variety of neurotoxins for therapeutic use. In 1968 he injected botulinum toxin type A into the intraocular muscles of primates (Koman et al. 1993). He initiated clinical use of botulinum toxin to treat strabismus in the 1970s. Later its use was expanded to treat dystonia and other movement disorders. The first clinical trial using botulinum toxin type A to treat spasticity in children with CP was reported by Koman and colleagues (1993). Since that time, there have been many studies published on the use of botulinum toxin to treat spasticity in children with cerebral palsy. Koman and

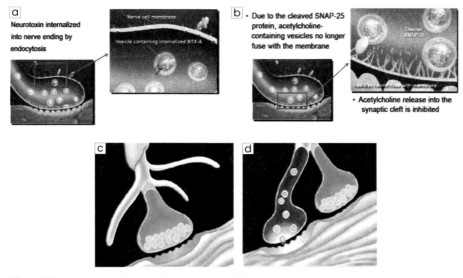

Figs. 16.5. Botulinum toxin's mechanism of internalization into a cell. (a) Neurotoxin internalized into nerve ending by endocytosis. (b) Due to the cleaved SNAP-25 protein, acetylcholine-containing vesicles no longer fuse with the membrane. Acetylcholine release into the synaptic cleft is inhibited. (c) After acetylcholine is blocked, collateral axonal sprouts develop. (d) The new sprout establishes a new neuromuscular injunction (NMJ). Eventually the original NMJ resumes function and the sprout regresses.

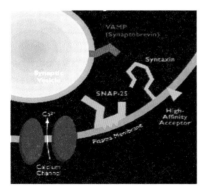

Fig. 16.6. Botulinum toxin type A cleaves SNAP-25 and type B cleaves VAMP, thus not allowing the release of acetylcholine from the synaptic vesicle.

colleagues (2000) again reported the efficacy of botulinum toxin type A to treat equinus foot deformity in a large multicenter placebo-control trial. Botulinum toxin has also been used to treat upper-extremity spasticity in cerebral palsy (Corry et al. 1997, Fehlings et al. 2000), hamstring spasticity (Corry et al. 1999) and gait disorder (Sutherland et al. 1996, Molenaers et al. 1999). Botulinum toxin injections in children with CP have been shown to be safe, with relatively few side-effects (Gormley et al. 2001a, b).

Similar to phenol blocks, botulinum toxin injections is a treatment for focal spasticity and not intended to treat generalized spasticity. Only three or four major muscle groups can be treated at any one time using the published dosing guidelines. If additional muscle groups need to be injected, then other treatment modalities or combinations of treatment with phenol blocks should be considered. Botulinum toxin should not be used alone to treat contracted muscles. Some adjunctive measures should be used to help relieve the contracture. Botulinum toxin can reduce spasticity but will not stretch the contracted muscle alone. As discussed in Chapter 12, muscles grow in response to stretch. The weakening effect of botulinum toxin on the muscle makes it easier to stretch. To reduce a muscle contracture, therefore, measures such as serial casting, splinting and/or range-of-motion exercises should be used in addition to botulinum toxin.

Botulinum toxin generally does not have a clinical effect for 1–3 days following the initial injection. Its maximum effect is approximately 1–2 weeks following the injections (Brin and Group 1997). Because of the delayed effect serial casting and other adjunctive measures are often times postponed until 7–14 days following the injections. Botulinum toxin diffuses quite readily within a muscle. Borodic and colleagues (1994) reported diffusion of up to 4.5 cm from the site injection in a rabbit model. For this reason botulinum toxin can be injected quite easily into the biggest bulk of a muscle and will diffuse quite readily to most of the neuromuscular junctions within that muscle. Neuromuscular junctions are generally concentrated in the middle of a muscle fiber. If a clinician knows the orientation of the fibers in a particular muscle, localization can be done easily. Studies have also shown that diluting botulinum toxin can increase its diffusion capacity (Shaari and Sanders 1993). A muscle can be localized by using motor point stimulation, electrical stimulation, electromyography, or palpation. Because of the diffusion capacity of botulinum toxin and the general ease of muscle localization, botulinum toxin injections can be carried out in a short period of time. Consequently, the injections in children with cerebral palsy are usually done in a clinic setting with or without conscious sedation. However, some centers do advocate using general anesthesia to reduce the trauma of the injections.

In children, botulinum toxin injections are dosed by body weight. The recommended published dose is 10–12 units/kg with a maximum dose of 400 units (Russman et al. 1997). Each major muscle group needs a sufficient amount of botulinum toxin to have a good clinical affect. That dose is usually a minimum of 2 units/kg in the arms and 3 units/kg in the leg. A maximum recommended dose per major muscle group in the arms is 4 units/kg, and 6 units/kg in the leg. Utilizing a relatively conservative dose within each major muscle group will help to avoid unintended local and systemic spread. The lethal dose in adult humans extrapolated from primate studies is 2500–3000 units (Schantz and Scott 1981). In juvenile monkey studies, the toxic dose is considered to be 33 units/kg and the lethal dose 39 units/kg (Scott and Suzuki 1988). Molenaers and colleagues (1999) have reported the use of botulinum toxin in children up to 29 units/kg body weight without significant side-effects. The above dosing guidelines are utilizing Botox (Allergan). Botox is botulinum toxin type A. An alternative preparation botulinum toxin type A is Dysport (Ipsen), which is available in Europe. Although both Botox and Dysport are botulinum toxin type A, their preparations and dosing guidelines are different. Therefore, they should not be considered interchangeable. Recently botulinum toxin type B has also become available for clinical use. This product known as Myobloc (Elan) has been used to treat dystonia, but there are no published reports on its use to treat spasticity in children with cerebral palsy.

Dosing in children is somewhat controversial since theoretically the same number of

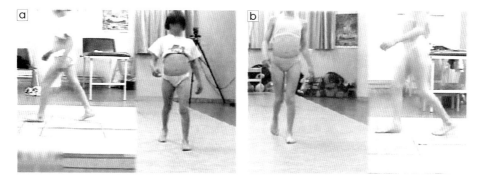

Fig. 16.7. Dr Molenaers' method. An illustration showing the effect of injecting multiple muscle groups with Botox at a single setting on the function of an 8-year-old girl with spastic diplegia. Under general anesthesia this girl underwent injection of multiple muscle groups (psoas, hamstrings and gastrocnemii bilaterally) with Botox. The total dose used was 26u/kg. To prevent overflow out of the muscle, care was taken to never inject more than 25 units at any one site and all injection sites were separated by a distance of 6 cm or more. A year later the right hip adductors, hamstrings and gastrocnemius were reinjected with a total dose of 12 u/kg of Botox. Following Botox injections the girl used appropriate daytime orthotics and went to physical therapy three times weekly. *See CD-Rom, Figure 16.7, for a dynamic illustration.* (a) Prior to Botox injection at age 8. She had had no orthopaedic treatment prior to this time. (b) Following Botox treatment at age 10 (20 months post the initial Botox injects and 15 months following the secondary Botox injections on the right side only). No treatment other than physical therapy and daytime orthotics had been employed in the interim.

neuromuscular junctions exist in a child's muscle as in an adult's. Thus it should follow that, regardless of the size or age of the patient, the same amount of botulinum toxin should be used to treat a specific spastic muscle. However, all current studies use dosing guidelines that correspond to body weight. It would seem prudent to adhere to these guidelines until further information is available.

The duration of botulinum toxin injections can vary. Studies in injections into lower-extremity muscles of ambulatory patients show that when sufficient doses are used, the duration effect is generally 4–8 months (Traboulsi and Maumenee 1990). Aggressive stretching, serial casting, and the use of splints (particularly night splints) and/or appropriate orthoses during the day will increase the duration of botulinum toxin's action. When using a multilevel approach such as that described by Molenaers and colleagues (1999, 2001), even longer duration effects can be seen. Molenaers used an approach in which the hip-flexor, adductors, hamstring and gastrocnemius muscles were injected simultaneously. To achieve an adequate clinical effect more than 20 units/kg of body weight were injected. The average duration of effect was 11 months. An aggressive rehabilitation program followed these injections that included stretching exercises, casting orthotic management and physical therapy (Fig. 16.7). If high doses of botulinum toxin are used to achieve multilevel effects, one should minimize the dose per injection site to 25 units and the total dose to approximately 6 units/kg for each major muscle group. Injecting too large a dose into any one injection site or muscle can lead to decreased toxin uptake in that particular muscle, thus increasing the risk of systemic side-effects. Factors that may decrease the duration of botulinum toxin effect include severe spasticity, fixed contractures, and/or a growth spurt.

Boyd and Graham (1999) stated that the risk of side-effects was approximately 5% in their patients. Most of these side-effects were minor and resolved quickly. Because botulinum toxin is a protein it can stimulate antibody formation, which in turn will increase toxin resistance. High doses and frequent injections of toxin increase this risk of developing neutralizing antibodies (Borodic et al. 1996). Long-term follow-up studies in patients treated with botulinum toxin for cervical dystonia indicate that resistance develops in approximately 5% of patients receiving Botox. (Greene et al. 1994). In a large open-label multicenter evaluation of children with CP, neutralizing antibodies were detected in 33 of 117 patients (28%) (Koman et al. 2001). Of these 33 patients, only seven were unresponsive to botulinum toxin injections. This indicates that the development of neutralizing antibodies does not necessary eliminate the clinical effect. Our experience at Gillette Children's Hospital has shown that patients can develop resistance over time even without neutralizing antibodies. Consequently, it would appear that we still have a relatively poor understanding of the mechanism of resistance to botulinum toxin injections. One of the reasons may be that the formulation of Botox has changed over the years. The original Botox contained 25 ng of neurotoxin complex protein per 100 units, whereas the current Botox formulation has approximately 5 ng of protein per 100 units. In our patient population at Gillette Children's Hospital, the decreased protein load seems to have decreased the development of Botox resistance. Some children will continue to develop resistance over time, but this resistance is less when the injection interval is longer and the total dose less. Current guidelines limit the injection interval to no more than every 3 months. Booster injections, in which a small amount of Botox is injected and than several weeks later additional amounts are injected, are discouraged. Our experience at Gillette Children's Hospital as well as that of other centers is that a patient can develop resistance to Botox in a certain body area such as the lower extremity, but still have a very good response to injections in the upper extremity. In addition, patients that have developed resistance over time can sometimes regain responsiveness when the injection interval is increased to more than 1 year. The reasons for this phenomenon are still unknown.

The given dosing limitations of both botulinum toxin injections and phenol blocks limits the number of muscle groups that can be injected, but by using a combination of phenol blocks and botulinum toxin injections, this can be overcome to some degree. Phenol blocks are commonly utilized in nerves such as the obturator and musculocutaneous nerves, which are comprised mainly of motor neurons with few sensory neurons. Conversely, botulinum toxin injections can be used in muscles that are innervated by highly mixed sensory motor nerves (such as the median or posterior tibialis nerves). Therefore, by using this combination method, small children can be treated with neurolytic blocks quite effectively. Botulinum toxin injections and phenol blocks also can be used as an adjunct to more global treatment such as orthopedic surgery, selective dorsal rhizotomy and/or intrathecal baclofen pumps. Typically, following these surgical procedures, a patient may still have a significant amount of spasticity in certain muscle groups. The hamstrings in particular may be spastic or minimally contracted following these procedures. In that case, neurolytic blocks can be used to optimize a patient's functional status by further decreasing tone/strength in these muscle groups. Neurolytic blocks also can be used to help maximize development, limit contractures

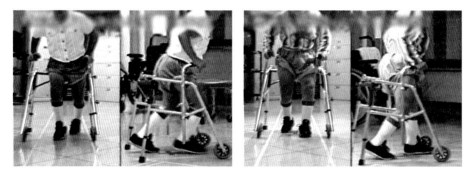

Fig. 16.8. Pre- and post-treatment example of a child with crouch gait and hamstring spasticity treated with a Botox at Gillette Children's Specialty Healthcare. *See CD-Rom, Figure 16.8, for a dynamic illustration.*

and/or reduce spasticity in a young child until such time as s/he is old and/or large enough for a specific surgical procedure. After surgical procedures have been completed as the child continues to grow and develop, neurolytic blocks can be used (particularly during adolescence), to treat recurrence of contractures and/or spasticity. Since there are no detrimental cumulative effects from botulinum toxin and phenol blocks, they can be utilized over the life span of a patient with spasticity.

Botulinum toxin injections, phenol blocks, and oral medications are a good addition to the spasticity management armamentarium. However, they should be considered an adjunct to other treatments and not as the sole treatment measure. Children with CP and spasticity are best treated when a combination of therapies are used. Accordingly, once a clinician understands the basic treatment principles, these interventions can be utilized in a highly effective manner with a minimal of side-effects (Fig.16.8).

Alternative treatments
Alternative treatments cover a broad range of healing philosophies, approaches and therapies that are generally not taught in standard medical-school curriculum, not used in hospitals, nor reimbursed by third-party payers. Also, they typically have not been proven or disproved by scientific method. Therefore, what is considered an alternative treatment often changes over time. Alternative interventions are often used because they are compatible with patients' values and beliefs. Often it is believed that alternative therapies are more natural and therefore have the potential of fewer side-effects (Astin 1998, Astin et al. 1998). People with chronic health conditions use alternative treatments more frequently than those who do not. It has been reported that 30%–70% of patients with chronic, recurrent or incurable conditions use alternative treatments (Kemper 2001, Mark and Barton 2001, Pitetti et al. 2001). It is not surprising, therefore, that individuals with cerebral palsy often make use of alternative therapies.

HYPERBARIC OXYGEN
Hyperbaric oxygen is approved in the treatment of crush injuries, carbon monoxide poisoning,

healing of problematic wounds and gas embolism. It has been advocated in the treatment of people with brain injury to increase the delivery of oxygen to the brain and benefit reversibly injured tissue. This is logical for acute brain injury, where some potentially viable but non-functioning tissue may exist. Rockswold and colleagues (1992) conducted a prospective study of the use of hyperbaric oxygen in the acute treatment of individuals with severe brain injury. They reported that survival was improved in the treated group, but functional outcome was not.

Cerebral palsy is by definition a static encephalopathy. As such it would be expected that there would not be an area of potentially reversible injury in the brain. Despite this, however, there has been a significant amount of publicity in the lay literature concerning the beneficial effect of hyperbaric oxygen for a number of conditions including CP. There have also been case reports in the medical literature about possible benefits as well. Montgomery et al. (1999) presented a case series of 25 children who showed improvements in some portions of the Gross Motor Function Measure (GMFM) and the Jebsen test of hand function. This led to a prospective, controlled study of the use of hyperbaric oxygen in CP. One hundred and eleven children with CP were randomly assigned to receive hyperbaric oxygen or slightly pressurized room air. The treatment group received 100% oxygen at 1.75 atmospheres for an hour for each treatment session. The control group received room air at 1.3 atmospheres, the lowest amount of pressure that could be perceived. This was necessary in order to blind the subjects to treatment. They received 40 treatments over a period of 2 months. Assessments included the GMFM, measures of language, orofacial structure and function, visuospatial and verbal working memory, and visual and auditory attention and the pediatric evaluation of disability inventory. Both groups showed improvement in some areas of function, but none of them were statistically significant. There was a statistically significantly greater incidence of ear problems in the group treated with hyperbaric oxygen. Their conclusion was that hyperbaric oxygen did not produce improvements in children with CP greater than those of their control group who were treated with slightly pressurized room air (Collet et al. 2001).

Studies to date do not show the benefit of hyperbaric oxygen for the treatment of CP. It is also associated with significant risks.

THRESHOLD ELECTRICAL STIMULATION

Electrical stimulation can be considered a standard part of medical practice. It is used to treat pain, augment bone- and wound-healing, and strengthen muscles. Threshold electrical stimulation differs from the type of stimulation typically used to strengthen muscles in that no muscle contraction results from this low-intensity stimulation that is at the sensory threshold. It is typically administered during sleep for at least 5 hours per night, at least 6 nights a week for 2–4 years. In theory, this stimulation causes an electromagnetic field that increases blood flow to the area which in turn causes the secretion of trophic hormones and provides increased sensory input in the absence of cortical inhibition. It is used to treat a wide variety of conditions, including CP. There have been case reports describing its effectiveness, including one that was a test/retest format including six children. This particular study showed improvement in testing that was not maintained when the treatment was discontinued (Pape et al. 1993, Pape 1997). One randomized placebo-controlled double-blind study has been done using this technique in children who have previously undergone selective dorsal rhizotomy. In this group of 44 children there was a statistically significant improvement noted in the GMFM but no change in spasticity, range of motion or strength (Steinbok et al. 1997). Some additional limited studies have shown increases in range of motion and motor control, but no discernible effect on motor function (Hazlewood et al. 1994, Sommerfelt et al. 2001).

In conclusion, threshold electrical stimulation may have some beneficial effects, does not have significant harmful effects, and is often used in conjunction with other therapies. Additional research is needed to prove or disprove its effectiveness.

CONDUCTIVE EDUCATION

Conductive education originated in Hungary at the Peto Institute. Conductors are involved in what is often referred to as a transdisciplinary approach. This technique involves the integration of educational and therapeutic approaches, with the ultimate goal of teaching and motivating the child to participate and function in society. Emphasis is on skills needed for independence, and teaching in small groups. Rhyme and song are used frequently and well as a relatively standard sequence of activities. It is highly structured and makes use of special equipment, like the ladder-back chair, but tries to avoid the use of orthoses (McKinlay 1990).

Some studies are beginning to emerge about the use of conductive education for children with CP. The classic inclusion criteria for participation in conductive education would exclude many with CP. Exclusion criteria include significant cognitive impairment, fixed contractures, poorly controlled epilepsy, visual problems, medical problems and severity of motor impairment (Bairstow et al. 1991). There have also been some studies comparing conductive education with "traditional" therapy intervention. These have generally included relatively small numbers of subjects and have involved comparison groups rather than randomization. Standardized assessment tools were used as well as videotapes reviewed by blinded reviewers. In general, both the groups receiving conductive education and the comparison groups have improved with no statistically significant differences (Catanese et al. 1995, Coleman et al. 1995, Spivack 1995, Reddihough et al. 1998).

To date, the limited studies available do not indicate that conductive education is superior to conventional intervention of a similar intensity.

ACUPUNCTURE

In a consensus statement developed by the National Institutes of Health, acupuncture has been noted to show promise in the treatment of a number of conditions. These conditions include postoperative pain, nausea and vomiting associated with chemotherapy, myofascial pain, osteoarthritis, low back pain, and headache (NIH 1997). One case series has been published concerning the use of acupuncture of the treatment of sialorrhea, a problem that is present in about 10% of children with CP. This involved tongue acupuncture for 10 children with persistent drooling daily for 5 weeks. Statistically significant improvement was noted in all of their measures, including a visual analog scale, drooling severity and drooling frequency. No side-effects were noted (Wong et al. 2001). Additional studies with controls would be helpful to assess treatment modality.

Adeli Suit

This system of treatment involves using the space suit originally designed to combat weightlessness in space for Russian cosmonauts. It is a system of elastic cords attached to a belt that delivers a vertical load to the body. Proponents of this therapy claim that in theory it increases proprioceptive input, decreases pathological signals and movements, improves bio-electric functions of muscles, and increases brain cortical activity and bone density. It is suggested that the suit may act as an orthosis that provides support for some joints, assistance to some motions that are weak, and resistance to some muscles. It is used as part of a system of exercises involving physical therapy for 5–7 hours a day, 5–6 days a week, for 4 weeks. No clinical trials have been reported as yet. Since it is not used in isolation, it will be difficult to evaluate the effect of the suit alone.

In my clinical practice, I follow two children who have traveled to Poland for this treatment at the Euromed Rehabilitation Center. Feedback that I have received from these two children and their parents indicate that they believe that there was a transient increase in mobility, but no functional change in their level of motor function.

Summary of Alternative Therapies

As long as there are chronic conditions that cannot be cured, there will always be an interest in pursuing alternative therapies. In order to assist our patients and their families in their considerations of whether or not to pursue these interventions, it is imperative that we keep the child's well-being at the center of all considerations, educate ourselves, and keep communication open and honest. When alternative treatments are proposed, we can help the family to look at the safety of the intervention, and help them determine whether or not anything is known about the efficacy/safety of the treatment in question. We should also urge them to continue with treatments that are known to have a beneficial effect. Finally, in the long term it would also be useful if respected treatment centers participated in well-structured clinical trials of alternative interventions in order to provide the objective data necessary to prove or disprove their efficacy.

REFERENCES

Alonso RJ, Mancall EL. (1991) The clinical management of spasticity. *Semin Neurol* **11:** 215–219.
Anderson J, Campbell SK, Gardner HG. (1992) Correlates of physician utilization of physical therapy. *Int J Technol Assess Health Care* **8:** 10–19.
Aoki K. (2001) Pharmacology and immunology of botulinum toxin serotypes. *Neurology* **248:** 3–10.
Aoki K, Guyer B. (2001) Botulinum toxin type A and other botuoinum toxin serotypes: a comparative review of biochemical and pharmacological actions. *Eur J Neurol* **8:** 21–29.
Astin JA. (1998) Why patients use alternative medicine: results of a national study. *J Am Med Assoc* **279:** 1548–1553.
Astin JA, Marie A, Pelletier KR, Hansen E, Haskell WL. (1998) A review of the incorporation of complementary and alternative medicine by mainstream physicians. *Arch Intern Med* **158:** 2303–2310.
Badell A. (1991) The effects of medications that reduce spasticity in the management of spastic cerebral palsy. *J Neurologic Rehabil* **5:** S13–S14.

Bairstow P, Cochrane R, Rusk I. (1991) Selection of children with cerebral palsy for conductive education and the characteristics of children judged suitable and unsuitable. *Dev Med Child Neurol* **33:** 984–992.

Bakheit AM. (1996a) Effective teamwork in rehabilitation. *Int J Rehabil Res* **19:** 301–306.

Bakheit AMO. (1996b) Management of muscle spasticity. *Crit Rev Phys Med Rehabil* **8:** 235–252.

Barry MJ. (1996) Physical therapy interventions for patients with movement disorders due to cerebral palsy. *J Child Neurol* **11:** S51–S60.

Barry MJ. (2001) Evidence-based practice in pediatric physical therapy. *PT Magazine* **11:** 38–51.

Bell KJ, Ounpuu S, DeLuca PA, Romness MJ. (2002) Natural progression of gait in children with cerebral palsy. *J Pediatr Orthop* **22:** 677–682.

Bly L. (1991) A historical and current view of the basis of neurodevelopmental treatment. *Pediatr Phys Ther* **3:** 131–135.

Bobath K, Bobath B. (1984) The neuro-developmental treatment. In: Scrutton D, editor. *Management of Motor Disorders in Children with Cerebral Palsy.* London: Spastics International Medical Publications.

Borodic G, Ferrante R, Pearce L, Smith K. (1994) Histologic assessment of dose related diffusion and muscle fiber reponse after therapeutic botulinum A toxin injections. *Mov Disord* **9:** 31–39.

Borodic G, Johnson E, Goodnough M, Schantz E. (1996) Botulinum toxin therapy, immunologic resistance, and problems with available materials. *Neurology* **46:** 26-29.

Boyd R, Graham H. (1999) Objective measurement of clinical findings in the use of botulinum toxin type A for the management of children with cerebral palsy. *Eur J Neurol* **6:** S23–S35.

Brin M, Spasticity Study Group (1997) Spasticity: etiology, evaluation, management and the role of botulinum toxin type A. *Muscle Nerve Suppl* **6:** S208–S220.

Butler C, Darrah J. (2001) Effects of Neurodevelopmental Treatment (NDT) for cerebral palsy: an AACPDM evidence report. *Dev Med Child Neurol* **43:** 778–790.

Campbell S, Anderson J, Gardner G. (1990) Physicians' belief on the efficacy of physical therapy in the management of cerebral palsy. *Pediatr Phys Ther* **3:** 169–173.

Carmick J. (1993) Clinical use of neuromuscular electrical stimulation for children with cerebral palsy. Part I: lower extremity. *Phys Ther* **73:** 505–513.

Catanese AA, Coleman GJ, King JA, Reddihough DS. (1995) Evaluation of an early childhood programme based on principles of conductive education: the Yooralla project. *J Paediatr Child Health* **31:** 418–422.

Chambers H. (1997) The surgical treatment of spasticity. *Muscle Nerve Suppl* **6:** S121.

Chan CH. (1990) Dantrolene sodium and hepatic injury. *Neurology* **40:** 1427–1432.

Cherry DB. (1980) Review of physical therapy alternatives for reducing muscle contracture. *Phys Ther* **60:** 877–881.

Coleman GJ, King JA, Reddihough DS. (1995) A pilot evaluation of conductive education-based intervention for children with cerebral palsy: the Tongala project. *J Paediatr Child Health* **31:** 412–417.

Collet J-P, Vanasse M, Marois P, Amar M, Goldberg J, Lambert J, Lassonde M, Hardy P, Fortin J, Tremblay SD, Montgomery D, Lacroix J, Robinson A, Majnemer A, Group H-CR. (2001) Hyperbaric oxygen for children with cerebral palsy: a randomised multicentre trial. *Lancet* **357:** 582–586.

Corry I, Cosgrove A, Walsh E, McClean D, Graham H. (1997) Botulinum toxin A in the hemiplegic upper limb: a double-blind trial (Class A). *Dev Med Child Neurol* **39:** 185–193.

Corry I, Cosgrove A, Duffy C, Taylor T, Graham H. (1999) Botulinum toxin A in hamstring spasticity. *Gait Posture* **10:** 206–210.

Cosgrove A, Corry I, Graham J. (1994) Botulinum toxin in the management of the lower limb in cerebral palsy. *Dev Med Child Neurol* **36:** 386–396.

Cutter NC, Scott DD, Johnson JC, Whiteneck G. (2000) Gabapentin effect on spasticity in multiple sclerosis: a placebo-controlled, randomized trial. *Arch Phys Med Rehabil* **81:** 164–169.

Dall JT, Harmon RL, Quinn CM. (1996) Use of clonidine for treatment of spasticity arising from various forms of brain injury: a case series. *Brain Inj* **10:** 453–458.

Damiano DL, Abel MF. (1998) Functional outcomes of strength training in spastic cerebral palsy. *Arch Phys Med Rehabil* **79:** 119–125.

Damiano DL, Kelly LE, Vaughn CL. (1995a) Effects of quadriceps femoris muscle strengthening on crouch gait in children with spastic diplegia. *Phys Ther* **75:** 658–671.

Damiano DL, Vaughan CL, Abel MF. (1995b) Muscle response to heavy resistance exercise in children with spastic cerebral palsy. *Dev Med Child Neurol* **37:** 731–739.

Damiano DL, Abel MF, Pannunzio M, Romano JP. (1999) Interrelationships of strength and gait before and after hamstrings lengthening. *J Pediatr Orthop* **19:** 352–358.

Damiano DL, Martellotta TL, Sullivan DJ, Granata KP, Abel MF. (2000) Muscle force production and functional performance in spastic cerebral palsy: relationship of cocontraction. *Arch Phys Med Rehabil* **81:** 895–900.

Damiano DL, Martellotta TL, Quinlivan JM, Abel MF. (2001a) Deficits in eccentric versus concentric torque in children with spastic cerebral palsy. *Med Sci Sports Exerc* **33:** 117–122.

Damiano DL, Quinlivan J, Owen BF, Shaffrey M, Abel MF. (2001b) Spasticity versus strength in cerebral palsy: relationships among involuntary resistance, voluntary torque, and motor function. *Eur J Neurol* **8** (suppl. 5)**:** 40–49.

Damiano DL, Dodd K, Taylor NF. (2002) Should we be testing and training muscle strength in cerebral palsy? *Dev Med Child Neurol* **44:** 68–72.

Davidoff RA. (1985) Antispasticity drugs: mechanisms of action. *Ann Neurol* **17:** 107–116.

Dimitrijevic MR. (1995) Evaluation and treatment of spasticity. *J Neurol Rehabil* **9:** 97-110.

Dunevsky A, Perel AB. (1998) Gabapentin for relief of spasticity associated with multiple sclerosis. *Am J Phys Med Rehabil* **77:** 451–454.

Easton J, Ozel T, Halpern D. (1984) Intramuscular neurolysis for spasticity in children. *Arch Phys Med Rehabil* **60:** 156–158.

Fehlings D, Rang M, Glazier J, Steele C. (2000) An evaluation of botulinum-A toxin injections to improve upper extremity function in children with hemiplegia cerebral palsy. *Pediatrics* **137:** 331–337.

Glenn M. (1990) Nerve blocks. In: Glenn M, Whyte J, editors. *The Practical Management of Spasticity in Children and Adults.* Philadelphia: Lea and Febiger. p 230.

Gormley ME. (1999) The treatment of cerebral origin spasticity in children. *NeuroRehabilitation* **12:** 93–103.

Gormley M, Gaebler-Spira D, Delgado M. (2001a) Use of botulinum toxin type A in pediatric patients with cerebral palsy: a three center retrospective chart review. *Child Neurol* **16:** 112–118.

Gormley ME, Krach LE, Piccini L. (2001b) Spasticity management in the child with spastic quadriplegia. *Eur J Neurol* **8** (suppl. 5): 127–135.

Gracies JM, Nance P, Elovic E, McGuire J, Simpson DM. (1997) Traditional pharmacological treatments for spasticity. Part II: general and regional treatments. *Muscle Nerve Suppl* **6:** S92–S120.

Greene P, Fahn S, Fahn BD. (1994) Development of resistance to botulinum toxin type A in patients with torticollis. *Mov Disord* **9:** 213–217.

Gruenthal M, Mueller M, Olson WL, Priebe MM, Sherwood AM, Olson WH. (1997) Gabapentin for the treatment of spasticity in patients with spinal cord injury. *Spinal Cord* **35:** 686–689.

Guiliani CA. (1991) Dorsal rhizotomy for children with cerebral palsy: supports for concepts of motor control. *Phys Ther* **71:** 248–259.

Hazlewood ME, Brown JK, Rowe PJ, Salter PM. (1994) The use of therapeutic electrical stimulation in the treatment of hemiplegic cerebral palsy. *Dev Med Child Neurol* **36:** 661–673.

Herman R, D'Luzansky SC. (1991) Pharmacologic management of spinal spasticity. *J Neurol Rehabil* **5:** S15–S20.

Howle J. (1999) Decision making in pediatric neurologic physical therapy. In: Campbell SK, editor. *The Guide to Physical Therapy Practice.* American Physical Therapy Association. p 27.

Johnson DC, Damiano DL, Abel MF. (1997) The evolution of gait in childhood and adolescent cerebral palsy. *J Pediatr Orthop* **17:** 392–396.

Kao I, Drachman D, Price D. (1976) Botulinum toxin: mechanism of presynaptic blockade. *Science* **193:** 1256–1258.

Kaplan MS. (1997) Tizanidine: another tool in the management of spasticity. *J Head Trauma Rehabil* **12:** 93–97.

Katz RT. (1988) Management of spasticity. *Am J Phys Med Rehabil* **667:** 108–116.

Kemper KJ. (2001) Complementary and alternative medicine for children: does it work? *Arch Dis Child* **84:** 6–9.

Koman LA, Mooney JF 3rd, Smith B, Goodman A, Mulvaney T. (1993) Management of cerebral palsy with botulinum-A toxin: preliminary investigation. *J Pediatr Orthop* **13:** 489–495.

Koman LA, Mooney JF, 3rd, Smith BP, Walker F, Leon JM. (2000) Botulinum toxin type A neuromuscular blockade in the treatment of lower extremity spasticity in cerebral palsy: a randomized, double-blind, placebo-controlled trial. BOTOX Study Group. *J Pediatr Orthop* **20:** 108–115.

Koman L, Brashear A, Rosenfeld S, Chambers H, Russman B, Rang M, Root L, Ferrari E, Garcia De Yebenes P, Smith B, Turkel C, Walcott J, Molly P. (2001) Botulinum toxin type A neuromuscular blockade in the treatment of equinus foot deformity in cerebral palsy: a multicenter, open-label clinical trial. *Pediatrics* **108:** 1062–1071.

Kottke FJ. (1980) From reflex to skill: the training of coordination. *Arch Phys Med Rehabil* **61:** 551–561.

270

Kriel RL, Krach LE, Hoff DS, Gormley ME Jr, Jones-Saete C. (1997) Failure of absorption of baclofen after rectal administration. *Pediatr Neurol* **16:** 351–352.

Little J, Merritt J. (1988) Spasticity and associated abnormalities of muscle tone. In: DeLisa J, editor. *Rehabilitation Medicine: Principles and Practice.* Philadelphia: JB Lippincott. p 430–447.

MacPhail HE, Kramer JF. (1995) Effect of isokinetic strength-training on functional ability and walking efficiency in adolescents with cerebral palsy. *Dev Med Child Neurol* **37:** 763–775.

Mahajan D, Desiraju T. (1988) Alterations of dendritic branching and spine density of hippocampal CA3 pyramidal neurons induced by operant conditioning in the phase of brain growth spurt. *Exp Neurol* **100:** 1–15.

Mandac BR, Hurvitz EA, Nelson VS. (1993) Hyperthermia associated with baclofen withdrawal and increased spasticity. *Arch Phys Med Rehabil* **74:** 96–96.

Mark JD, Barton LL. (2001) Integrating complementary and alternative medicine with allopathic care in the neonatal intensive care unit. *Altern Ther Health Med* **7:** 136, 134–135.

Mayer NH. (1991) Functional management of spasticity after head injury. *J Neurol Rehabil* **5:** S1–S4.

McKinlay M. (1990) Conductive education in Hungary and Britain. *Health Visitor* **63:** 298–300.

Merritt JL. (1981) Management of spasticity in spinal cord injury. *Mayo Clin Proc* **56:** 614–622.

Middleton JW, Siddall PJ, Walker S, Molloy AR, Rutkowski SB. (1996) Intrathecal clonidine and baclofen in the management of spasticity and neuropathic pain following spinal cord injury: a case study. *Arch Phys Med Rehabil* **77:** 824–826.

Milla PJ, Jackson ADM. (1977) A controlled trial of baclofen in children with cerebral palsy. *J Int Med Res* **5:** 398–404.

Molenaers G, Desloovere K, Eyssen M, Decat J, Jonkers I, De Cock P. (1999) Botulinum toxin type A treatment of cerebral palsy: an integrated approach. *Eur J Neurol* **6:** S51–S57.

Molenaers G, Desloovere K, De Cat J, Jonkers I, De Borre L, Pauwels P, Nijs J, Fabry G, De Cock P. (2001) Single event multilevel botulinum toxin type A treatment and surgery: similarities and differences. *Eur J Neurol* **8** (suppl. 5): 88–97.

Montgomery D, Goldberg J, Amar M, Lacroix V, Lecomte J, Lambert J, Vanasse M, Marois P. (1999) Effects of hyperbaric oxygen therapy on children with spastic diplegic cerebral palsy: a pilot project. *Undersea Hyperb Med* **26:** 235–242.

Morrison J, Matthews D, Washington R, Fennessey P, Harrison L. (1991) Phenol motor point blocks in children: plasma concentrations and cardiac dysrhythmias. *Anesthesiology* **75:** 359–362.

Mueller ME, Gruenthal M, Olson WL, Olson WH. (1997) Gabapentin for relief of upper motor neuron symptoms in multiple sclerosis. *Arch Phys Med Rehabil* **78:** 521–524.

Nance PW. (1997) Tizanidine: an alpha2-agonist imidazoline with antispasticity effects. *Todays Ther Trends* **15:** 11–25.

NIH (1997) *Acupuncture.* NIH Consensus Statement, November 3–5, **15:** 1–34.

O'Dwyer N, Neilson P, Nash J. (1989) Mechanisms of muscle growth related to muscle contracture in cerebral palsy. *Dev Med Child Neurol* **31:** 543–547.

Olney SJ, Wright MJ. (2000) Cerebral palsy. In: Campbell S, editor. *Physical Therapy for Children*, 2nd edn. Philadelphia: W.B. Saunders. p 554.

Palisano R, Rosenbaum P, Walter S, Russell D, Wood E, Galuppi B. (1997) Development and reliability of a system to classify gross motor function in children with cerebral palsy. *Dev Med Child Neurol* **39:** 214–223.

Pape K. (1997) Therapeutic Electrical Stimulation (TES) for the treatment of disuse muscle atrophy in cerebral palsy. *Pediatr Phys Ther* **9:** 110–112.

Pape KE, Kirsch SE, Galil A, Boulton JE, White MA, Chipman M. (1993) Neuromuscular approach to the motor deficits of cerebral palsy: a pilot study. *J Pediatr Orthop* **13:** 628–633.

Parziale JR, Akelman E, Herz DA. (1993) Spasticity: pathophysiology and management. *Orthopedics* **16:** 801–811.

Pinder RM, Brogden RN, Speight TM, Avery GS. (1977) Dantrolene sodium: a review of its pharmacological properties and therapeutic efficacy in spasticity. *Drugs* **13:** 3–23.

Pitetti R, Singh S, Hornyak D, Garcia SE, Herr S. (2001) Complementary and alternative medicine use in children. *Pediatr Emerg Care* **17:** 165–169.

Priebe MM, Sherwood AM, Graves DE, Mueller M, Olson WH. (1997) Effectiveness of gabapentin in controlling spasticity: a quantitative study. *Spinal Cord* **35:** 171–175.

Reddihough DS, King JA, Coleman G, Canatanese T. (1998) Efficacy of programmes based on Conductive Education for young children with cerebral palsy. *Dev Med Child Neurol* **40:** 763–770.

Remy-Neris O, Barbeau H, Daniel O, Boiteau F, Bussel B. (1999) Effects of intrathecal clonidine injection on spinal reflexes and human locomotion in incomplete paraplegic subjects. *Exp Brain Res* **129:** 433–440.

Rockswold GL, Ford SE, Anderson DC, Bergman TA, Sherman RE. (1992) Results of a prospective randomized trial for treatment of severely brain-injured patients with hyperbaric oxygen. *J Neurosurg* **76:** 929–934.

Rosales R, Arimura K, Takenaga S, Osame M. (1996) Extrafusal and intrafusal muscle effects in experimental botulinum toxin A injection. *Muscle Nerve* **19:** 488–496.

Russman B, Tilton A, Gormley M. (1997) Cerebral palsy: a rational approach to a treatment protocol, and the role of botulinum toxin in treatment. *Muscle Nerve Suppl* **6:** S181–S193.

Sachais BA, Logue JN, Carey MS. (1977) baclofen, a new antispastic drug. *Arch Neurol* **34:** 422–428.

Schantz E, Scott A. (1981) Use of crystalline type A boulinum toxin in medical research. In: Lewis G, editor. *Biomedical Aspects of Botulism*. New York: Academic Press. p 143–150.

Schantz E, Johnson E. (1992) Properties and use of botulinum toxin and other microbial neurotoxins in medicine. *Microb Rev* **56:** 80–99.

Schwartzman JS, Tilbery CP, Kogler E, Gusman S. (1976) Effects of lioresal in cerebral palsy. *Folha Med* **72:** 297–302.

Scott A, Suzuki D. (1988) Systemic toxicity of botulinum toxin by intramuscular injection in the monkey. *Mov Disord* **9:** 213–217.

Shaari C, Sanders I. (1993) Qualifying how location and dose of botulinum toxin injections affect muscle paralysis. *Muscle Nerve* **16:** 964–969.

Sommerfelt K, Markestad T, Berg K, Saetesdal I. (2001) Therapeutic electrical stimulation in cerebral palsy: a randomized, controlled, crossover trial. *Dev Med Child Neurol* **43:** 609–613.

Spira R. (1971) Management of spasticity in cerebral palsied children by peripheral nerve block with phenol. *Dev Med Child Neurol* **13:** 164–173.

Spivack F. (1995) Conductive Education Perspectives. *Infants Young Child* **8:** 75–85.

Steinbok P, Reiner A, Kestle JR. (1997) Therapeutic electrical stimulation following selective posterior rhizotomy in children with spastic diplegic cerebral palsy: a randomized clinical trial. *Dev Med Child Neurol* **39:** 515–520.

Sutherland D, Kaufman K, Wyatt M, Chamber H. (1996) Injection of botulinum A toxin into gastrocnemius muscle of patients with cerebral palsy: a 3D motion analysis study. *Gait Posture* **4:** 269–279.

Tardieu C, Lespargot A, Tabary C, Bret MD. (1988) For how long must the soleus muscle be stretched each day to prevent contracture? *Dev Med Child Neurol* **30:** 3-10.

Terrence CF, Fromm GH. (1981) Complications of baclofen withdrawal. *Arch Neurol* **38:** 588–589.

Terrence CF, Fromm GH, Roussan MS. (1983) baclofen: its effect on seizure frequency. *Arch Neurol* **40:** 28–29.

Traboulsi E, Maumenee I. (1990) Eye problems. In: Oski FA, editor. *Principles and Practice of Pediatrics*. Philadelphia: J.B. Lippincott. Chapter 34.

Weingarden SI, Belen JG. (1992) Clonidine transdermal system for treatment of spasticity in spinal cord injury. *Archives of Physical Medicine and Rehabilitation* **73:** 876–877.

Whyte J, Robinson KM. (1990) Pharmacologic management. In: Glenn M, Whyte J, editors. *The Practical Management of Spasticity in Children and Adults*. Philadelphia: Lea and Febiger. p 201–226.

Wiley ME, Damiano DL. (1998) Lower-extremity strength profiles in spastic cerebral palsy. *Dev Med Child Neurol* **40:** 100–107.

Wong V, Sun JG, Wong W. (2001) Traditional Chinese medicine (tongue acupuncture) in children with drooling problems. *Pediatr Neurol* **25:** 47–54.

Wood K. (1978) The use of phenol as a neurolytic agent: a review. *Pain* **5:** 205–229.

Young RR. (1994) Spasticity: a review. *Neurology* **44** (suppl.l 9): S12–S20.

Young RR. (1997) Current issues in spasticity management. *Neurologist* **3:** 261–275.

Young RR, Delwaide PJ. (1981) Drug therapy: spasticity. *New Engl J Med* **304:** 28–33.

17
ORTHOTICS AND MOBILITY AIDS IN CEREBRAL PALSY

James R. Gage and Deborah S. Quanbeck

The history of orthotics goes back many centuries. Orthotics probably found their original use in the treatment of fractures. Prior to his death in 370 BC, Hippocrates described the treatment of fractures with closed reduction and splinting in great detail. He stressed that for complete immobilization of the bone in question, the device had to include both the proximal and the distal joints. He also emphasized that pressure points should not be placed over bony prominences.

Ambrose Paré (1510–90) wrote a book that dealt entirely with orthoses, prostheses and other assistive devices. In addition to corsets and fracture braces, he described shoe modifications for talipes equinovarus.

Nicholas André, to whom we owe both the name and symbol of the orthopaedic profession, was a professor of medicine at the University of Paris in the middle of the 18th century. His major interest was in the correction of deformities in children, and he relied heavily on orthoses.

Over the next century, orthotics continued to grow as a major tool for bonesetters and physicians interested in deformity correction. According to Bunch (1985), in the 19th century "the relationship between bonesetters and bracemakers became increasingly close, and a personal bracemaker was part of every 'orthopaedic office'". Perhaps the most famous of these was Hugh Owen Thomas (1834–91), a Welsh bonesetter who was the inventor of many or the orthotic and prosthetic devices that are still in use today.

Winthrop Morgan Phelps, an orthopaedist who practiced in the first half of the 20th century, started his career at Yale but later moved to Johns Hopkins University in Baltimore. He had a keen interest in cerebral palsy, and although he was an orthopaedic surgeon, advocated bracing rather than surgery as the primary method of controlling deformity in this condition.

In the first half of the 20th century, braces were constructed primary from leather and metal. As such, they were heavy and cumbersome. Plastic was introduced after World War II, but did not come into common orthotic use until the 1970s. Currently most orthotics are made of a hard and durable plastic known as polypropylene, although other plastics are in use as well. However, the search continues for strong, durable and extremely lightweight composite materials, e.g. carbon fiber, which may prove to be even better-suited to these applications (Heim et al. 1997).

Orthotics are named from the joints they control. Thus an HKAFO (hip–knee–ankle–foot orthosis) would have to exert some control on all of the joints named. As such, it would

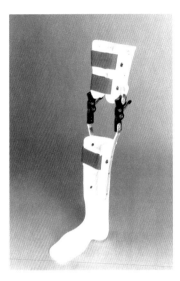

Fig. 17.1. A KAFO. KAFOs were widely prescribed in the past. However, in addition to being cumbersome, they have been shown to interfere with balance and greatly increase the energy cost of walking. With a combination of appropriate surgery, rehabilitation and below-knee bracing, the need for KAFOs can almost always be eliminated.

consist of some type of long-leg orthosis attached via some type of hip joint/hinge to a pelvic band or belt. For practical purposes, HKAFOs are virtually never used in individuals with cerebral palsy who are ambulatory. KAFOs (long-leg braces) are used in very rare instances, and ankle–foot orthoses (AFOs) and foot orthotics (FOs) are used commonly.

Thirty years ago, in an effort to control the secondary (growth) deformities of muscle and bone, HKAFOs and KAFOs made of leather and metal were commonly prescribed for ambulatory children with cerebral palsy (Fig. 17.1). Gradually, however, it was recognized that they were not helpful and that, in fact, most children refused to wear them. In fact, we know now that a long leg brace is a great hindrance to ambulation in that it interferes with balance, blocks knee flexion in swing phase (thereby compounding the child's difficulties with foot clearance), and greatly increases the energy cost of walking. In addition, now that we have a better understanding of cerebral palsy and gait, we have learned that most of the deformities that we previously tried to control with KAFOs can be managed with appropriate surgical correction of fixed deformities and an AFO or foot orthotic.

Purpose of an orthosis
An effective orthosis ought to: (1) protect a part, (2) prevent future deformity, and/or (3) improve function. Therefore every time a caregiver sees a child with cerebral palsy s/he should ask her/himself whether the orthosis is serving one or more of the three purposes listed above. If the answer is "no", the device should be discontinued. A knee orthosis prescribed for a football player following a cruciate injury would be an example of "protecting a part". A rigid AFO night-splint, which is worn in conjunction with a knee immobilizer during the hours of sleep, is a good example of an orthosis used to "prevent future deformity", as it is intended to maintain the gastrocnemius and soleus on mild stretch and thereby encourage their growth. Since this book is about ambulation, an example of an orthosis that "improves function" would be any orthotic device prescribed to improve the child's ability

to walk. An orthosis prescribed for this reason, however, is probably the most difficult to order. This is because if it is to be effective, the prescribing physician must understand the specific purpose for which the orthotic device is intended. Sadly, that is usually not the case. In that regard, our best advice would be to go back to Chapter 4 and review the priorities of normal gait: (1) stability in stance, (2) clearance in swing, (3) pre-position of the foot at initial contact, (4) adequate step length, and (5) energy conservation. It is for these reasons that an orthosis is usually prescribed.

Although it is known that an AFO will actually increase the oxygen cost of walking in an unaffected individual (Fowler et al. 1993, Waters and Mulroy 1999), in a child with cerebral palsy an appropriate foot orthosis can provide stability in stance and thus greatly improve stability. That improvement in stability often translates into better balance, faster gait velocity and a lower energy cost as well (Abel et al. 1998, Maltais et al. 2001, White et al. 2002). However, whether or not an orthosis can actually reduce muscle tone, as some have claimed, is questionable (Harris and Riffle 1986, Crenshaw et al. 2000). A leaf-spring brace may be adequate to prevent foot drop and/or control varus positioning of the foot in swing and at initial contact, which in turn may reduce the child's incidence of tripping and/or falling. Similarly, a floor-reaction type of AFO, so long as the prerequisites for its use have been met, may prevent crouch gait. However, even if the indications for the orthotic device are understood and the orthosis is prescribed for the correct reasons, the prescribing physician must realize that the brace will not perform its intended purpose unless the prerequisites for its use have been met. Consequently, we need to look briefly at a few of these prerequisites.

Control of dynamic deformities

In general, orthotics are useful for controlling *dynamic* as opposed to *static* deformities. Assume, for example, that you see a child with a fixed hindfoot varus deformity and prescribe a foot orthosis. Unfortunately, the prerequisite for an orthosis (i.e. dynamic deformity) is not present, and so the orthotic could never function as intended. Let us suppose further that the child undergoes orthopaedic surgery, following which the foot can be appropriately positioned when the child is at rest. Nevertheless, because of residual dynamic muscle imbalance, when walking the foot assumes an equinovarus deformity in late swing. Furthermore, this dynamic deformity places the foot in a position of instability at initial contact. At this point an appropriate orthosis is required. For the reasons discussed below, if the child happened to have diplegia, an appropriately "tuned" leaf-spring orthosis might be an ideal prescription (Õunpuu et al. 1996). On the other hand, in a child with fairly severe hemiplegia who had both gastrocnemius and soleus involvement, a hinged AFO might be required to control the deformity (Romkes and Brunner 2002). Finally, if following surgical correction of the fixed deformity the foot retained a normal position in swing and the dynamic varus occurred only in stance phase, an SMO or UCBL might be adequate to control the deformity (see below).

LEVER-ARM DYSFUNCTION

Lever-arm dysfunction will prevent an orthotic from functioning optimally (Butler et al. 1992). Because we are bipeds, we have feet (as opposed to hooves or paws). As such, as we move forward we walk out along the length of our foot in much the same way an individual walks out into a lake along the length of a dock or pier. If an individual with "malignant malalignment syndrome" (the combination of internal femoral and external tibial torsion—see Fig. 12.11 and its associated text) walks north, his right knee is going roughly northwest and his right foot northeast. As a result, he is unable to progress forward along the length of his foot. Instead his body weight will exit the foot's base of support on the medial side of the midfoot. Consequently, he is forced to transfer weight to the other foot more quickly than intended, i.e. take a shorter step length. If associated valgus of the hindfoot is present, support will be lost even sooner. In a situation such as this, attempting to brace the dynamic foot valgus might improve the situation slightly, but obviously it will not solve the major problem that stems from the rotational malalignment (Saraph et al. 2001).

FIXED JOINT CONTRACTURES
Fixed joint contractures act to prevent the normal/needed excursion for which the joint was intended. In that regard they also introduce gait deviations such as a short step length. However, fixed contractures of the knee, hip and/or ankle will also interfere with *second rocker* (see Chapter 4), and by so doing reduce or eliminate the plantarflexion/knee-extension (PF/KE) couple. This in turn will prevent a floor-reaction type of AFO from functioning optimally. On the basis of this, it should now be apparent to the reader that the prerequisites of a floor-reaction type of AFO include (1) correction of lever-arm dysfunction, and (2) correction of fixed joint contractures.

Orthosis manufacture
For an orthosis to function effectively, it must be made correctly. An orthosis is only as good as the foot-mold upon which it is based, and sadly some orthotists have a tendency to mold the foot where it rests rather than in the position in which it will function optimally. Additionally, orthotics (particularly foot orthotics, FOs) must encompass enough of the foot to maintain the correction in weightbearing. Furthermore, the material from which they are fabricated needs to be soft enough to distribute pressure, but firm enough to maintain correction. An orthosis that is too flexible may be very comfortable, but may not control the deformity sufficiently to be effective (Suzuki et al. 2000). If orthotists routinely remembered that pressure is equal to force divided by the area over which it is distributed (P = F/A), the small, rigid orthotics that do little more than produce blisters and calluses would disappear rapidly. There is little difficulty in getting a child to wear an orthotic that is comfortable and that provides the intended benefit. Children are quick to perceive benefit and will soon refuse to wear a device that is painful and/or does not improve their ability to walk.

This is the type of reasoning that must go on whenever an orthosis is prescribed to improve function, and as should now be apparent to the reader, this type of reasoning is cannot occur without an adequate knowledge of normal and pathological gait.

Types of orthoses
The major types of below-knee orthotics that are currently used to improve function in gait

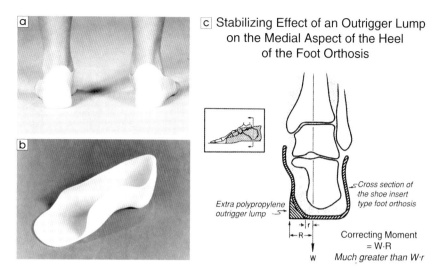

Fig. 17.2. (a) An example of planovalgus feet that are well controlled by UCBLs. The heels are adequately contained to prevent valgus and the medial wall is high enough to provide adequate support. It is important to remember that if the deformity of the foot is not fully corrected when the mold is taken, the orthosis will never be satisfactory. (b) A UCBL fitted with a "Gillette wedge" on the bottom of the heel. This is a wedge on the medial or lateral side of the heel that makes use of the ground reaction force to generate a corrective moment against valgus or varus deformities. (c) Stabilizing effect of an outrigger wedge on the medial aspect of the heel. In order to be effective, the medial wall has to be high and malleable enough to distribute pressure. The heel and arch are well molded.

are listed below. These orthoses are made of lightweight plastic (usually polypropylene) and are designed to fit inside a conventional shoe. Going from least to most control, these include the following.

FOOT ORTHOTICS

Foot orthotics exert their effect in stance phase and do little or nothing during swing. These orthoses find their principle use in restoring stability in stance for individuals who have functional varus or valgus deformities during the stance phase of gait. There are basically two types. (1) The *UCBL* (University of California Biomechanics Laboratory) is an in-shoe plastic slipper that controls functional varus and valgus deformities and, to some degree, supple malalignment of the hindfoot and midfoot (Fig. 17.2). They derive their name from Dr Vern Inman, the professor of orthopaedics at the University of California at Berkeley who first proposed their use. (2) The *SMO* (supramalleolar orthoses) (Fig. 17.3) is rather more encompassing and covers about the same area as a high top shoe. In addition to doing a better job of controlling varus/valgus deformities in stance, in our experience they seem to lessen foot-drop in swing to some degree.

FLEXIBLE ANKLE–FOOT ORTHOSIS

As stated earlier, if a dynamic deformity is present only in stance phase, an FO will suffice.

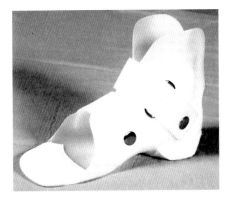

Fig. 17.3. A thin, well-fitting SMO. To provide comfort and allow the use of "normal" shoes, the orthotic should be as thin and soft as possible to distribute pressure, while maintaining enough stiffness to control the deformity. It is important to encompass the foot to provide the needed "wraparound" support. The trim-lines allow free plantarflexion/dorsiflexion, while the medial and lateral extensions provide good varus valgus control. The heel and bottom are flat, such that when the orthosis is placed on a level surface, it will rest in an appropriate position even when the child is not wearing it.

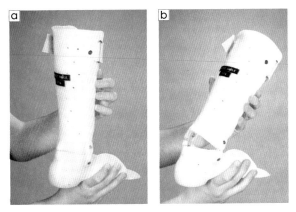

Fig. 17.4. (a, b) Hinged AFO. The standard hinged AFO allows free dorsiflexion, but prohibits plantiflexion. For that reason, it is often useful in controlling dynamic deformity in children with hemiplegia, but promotes crouch gait in children with diplegia (see text for an explanation as to why this is true).

An AFO is necessary to control a dynamic deformity that is present in swing phase. Again, there are two basic designs: the hinged AFO, and the leaf-spring AFO.

The hinged AFO (Fig. 17.4a) normally has an ankle hinge that blocks plantiflexion but allows free dorsiflexion. In general, the orthopaedic staff here at Gillette Children's Hospital does not feel they are useful for children with spastic diplegia, although they do serve a role in some children with hemiplegia. Many physical therapists and PM&R physicians use hinged AFOs extensively, however, because they feel that children with diplegia are more functional in them. In the short term that may be true, but in the long term they encourage crouch gait. If one recalls the growth principles discussed in Chapter 12, the reason for this becomes obvious. Soleus contraction is totally blocked at the ankle by the 90° plantarflexion stop. However, because the hinge allows free dorsiflexion, the soleus muscle is stretched with each step the child takes. Stretch is the muscle's stimulus for growth; hence with physiologic stretching, a growing child's muscle will add sarcomeres and elongate in length. As it becomes longer, however, the soleus has less and less ability to restrain the forward progression of the tibia in second rocker, and so the child soon starts to walk with excessive knee flexion in stance. Depending on the magnitude of that knee flexion, the PF/KE couple will be reduced or eliminated altogether. Recall that the gastrocnemius acts to assist the soleus at push-off in terminal stance. However, it too finds its action blocked at the ankle.

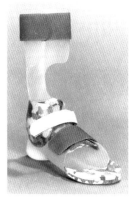

Fig. 17.5. Leaf-spring AFO. A properly "tuned" leaf-spring orthosis will control foot position in swing, but still allow some ankle mobility in stance. The problem is that today's plastics fatigue with repetitive bending stress. The world is still waiting for the "ideal hinge", which would fully control foot position in swing while still allowing free ankle mobility in stance.

But because the gastrocnemius crosses the knee as well as the ankle, the muscle is still free to act at the upper joint. Consequently the action of the gastrocnemius is now restricted to knee flexion, which becomes progressively easier to accomplish as the PF/KE couple lessens. In addition, so far as muscle length is concerned, since knee flexion and ankle dorsiflexion counterbalance each other, the gastrocnemius has much less growth stimulus than the soleus. Accordingly over time the soleus elongates, the gastrocnemius stays at length or may actually become contracted, and crouch gait progressively increases. Therefore it is our opinion that even in the short term there are better ways to obtain functionally good results than a hinged AFO.

The leaf-spring AFO is a one-piece, short-leg brace that is usually fabricated with the ankle in 5°–10° of dorsiflexion. The orthosis itself can then be ground back at the ankle to allow the desired amount of flexion/extension mobility. We usually order this brace with a "thin, foot-wrap, UCBL bottom" to provide better varus/valgus control (Fig. 17.5). The degree of flexion-extension mobility depends upon how much of the plastic has been ground away at the ankle joint. However, the orthosis remains quite rigid to varus/valgus stresses. This brace can be used to control functional equinus and/or varus/ valgus malpositions during the swing phase of gait. In so doing, it acts to pre-position the foot appropriately in terminal swing. It will also help to control dynamic equinus in stance to some degree. The greater the equinus moment, however, the more rigid the ankle needs to be. In addition, the integrity of the plastic degrades over time, so that the leaf-spring may eventually break or become inadequate to maintain appropriate foot position. Therefore what we are looking for is a device that will control the position of the foot in swing phase, initial contact, and during loading response, but leave the ankle completely unencumbered during midstance and terminal stance. Unfortunately we have no information to suggest that this particular orthosis has yet been invented.

RIGID ANKLE–FOOT ORTHOSIS
The rigid ankle–foot orthosis is very similar to the leaf-spring orthosis except that the ankle is molded in a neutral position and is left rigid (Fig. 17.6). This orthosis is used to manage stance phase deformities (varus, valgus or equinus) that are too strong to be controlled by

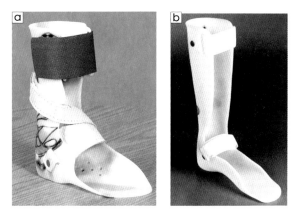

Fig. 17.6. Solid ankle AFOs. (a) Solid ankle dynamic ankle–foot orthosis (DAFO), used to manage stance phase deformities (varus, valgus or equinus), which are too strong to be controlled by a leaf-spring AFO. The more dynamic deformity present, the more rigidity that is required. This is the dynamic type, which is not as tall, has a more intimate fit, and is made of a thinner, more yielding material for better patient comfort. (b) Standard solid ankle AFO; this orthosis comes up higher on the child's calf and is more rigid. There is always a trade-off between functional movement and adequate control of the deformity. In a rigid, solid-ankle design, a rocker can sometimes be employed on the sole of the shoe to mimic the functional effect of the normal foot-rockers.

a leaf-spring AFO. The major drawback of this brace is the same as the hinged AFO in that it completely blocks the acceleration forces of third rocker and so any power that the posterior calf musculature might deliver in terminal stance is lost. Crouch gait is less likely, however, since ankle dorsiflexion is blocked as well. The "rolling motion" produced by the three stance-phase rockers (see Chapter 4) is also lost. However, this can be restored to some degree by putting a rocker sole on the patient's shoe (Meadows et al. 1980, Meadows 1984).

FLOOR-REACTION ANKLE–FOOT ORTHOSIS
The first prototype of this orthosis was made at Newington Children's Hospital in 1983 as a modification of the Saltiel brace (Saltiel 1969). There are currently three different designs of this orthosis. The first is a one-piece, rigid ankle design (Fig. 17.7a), the second is a rigid ankle design with a removable anterior shell, and the third is a rear-entry, hinged design (Harrington et al. 1984). This rear-entry, hinged ankle–foot orthosis was designed by Al Masunis, an engineer at Newington Children's Hospital, and has been in use since the beginning of 1990 (Fig. 17.7b). Its major advantages are that it controls second rocker, but does not interfere with first rocker (weight acceptance) or third rocker (acceleration), whereas the two earlier designs essentially eliminate ankle motion in stance (Fig. 17.8). Furthermore, in our opinion, it is more effective than the earlier models in preventing crouch gait, and according to our patients who use it, it is also much more comfortable. This AFO has two major disadvantages, however. First, it is bulky and difficult to fit into a shoe; secondly it does not prevent equinus in swing, although an elastic extension aid could be attached to the orthosis for this purpose.

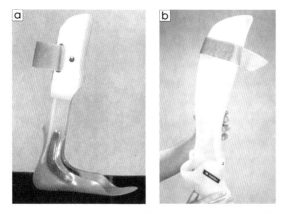

Fig. 17.7. The rear-entry, hinged floor-reaction orthosis, compared with a solid ankle floor-reaction orthosis (FRO). Both of these devices are comfortable and can of control crouch secondary to soleus weakness, providing the pre-requisites for their use have been met (see caption for Fig. 17.8). The hinged model allows soleus contraction whereas the solid-ankle type does not. The major disadvantages of the hinged FRO device are that it is too large to fit easily into a shoe, and since the heel is not fully contained, it does not control pes valgus well. More rigid, thin, lightweight materials (such as carbon composites) may solve this problem.

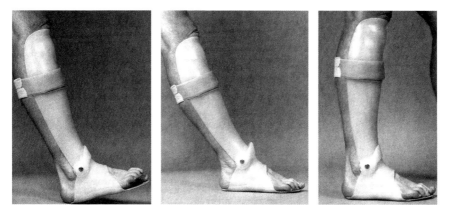

Fig. 17.8. An individual walking in a hinged floor-reaction orthosis. Notice that the device blocks dorsiflexion and so provides a PF/KE couple while still allowing plantarflexion for propulsion in terminal stance. There are prerequisites for using this orthosis: (1) the foot and knee are appropriately aligned, (2) the knee extends fully, (3) a significant hip-flexion contracture is not present, and (4) pes valgus is minimal.

Orthoses: conclusions

As you read the final chapters of this book, which deal with the specifics of treatment of the various types of cerebral palsy, the reader will discover that the prerequisites of bracing change with time. Figure 21.6 illustrates this. Following surgical correction of his lever-arm disfunction and appropriate lengthening of his contracted hamstring and psoas muscles, his soleus and vasti muscles were still too long. Accordingly, he was placed in rear-entry, floor-reaction AFOs, which provided him with enough support to walk in a fully upright position. Meanwhile he was in the midst of his adolescent growth spurt and hence over a relatively short time (6–9 months), his long bones grew sufficiently to re-tension the elongated muscles. During that time he was also working diligently in a rehabilitation program. As a result, 9 months after surgery, the floor-reaction AFOs were no longer needed. In fact, had he continued to wear them, within a relatively short time, he probably would have developed genu recurvatum. However, a child with spastic diplegia such as this boy usually has ongoing muscle imbalance between the relatively weak tibialis posterior and the stronger peroneals, such that dynamic pes valgus continues to be a problem. To prevent this, when the floor-reaction AFOs are discontinued, we feel it is prudent to prescribe a set of UCBLs. This then answers the final question that is often asked regarding orthotics, "How long should orthoses be continued?"

The answer is, "As long as they are fulfilling the purpose for which they were prescribed." Unfortunately, it is sometimes difficult or impossible to determine that without assessing the child's gait in the motion analysis laboratory with and without the orthotic devices. When this is done, and the child's barefoot walk is compared to the one in which he was wearing his orthoses, it is often discovered that the braces improve not only the appearance of gait, but the gait velocity and energy cost as well. This finding is also strongly supported by the literature (Rethlefsen et al. 1999). Because of this, it is our feeling that orthotics are an integral part of the post-surgical treatment. Their principle role is to control dynamic deformities during gait, and as such they play a vital role in the overall treatment outcome. It is our personal feeling, therefore, that we should not penalize that outcome by insisting on comparing pre-treatment status to post-treatment outcomes under identical conditions, e.g. barefoot to barefoot. Appropriate orthotics contribute a great deal to the overall result. Therefore we should not hesitate to include them in the final outcome evaluation.

Mobility aids

Walkers, crutches, canes and other mobility devices are prescribed for difficulties with balance rather than weakness. Typically an individual with cerebral palsy who uses mobility aids does so because of issues with balance, not strength (Fig. 17.9). The recovery period immediately following surgery is an exception to this, as in that instance weakness is also a significant component of the problem. Nevertheless, mobility aids are always a compromise as they have been shown to increase the cost of walking significantly (see Chapter 10) (Waters et al. 1978, Koop et al. 1989, Waters and Mulroy 1999).

The type of mobility aid selected depends on the severity of the child's balance difficulties. As a general rule, children with spastic diplegia who require mobility aids typically can be taught to ambulate with Lofstrand crutches (which are far preferable), whereas children with spastic quadriplegia frequently require a walker. Wheeled walkers, although slightly less stable, are far superior to pick-up walkers. In the former, walking is a continuum, whereas in the latter, walking becomes a series of stops and starts. Similarly, we feel that posterior rollator walkers are much better than those that are anterior. The literature supports this as well. Several authors have found that step length, single support and double support time were significantly better in a posterior (as compared to an anterior) walker. Flexion angles of the trunk, hip and knee were lower using a posterior walker as

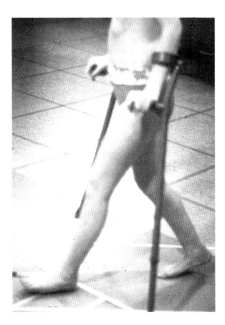

Fig. 17.9. Child walking with Lofstrand crutches. Forearm crutches are ideal for children who need minimal assistance with balance. They are minimally encumbering and provide an adequate balance assist to the individual while still allowing a relatively upright stance during gait. They also permit a much more "fluid" gait than devices such as quad canes.

well. Finally, gait analysis data and oxygen consumption measurements indicated that the posterior walker has more advantages in terms of upright positioning and energy conservation than the anterior walker (Logan et al. 1990, Greiner et al. 1993, Park et al. 2001). By contrast, Mattsson and Anderson (1997) did not find a significant difference in the parameters they measured, although they did note that children preferred posterior walkers.

When a child begins ambulation following surgery, s/he usually starts in parallel bars. We progress to a rollator walker as soon as the child is able to do so, sometimes as soon as a few weeks after surgery. However, the leap from a walker to Lofstrand crutches is a much longer one, as a child usually cannot progress to crutches until s/he has regained adequate strength to do so. In general, this takes at least 2–3 months from the time of surgery. Although many physical therapists like quad canes, we do not. As with pick-up walkers, we find that quad canes seem to *"arrest gait"*, and the fluidity or "flow of walking" disappears when they are used. Therefore our usual program is parallel bars progressing to a posterior rollator walker, to two Canadian crutches, to a single crutch, and finally to independent ambulation. We permit our patients to progress through this program as rapidly as their strength and balance will allow. So far as aids are concerned, we can usually eventually get a child to walk with either the same or with less support than he had preoperatively. However, with many of the children we treat, balance is sufficiently impaired that they will require a rollator walker or crutches permanently.

Although we cannot cite specific studies and currently do not have sufficient data to prove this, our empiric experience suggests that a child with adequate balance who undergoes multiple lower-extremity procedures (MLEP) to improve gait prior to his/her adolescent growth spurt, stands a good chance of reducing or discarding altogether his/her mobility aids; a child with the same degree of balance impairment operated upon during puberty will usually continue to walk with the same mobility aids post-surgery; and a young man or woman who has MLEP after puberty, even with adequate balance, will frequently add mobility aids (usually Lofstrand crutches). In the latter case, the individual normally will demonstrate improved gait parameters and speed, and will usually state that s/he feels that her/his ability to walk is significantly improved. Nevertheless, the individual seems unable to fully adapt to her/his new body position in space and continues to have a "fear of falling". In our experience, this phenomenon has occurred with enough frequency that we now routinely warn our older patients, prior to their surgery, that this problem may occur.

REFERENCES

Abel MF, Juhl GA, Vaughan CL, Damiano DL. (1998) Gait assessment of fixed ankle–foot orthoses in children with spastic diplegia. *Arch Phys Med Rehabil* **79:** 126–133.

Bunch WH. (1985) Introduction to orthotics. In: Pedegana LR, editor. *Atlas of Orthotics,* 2dn edn. St Louis: C.V. Mosby. p 3–5.

Butler PB, Thompson N, Major RE. (1992) Improvement in walking performance of children with cerebral palsy: preliminary results. *Dev Med Child Neurol* **34:** 567–576.

Crenshaw S, Herzog R, Castagno P, Richards J, Miller F, Michaloski G, Moran E. (2000) The efficacy of tone-reducing features in orthotics on the gait of children with spastic diplegic cerebral palsy. *J Pediatr Orthop* **20:** 210–216.

Fowler PT, Botte MJ, Mathewson JW, Speth SR, Byrne TP, Sutherland DH. (1993) Energy cost of ambulation with different methods of foot and ankle immobilization. *J Orthop Res* **11:** 416–421.

Greiner BM, Czerniecki JM, Deitz JC. (1993) Gait parameters of children with spastic diplegia: a comparison of effects of posterior and anterior walkers. *Arch Phys Med Rehabil* **74:** 381–385.

Harrington ED, Lin RS, Gage JR. (1984) Use of the anterior floor reaction orthosis in patients with cerebral palsy. *Bull Orthot Prosthet* **37:** 34–42.

Harris SR, Riffle K. (1986) Effects of inhibitive ankle–foot orthoses on standing balance in a child with cerebral palsy. A single-subject design. *Phys Ther* **66:** 663–667.

Heim M, Yaacobi E, Azaria M. (1997) A pilot study to determine the efficiency of lightweight carbon fibre orthoses in the management of patients suffering from post-poliomyelitis syndrome. *Clin Rehabil* **11:** 302–305.

Koop S, Stout J, Starr R, Drinken W (1989) Oxygen consumption during walking in normal children and children with cerebral palsy. *Dev Med Child Neurol* **31** (suppl. 59): 6. (Abstract.)

Logan L, Byers-Hinkley, K, Ciccone CD. (1990) Anterior versus posterior walkers: a gait analysis study. *Dev Med Child Neurol* **32:** 1044–1048.

Maltais D, Bar-Or O, Galea V, Pierrynowski M. (2001) Use of orthoses lowers the O(2) cost of walking in children with spastic cerebral palsy. *Med Sci Sports Exerc* **33:** 320–325.

Mattsson E, Andersson C. (1997) Oxygen cost, walking speed, and perceived exertion in children with cerebral palsy when walking with anterior and posterior walkers. *Dev Med Child Neurol* **39:** 671–676.

Meadows B (1984) *The influence of polypropylene ankle–foot orthoses on the gait of cerebral palsied children.* PhD dissertation, School of Engineering, University of Strathclyde, Glasgow.

Meadows CB, Anderson DM, Duncan LM, Sturrock MBT. (1980) *The Use of Polypropylene Ankle–Foot Orthoses in the Management of the Young Cerebral Palsied Child.* Dundee: Broughty Ferry.

Õunpuu S, Bell KJ, Davis 3rd RB, DeLuca, PA. (1996) An evaluation of the posterior leaf spring orthosis using joint kinematics and kinetics. *J Pediatr Orthop* **16:** 378–384.

Park ES, Park CI, Kim JY. (2001) Comparison of anterior and posterior walkers with respect to gait parameters and energy expenditure of children with spastic diplegic cerebral palsy. *Yonsei Med J* **42:** 180–184.

Rethlefsen S, Tolo VT, Reynolds RA, Kay R. (1999) Outcome of hamstring lengthening and distal rectus femoris transfer surgery. *J Pediatr Orthop B* **8:** 75–79.

Romkes J, Brunner R. (2002) Comparison of a dynamic and a hinged ankle–foot orthosis by gait analysis in patients with hemiplegic cerebral palsy. *Gait Posture* **15:** 18–24.

Saltiel J. (1969) A one-piece, laminated, knee locking, short leg brace. *Bulletin Orthot Prosthet* **23:** 68-75.

Saraph V, Zwick EB, Steinwender C, Steinwender G, Linhart W. (2001) Conservative management of dynamic equinus in diplegic children treated by gait improvement surgery. *J Pediatr Orthop B* **1:** 287–292.

Suzuki N, Shinohara T, Kimizuka M, Yamaguchi K, Mita K. (2000) Energy expenditure of diplegic ambulation using flexible plastic ankle foot orthoses. *Bull Hosp Jt Dis* **59:** 76–80.

Waters RL, Mulroy S (1999) The energy expenditure of normal and pathologic gait. *Gait Posture* **9:** 207–231.

Waters RL, Hislop HJ, Perry J, Antonelli D. (1978) Energetics: application to the study and management of locomotor disabilities. Energy cost of normal and pathologic gait. *Orthop Clin North Am* **9:** 351–356.

White H, Jenkins, J, Neace WP, Tylkowski C, Walker J. (2002) Clinically prescribed orthoses demonstrate an increase in velocity of gait in children with cerebral palsy: a retrospective study. *Dev Med Child Neurol* **44:** 227–232.

18
SPASTICITY REDUCTION

Leland Albright, Warwick J. Peacock and Linda E. Krach

Introduction by James R. Gage

In Chapter 12 we pointed out that children with cerebral palsy have a spectrum of deformities. The primary abnormalities (loss of selective motor control, problems with balance, and abnormal tone) can be reduced to some extent, but cannot currently be corrected. Because these primary problems interfere with the growth process, however, they act to generate the secondary problems (bony deformities and muscle contractures) which are so functionally devastating to these children. Spasticity, which is the primary tone abnormality present in children with diplegia and hemiplegia, is particularly troublesome.

When we discussed abnormal central nervous system tone in Chapter 12, we indicated that spasticity has several deleterious effects on growth and locomotion. (1) Spasticity acts like a brake on the system and this drag on movement increases energy consumption. A child with spasticity is in the same sort of predicament as the Tin Man in *The Wizard of Oz*, who could not move effectively until his joints were oiled. (2) Spasticity interferes with the voluntary control of movement, and can be compared with static interference on the radio, insofar as voluntary motor control can be likened to the radio broadcast, and spasticity can be likened to the static. If the static can be eliminated, even a distant station can be heard quite clearly. On the other hand, eliminating the static is of no help whatsoever if there is no underlying signal, i.e. there is nothing being broadcast. (3) Spasticity inhibits the effectiveness of stretch on muscles during normal activities, and by so doing inhibits muscle growth. (4) Spasticity induces excessive/abnormal torques on long bones during growth, which in turn leads to torsional deformities via the *Star Wars* principle: "May the force be with you!"

In short, spasticity, in conjunction with abnormal selective motor control and balance, leads to a cascade of abnormal growth events that terminates with a combination of bony deformities (hip subluxation/dislocation, abnormal long-bone torsions, and/or foot deformities) and abnormal muscle lengths (usually contracture of hip- and knee-flexors plus the gastrocnemius in conjunction with excessive length of hip extensors and the three monoarticular muscles of the quadriceps—vastus medialis, intermedius and lateralis) (Fig. 18.1).

As will be discussed in Chapters 19–22, correction of these secondary deformities (those associated with abnormal growth forces) can usually be accomplished without too much difficulty, but maintenance of the correction is a major problem in the growing child. Thus spasticity reduction, via selective dorsal rhizotomy (SDR) or an intrathecal baclofen (ITB) pump, not only acts to lessen the deformities of growth, but also minimizes the

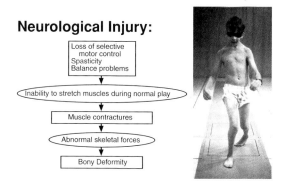

Neurological Injury:

Loss of selective
motor control
Spasticity
Balance problems

↓

Inability to stretch muscles during normal play

↓

Muscle contractures

↓

Abnormal skeletal forces

↓

Bony Deformity

Fig. 18.1. The cascade of deformities in spastic diplegia. Left: the cascade of deformities begins with the primary abnormalities, which arise directly from the CNS injury and lead to the secondary (growth deformities). Right: the boy's gait demonstrates the muscle contractures and bony deformities that are the end result. Note that spasticity (underlined) is one of the primary abnormalities of neurological injury. Permanent spasticity reduction allows us block some of this cascade effect and so prevent future deformity.

chance of recurrence once they have been corrected.

When the Motion Analysis Laboratory opened at Newington Children's Hospital in 1981, there were no effective treatments for the primary problems of cerebral palsy beyond a few oral medications and physical therapy. Orthopaedic correction of all deformities was the norm, and postoperative stiffness and rapid recurrence of deformity were common sequelae. Then in 1986, Dr Warwick Peacock—who had recently immigrated to the United States from South Africa—introduced a new treatment for spasticity, SDR. When I first heard of this procedure I was highly skeptical. In 1986, however, when I met Dr Peacock and reviewed a videotape of his preoperative and postoperative outcomes, my skepticism quickly turned to credulity.

In the years that followed, there has been a great deal of debate as to whether rhizotomy and/or the ITB pump are useful in the treatment of cerebral palsy. Fortunately, three separate randomized clinical trials—the first in Vancouver by Steinbok et al. (1997), the second in Seattle by McLaughlin et al. (1998), and the third in Toronto by Wright and colleagues (1998)—have done much to answer this question. All three studies showed a significant reduction in spasticity, although there was a difference between the three studies with respect to the functional outcome. The Vancouver and Toronto studies noted a significant advantage for functional outcome, whereas the Seattle study did not. However, a meta-analysis of three papers published in 2002 concluded that there was a significant reduction of spasticity in the pooled results of the children studied who had had the combination of selective dorsal rhizotomy and physical therapy, with a mean reduction of Ashworth score of 1.2 (Wilcoxon P<0.001) (McLaughlin et al. 2002). In addition, the meta-analysis also revealed a significant reduction in GMFM score of +4.0 (P=0.008). It is interesting that in all three studies there was also a "consistent and statistically significant (P=0.0002) inverse correlation between the baseline GMFM-66 score and the percent of dorsal root tissue transected."

Even given that the studies referenced above demonstrate that selective dorsal rhizotomy

287

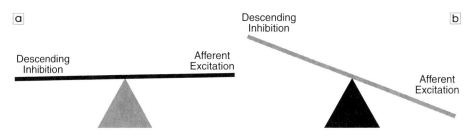

Fig. 18.2. (a) Normal balance of spinal circuits. In a neurologically normal individual, afferent excitation from the spinal circuits is balanced by descending inhibition from the central nervous system. (b) Graphic illustration of the imbalance of spinal circuits in spastic cerebral palsy. Due to the loss of central nervous system inhibition, normal balance of the spinal circuits is lost. Balance can be restored by either SDR or the ITB, but they act on opposite ends of the teeter-totter (see-saw). Rhizotomy eliminates some of the afferent impulses to the brain and so reduces afferent excitation, whereas the baclofen pump increases afferent inhibition by substituting baclofen (chlorophenyl-gamma amino butyric acid, an agonist of the inhibitory neurotransmitter, GABA), for GABA in the receptors of spinal-cord neurons.

does significantly reduce spasticity and enhance function, there is still an ongoing debate as to whether spasticity reduction and orthopaedics are simply two different pathways to the same goal. However, to the reader, who by this time has gained some understanding as to how the primary and secondary problems of cerebral palsy are related, the answer should be obvious. Spasticity reduction and orthopaedics are complementary, since the former minimizes one of the primary disorders (spasticity) and the latter corrects the secondary deformities of muscle and bone.

We know now that SDR works well to reduce spastic tone, but does not affect so called "extrapyramidal tone" (which probably represents abnormal tone emanating from basal ganglia injury). Fortunately, the ITB pump can be used in children with mixed tone. Consequently, each method has its advantages and disadvantages.

Selective dorsal rhizotomy is a one-off procedure, and if it works it essentially solves the problem of spasticity. In the case of a good outcome, this "permanency" is an advantage. Unfortunately, however, if the procedure produces adverse results, the major disadvantage is that there is no way they can be undone.

The ITB pump has the advantage of not being permanent. Hence, if an adverse outcome arises as a result of pump implantation, the pump can be discontinued or the baclofen dose modified. The downside of "non-permanency" is that the pump must be refilled at roughly 3-month intervals and, as such, it is expensive to maintain. Furthermore, the batteries (and hence the pump itself) must be replaced every 7 years, and there is an appreciable complication rate. All of this will be discussed more completely in the sections devoted to SDR and the ITB pump that follow.

We currently employ SDR for candidates who fully meet the criteria (born preterm, with spastic diplegic involvement, pure spasticity, and good preservation of selective motor control and balance), and use ITB with children who have significant spasticity but who do not meet the rigid criteria listed above (Fig. 18.2). In both cases we use the procedures in conjunction with orthopaedic correction of lever-arm dysfunction (bony deformity) and

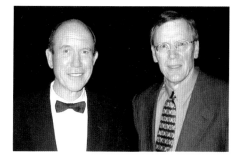

Fig. 18.3. Dr Warwick Peacock (left) and Dr Leland Albright (right). Both men have made enormous contributions to the treatment of cerebral palsy. In 1986 Dr Peacock introduced the SDR to the United States, and in the early 1990s Dr Albright pioneered the use of the baclofen pump for spasticity reduction in children.

residual muscle contractures. However, once spasticity is reduced, muscle contractures can usually be prevented or corrected with the combination of good physical therapy and a daily program of passive stretching. This can be augmented, if necessary, with botulinum toxin and stretching casts. Orthopaedic lengthenings of muscle contractures are done only if the more conservative treatment modalities fail. It is our opinion that, in general, orthopaedic lengthening of muscle should be done "at last" and not "at first". Using this type of combined approach to management, we now have many children whom we have brought to maturity with good bony alignment, stable feet and normal muscle length, without having to resort to orthopaedic lengthening of muscles.

I consider myself very privileged to know personally the two men who introduced these treatment modalities, and to count them as friends. We are all fortunate that Drs Peacock and Albright have agreed to contribute to this chapter, describing their particular contributions to the treatment of cerebral palsy.

Intrathecal baclofen for spasticity

PHARMACOLOGY OF ORAL AND INTRATHECAL BACLOFEN

Baclofen, chlorophenyl-gamma amino butyric acid, is an agonist of the inhibitory neurotransmitter, $GABA_b$. Baclofen was synthesized because GABA itself is strongly polar and hydrophilic, and does not penetrate the blood–brain barrier. Baclofen is absorbed rapidly and well from the alimentary tract, achieving peak blood levels 2 hours after an oral dose (Faigle and Keberle 1972). The serum half-life of orally administered baclofen is 3.5 hours. Baclofen crosses the blood–brain barrier better than GABA, but relatively poorly: oral baclofen doses of 30–60 mg are associated with CSF levels of 12–96 ng/ml, whereas ITB doses of 400 μg are associated with CSF levels of 396 mg/ml (Sallerin-Caute et al. 1991). In spite of the poor CNS penetration, oral baclofen given in therapeutic doses is often associated with decreased concentration or lethargy. Oral baclofen in therapeutic dosage reduces spasticity mildly, e.g. by about one grade on the Modified Ashworth scale.

Baclofen administered into the lumbar CSF as a bolus dose distributes within CSF and migrates into the superficial layers of the spinal cord where it, in essence, replaces deficient GABA that should have been released by descending inhibitory impulses. The effects of a bolus ITB dose on spasticity begin within 1–2 hours, are maximal at about 4 hours and cease within 8–12 hours. The half-life of ITB is 4 hours (Mueller et al. 1988). It is cleared at CSF clearance rates. ITB infusion is associated with minimal serum levels. In a series of six children receiving 77–400 µg ITB/day, serum levels were at or below the limit of quantification (10 ng/ml) in all patients (Albright and Shultz 1999).

Baclofen's site of action in treating dystonia is unknown. It may work at a spinal-cord level, decreasing the effect of descending excitatory impulses, or intracranially by inhibiting the excessively stimulated pre-motor and supplementary motor cortex (Albright et al. 2001).

PATIENT SELECTION AND INDICATIONS FOR ITB
Ideally, patients are evaluated for ITB by a multidisciplinary team, including neurology, neurosurgery, occupational therapy, orthopaedics, physiatry, physical therapy and social work. It is important for patient and family goals to be clearly established before any treatment recommendation is given, and if the recommendation is for ITB, it is important for the patient and family to hear the estimations of the evaluating team as to how ITB might help the patient to achieve their goals.

ITB is indicated for spasticity and dystonia. In patients with spasticity of cerebral origin, ITB is recommended to treat moderate or severe spasticity (Ashworth scores of 3–5), which is usually generalized and involves the upper and lower extremities. That spasticity is either impeding care, impeding function or causing musculoskeletal contractures, and has been treated (ineffectively) with multiple oral medications before ITB is recommended.

Most candidates for ITB are 4 years of age or older because of the size of the current pumps. However, I have inserted a pump into a 9-month-old child, weighing 18 lb, with severe hypertonicity after near-drowning. The limitation for pump placement is size, not age.

ITB is also indicated for generalized, severe dystonia. Usually this is dystonia that is secondary to cerebral palsy or traumatic brain injury, but it has been used to treat dystonia of other causes (Albright 1999). ITB is also effective in treating children with diffuse hypertonicity and opisthotonic posturing after near-drowning or other anoxic events.

As a general rule, ITB does not significantly decrease athetosis or chorea, and it certainly has no effect on tremor or ataxia. ITB is relatively contraindicated in children with spasticity of the extremities that is associated with hypotonia of the neck and trunk. If they are treated with a pump, the extremities loosen but the hypotonia worsens and function may decrease; however, sometimes the extremity tightness is severe enough to warrant the cervical/trunk worsening. The presence of a gastrostomy tube is not a contraindication to pump insertion and does not appear to increase the risk of a pump infection.

SCREENING
Nearly all people with either spasticity or dystonia are tested for their response to ITB before a pump is inserted. It may be reasonable to insert a pump without a screening trial for the unusual child with severe spasticity or dystonia who has failed all oral medications and has had a spine fusion. Insertion of a screening dose or of an intrathecal catheter for screening infusion in these children often requires intraoperative drilling of the fusion mass and if that is to be done, it may be reasonable to go ahead and insert the pump and intrathecal catheter. Because approximately 90% of such children respond to ITB, I have occasionally inserted pumps without confirming efficacy first.

The purpose of screening people with spasticity is to determine if ITB decreases spasticity in the legs, not to determine if the bolus test dose improves spasticity in the arms (although it may) or if it improves function. If function improves in either arms or legs after a bolus dose, there is a good likelihood that function will improve if the patient receives continuous ITB infusion, but the corollary is not true; if function does not improve during a test dose, it may well improve during chronic infusion.

The purpose of screening people with dystonia is to determine if ITB decreases dystonia diffusely. Children with mixed spasticity and dystonia can be screened with a bolus injection but those with predominantly or exclusively dystonia are usually screened with a continuous infusion via an intrathecal catheter, because dystonia response rates to screening infusions are higher than to screening bolus doses.

BOLUS SCREENING INJECTIONS

Response of spasticity to ITB is tested by bolus injections that are given via a lumbar puncture. Doses of 25 µg may be used to test children weighing less than 40 lb (although 50 µg might be used if the spasticity were severe) and doses of 50 µg are used in those weighing more. Muscle tone in the extremities is graded on the Modified Ashworth Scale before the injection, then at 2-hour intervals afterward for 8 hours. Children are monitored with pulse oximetry during the evaluation. A decrease of one point or more in mean Ashworth scores in the lower extremities is considered to be clinically significant, in which case the pump is often inserted the following day. Side-effects of the lumbar puncture (headache, nausea) are common, but side-effects from the test dose (lethargy, confusion) are rare and transient, subsiding in 2–4 hours.

The response rate of patients with cerebral spasticity to 50 µg bolus injections was 75% in a randomized prospective double-blind multi-institution study (Gilmartin et al. 2000). In our experience, nearly all patients with pure spasticity respond to bolus doses of 50–100 µg. Patients who do not respond often have unrecognized concomitant dystonia. Because the response rate to bolus injections is so high, few centers now utilize placebo injections during screening, except for investigational studies.

The response rate of patients with dystonia to bolus screening doses is considerably lower. In a review of the literature of patients screened with bolus doses, 24/46 (52%) responded (Albright 1999). This low rate probably reflects the small amount of baclofen that would get into the cervical region or the intracranial subarachnoid space after a lumbar bolus injection.

CONTINUOUS SCREENING INFUSIONS

Infusion screening is done by a micro-infusion pump on the bedside that is connected to an intrathecal catheter. Intrathecal catheters should probably be inserted in the operating room to decrease the risk of catheter infection. Catheters are inserted via a Tuohy needle (inserted at as oblique an angle as feasible) and advanced up to the mid-cervical area, then either tunneled subcutaneously to exit the skin and connected to the external micro-infusion pump, or tunneled anteriorly and connected to a subcutaneous Mediport or Bard port. A Huber needle can be inserted percutaneously into the port and connected to the micro-

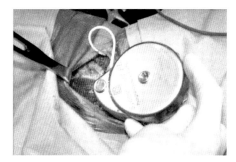

Fig. 18.4. A baclofen pump. An illustration of a pump being inserted into a right abdominal subfascial pocket. Orientation is with the child's head to the right.

infusion pump. Infusion doses begin at ~200 µg/day and increase by 50 µg every 8 hours until (1) the mean dystonia score decreases by 25% or more on the BAD scale (Barry et al. 1999), (2) unacceptable side-effects (such as obtundation) occur, or (3) a dose of 900 µg/day is reached without a significant response.

Response rates of secondary dystonia to screening infusions are about 90%, and often occur when the infusion rate is 400–600 µg/day, substantially higher than doses to which spasticity responds.

PUMP IMPLANTATION

There are two commercial pump manufacturers, Medtronic and Arrow. Medtronic makes battery-powered pumps that are externally adjustable by a computer and microwave telemetry. Medtronic pump reservoirs hold either 10 or 18 ml and the battery lasts 7–8 years. The Arrow pump is gas-powered and runs indefinitely. It is available with reservoirs of 20, 40 or 60 ml. The rate of infusion of Arrow pumps is fixed, but the infusion dosage can be altered by changing the concentration of baclofen in the pump. In treating spasticity and dystonia associated with cerebral palsy, the Medtronic pump is used more commonly because of the frequent need for dose adjustments.

Pumps are inserted under general anesthesia in operations that last for 60–90 minutes. Patients are positioned in a lateral position, most often with the right side up. Pumps are inserted through a subcostal incision and secured into surgically created pockets located either superficial to external fascia of the external oblique and rectus abdominis muscles, in people with substantial subcutaneous tissue (e.g. 2 cm or more), or below the fascia, in people with little subcutaneous tissue (the majority of children with cerebral palsy) (Fig. 18.4) (Kopell et al. 2001). Posteriorly, catheters are inserted obliquely via Touhy needles into the thecal sac and advanced cephalad under fluoroscopic guidance. The position of the catheter tip varies with the clinical indication for ITB. For the few subjects with spastic paraparesis, the tip is positioned at ~T10. For those with spastic quadriparesis, the tip is positioned at C7–T3. For those with dystonia of the upper and lower extremities, I position the catheter at about C4–C5 (Fig. 18.5). Insertion of the intrathecal catheter into persons who have undergone spine fusion requires either insertion of the Touhy needle below the fusion mass, drilling a small tunnel through the fusion mass at ~L2–L3 to access the dura or tunneling the catheter subcutaneously to the cervical region above the fusion and inserting it into the intradural space via a small laminectomy.

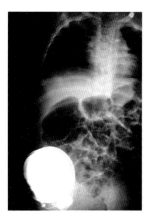

Fig. 18.5. Roentgenogram of pump and catheter. Radiograph demonstrating the pump and intrathecal catheter positioned in the mid-cervical region for a child with dystonia.

ITB COMPLICATIONS/COMPLICATION AVOIDANCE

In a multicenter study of ITB for spastic cerebral palsy, ITB was associated with adverse events such as headache, nausea, hypotonia or somnolence in 42/51 patients, and with device related events such as infections, catheter problems or CSF leaks in 30/46 patients (Gilmartin et al. 2000). In general, ITB therapy is associated with three main complications: infections, catheter malfunctions and CSF leaks. Infections develop in 10%–20% of cases and occur mostly within three months after pump insertion. They are caused most often by staphylococcus aureus and cause fever, swelling, erythema of the incisions, and drainage through the incisions. Infections may be limited to the pump or extend into the CSF. The diagnosis is confirmed by culture of fluid around the pump and of CSF drawn through the side port of the pump. Treatment almost always involves removal of the pump and intrathecal catheter, although rarely, the infection can be eradicated by intravenous and intrapump antibiotics (Galloway and Falope 2000). Infections occur in spite of multiple prophylactic measures, including administration of antibiotics during pump surgery, irrigation of wounds with antibiotics, and administration of antibiotics for 2–3 days postoperatively.

Catheter problems occur in up to 25% of cases and include disconnection, leak through the catheter wall, and migration out of the thecal sac, kinking, and occlusion of the catheter tip. Build-up of granulation tissue around the catheter tip has been reported in adults with pumps infusing morphine, but not in children or adults receiving ITB. Catheter malfunctions require replacement of the affected portion of the catheter. Recent data indicate that the two-piece catheter (Medtronic 8711) has fewer complications (11%) than the one-piece catheter (Medtronic 8709) (26%).

CSF leaks result from CSF tracking along the catheter from the site where it penetrates the thecal sac. Leaks occur in 10%–15% of patients, and occur more frequently in people with dystonia than with spasticity. Inserting the Touhy needle into the sac obliquely, at an angle more parallel to the spinal axis than would be used to do a conventional spinal tap, may diminish the frequency of leaks. CSF leaks are treated with bed-rest, an abdominal binder and at times by insertion of a lumbar drain for external CSF drainage for 3–7 days. In cases of recurrent or persistent CSF leaks, treatment involves surgical exposure of the catheter and application of a purse-string suture (perhaps supplemented with fibrin glue) around the catheter where it penetrates the dura.

Seizure frequency is affected rarely by ITB (Gilmartin et al. 2000). Although many children with cerebral palsy have seizures, the frequency of those seizures does not seem to be significantly altered—either increased or decreased—by ITB therapy.

The course of scoliosis after ITB is unclear, but is probably not increased.

CHRONIC CARE OF INDIVIDUALS WITH BACLOFEN PUMPS

After pump insertion, ITB doses are adjusted frequently (often daily) until there is an appreciable improvement in spasticity or dystonia, and then may be adjusted whenever the patient returns for pump refill. Doses for spasticity are adjusted upward by 10%–20% until the effects are near the desired goal, and then are fine-tuned with changes of 5–20 µg. Doses for dystonia may be adjusted by larger increments, e.g. 50 µg, until the effects are near the desired goal, and then fine-tuned with smaller changes, e.g. 20–30 µg/day.

Pumps are refilled at intervals ranging from 3 weeks to 5 months, with an average of every 3 months. Refill frequency varies with the pump reservoir size, the baclofen concentration (500–2000 µg/ml) and the infusion dosage. Refills are done percutaneously via a Huber needle inserted into the septum in the center of the pump. Few children need topical anesthesia with EMLA cream or ethylene chloride before the refills.

ITB OVERDOSAGE

ITB overdoses are almost never due to pump malfunction but rather to iatrogenic maneuvers, most commonly attempts to evaluate patency of the catheter. Mild ITB overdoses cause only lethargy and hypotonia, will clear within a few hours, and do not need to be treated—although some physicians give 1–2 mg doses of physostigmine in these circumstances. Large ITB overdoses result in coma and in hyptonia that requires assisted ventilation. Such overdoses are treated by intubation, turning off the pump, and at times by barbitaging 10–20 ml of normal saline into CSF several times. Baclofen is not neurotoxic; once the excess baclofen is metabolized (in 24–48 hours), muscle tone returns to baseline and the infusion typically resumes.

ITB WITHDRAWAL

Baclofen withdrawal after chronic ITB infusion can be a serious problem and severe cases have the potential to be life-threatening (Coffey et al. 2002). The most common symptoms of withdrawal are hypertonicity and itching, followed by fever, confusion, and rarely by psychosis or hallucinations. Severe cases of baclofen withdrawal may result in rapidly increasing spasticity and spasms as well as severe itching or paresthesias, malaise and seizures. In addition, body temperature is often elevated as a result of the intense muscle activity. Symptoms of withdrawal are more likely to result from an abrupt cessation of infusion, such as that due to a catheter break or dislodgement, than to the pump reservoir running dry. As soon as ITB withdrawal is suspected, the patient should be given oral baclofen, usually 20 mg t.i.d., which is continued until the infusion resumes. By providing the individual with oral baclofen and a benzodiazepine during the workup, the severity of baclofen withdrawal can be greatly reduced, but prompt action is still necessary to reestablish the delivery of baclofen to the intrathecal space.

ITB Treatment Outcomes

Spasticity

Continuous ITB infusion decreases spasticity in the upper and lower extremities, and reduces clonus and muscle spasms (Butler and Campbell 2000). The efficacy has been demonstrated in both single- and multi-institution studies, in screening studies done in a double-blind manner as well as in long-term follow-up studies done retrospectively. In a multicenter study, 39 months after pump implantation lower-extremity tone (Ashworth) decreased from 3.6 to 1.9 and upper-extremity tone decreased from 2.6 to 1.5 (Gilmartin et al. 2000). Reported effects of ITB on the lower extremities have usually been more pronounced than upper extremity effects because most intrathecal catheters have been positioned in the T10–T12 region, so that the resulting baclofen concentration is higher in the lumbar region of the spinal cord than in the cervical. When catheters are positioned higher, upper-extremity spasticity is reduced more (Grabb et al. 1999). Range of motion also appears to be increased, particularly in the lower extremities.

The effects of ITB on function have not been evaluated in a well-designed prospective, controlled study, except in a single subject reported by Almeida and colleagues (1997), who found improved spasticity (in eight results), improved quality of movement (in two measures), reduced functional limitations (in eight results) and greater social-role participation (in a single result). Butler and Campbell (2000) reviewed the 14 publications about ITB for spasticity, and graded the quality of each of those studies. The studies indicated that function is probably improved, including improved upper-extremity function, improved activities of daily living (ADL), and, in about one-third of individuals, improved speech and swallowing. Other improvements included better gait, overall function, self-care, positioning and ease of care. Although such changes are seen relatively frequently after pump insertion, there is at present no good method of determining before pump placement the functional changes that may occur afterward.

One of the indications for ITB therapy in spasticity is to decrease the development of musculoskeletal contractures. Data supporting the effectiveness of ITB in doing so are limited to one study, in which orthopedic intervention was thought to be necessary in 24 children prior to pump implantation, but was performed in only 10 of the children after pump implantation (Gerstzen et al. 1998). In our experience, many children have needed an orthopedic operation—often multilevel—after pump insertion, but no child who has had an orthopedic operation, e.g. a TAL, after pump insertion, has had to have it repeated. Gait analysis before and after ITB therapy has been reported (Moto et al. 2001). Gait appears to improve the most in children who ambulate without assistive devices.

Dystonia

The literature on ITB in dystonia is relatively limited. In the largest published series, 86 patients (71% with cerebral palsy) were offered treatment with ITB (Albright et al. 2001). Over 90% responded to screening and pumps were implanted in 77. Dystonia scores were significantly decreased at 3, 6, 12 and 24 months after implantation, compared with baseline scores. Dystonia scores were significantly lower in children whose intrathecal catheters were positioned above T4 than in those with catheters at T6 or below. Patients reported that quality of life and ease of care improved in 86% and speech improved in 33%.

Within the next two years, a pump one-third smaller than current models will be available from Medtronic with the same reservoir volume as the current size model. In contradistinction to the current models, which sometimes decrease the rate of infusion as the residual volume decreases to 2 ml, infusion with the next model will remain constant until the pump is nearly empty. The current intrathecal catheters are susceptible to disconnection, fracture and kinking. Catheters are being designed to decrease the frequency of those complications.

It is likely that progressively more patients in the US and Europe will be treated with ITB in the coming decade as its effects on spasticity and dystonia become better known. The substantial costs of the pump and medication will limit or prevent the use of ITB in developing nations.

Selective dorsal rhizotomy for the relief of spasticity

Cerebral palsy is a movement disorder produced by an insult to the immature brain. The underlying pathology remains static but the motor manifestations may change with time. Over the last four decades the incidence of cerebral palsy has remained fairly constant at about two cases per thousand livebirths (Stanley 1979, Evans et al. 1985). The spastic variety is the commonest. Spasticity or muscle hypertonus is characterized clinically by an increased resistance to passive movement, brisk deep-tendon reflexes, reduced range of movement and clonus. Spasticity is also associated with some degree of weakness, abnormal posture and movement patterns, and a tendency to develop musculoskeletal deformities. Many methods of treatment have been used in an attempt to reduce spasticity but when muscle hypertonus remains severe and interferes with movement patterns, especially in gait, rhizotomy has proven to be of value in carefully selected cases (Fasano et al. 1978, Peacock et al. 1987, Vaughan et al. 1988, Cahan et al. 1990, Stout et al. 1993, Steinbok et al. 1997).

PATHOPHYSIOLOGY
The neural mechanism involved in the maintenance of normal muscle tone was poorly understood until Sir Charles Sherrington (1898) performed his classic experiments in the 1890s. By transecting the midbrain of cats he produced a marked increase in muscle tone. If placed upright, the cats could indefinitely maintain a standing position due to the spasticity in their fore- and hindlimbs. Based on a belief that the posterior or dorsal roots of the spinal nerves played an important role in the maintenance of muscle tone and therefore spasticity, he exposed and divided all the spinal posterior nerve roots. To his amazement, the limb spasticity resolved. He then postulated that, because transection of the brainstem produced the spasticity, the interrupted descending tracts must have been an inhibitory factor in the control of muscle tone. As division of the posterior roots relieved the increased tone he felt that those roots must contain excitatory fibers which tended to elevate muscle tone and, in the absence of the inhibitory influence of the descending tracts, this excitatory influence would be unopposed resulting in spasticity.

In skeletal muscle, muscle spindles were identified which were responsive to stretch.

When a muscle spindle is stretched it sends an excitatory impulse via the posterior root to the anterior horn cell. The anterior horn cell then, in turn, sends an impulse out to the muscle via the anterior or motor root bringing about a force generating contraction. The anterior horn cell is also under the inhibitory influence of the descending motor tracts. Thus, through the posterior root, the muscle spindle has an excitatory effect on the anterior horn cell and the descending motor tracts have an inhibitory effect. When these two effects are appropriately balanced, muscle tone is normal. However, if the descending motor tracts are damaged as occurs with stroke, spinal cord injury or, as is found with cerebral palsy, there is a loss of inhibition and the excitatory influence from the muscle spindle is relatively unopposed resulting in a rise in muscle tone or spasticity.

Spasticity can be defined as a velocity dependent increase in resistance to passive stretch with a "clasp-knife" component associated with hyperactive deep-tendon reflexes. Along with weakness and decreased fine-motor control, spasticity is a predominant feature of the upper motor-neuron lesion. Upper motor neurons may be damaged at either the spinal or cerebral level. The other clinical feature often encountered is clonus at the ankle.

For a number of reasons range of motion of the affected joints becomes limited. First, as a result of dynamic tightness due to the increased muscle tone, range of movement is reduced. Secondly, because of the muscle hypertonus, sarcomeres are not added to the muscle during growth resulting in true shortening (Tabary et al. 1981, Ashby et al. 1987, Lee et al. 1987, Tardieu and Tardieu 1987). Thirdly, during active voluntary movement in a child with spastic cerebral palsy agonist muscle contraction initiates a hyperactive reflex response in the antagonist muscle groups (Knutsson and Martensson 1980, Corcos et al. 1986, Tardieu and Tardieu 1987). Thus, because of dynamic tightness, true shortening and co-contraction range of motion are reduced.

In the presence of skeletal growth, spasticity is also a deforming force. Because of the persistent influence of this muscle hypertonus in the growing child, torsional deformities of the long bones of the lower extremities (femur and tibia), foot deformities and/or scoliosis may develop (Samilson 1975, Lance 1980).

Studies have also shown that movement carried out in the presence of spasticity requires more energy than when muscle tone is normal. There is also evidence to show that energy costs are reduced when muscle hypertonicity is reduced (Lundberg 1975, Waters et al. 1978, Stout et al. 1993).

HISTORY OF SELECTIVE RHIZOTOMY FOR SPASTICITY
In 1913, Foerster described 159 cases of posterior rhizotomy performed in patients with severe spasticity. Eighty-eight of these were performed on patients who had "congenital spastic paraplegia". He divided the entire posterior roots from the second lumbar level to the second sacral with sparing of the posterior root at the fourth lumbar level. This root was spared in an attempt to preserve power in the knee-extensor muscles. He used intraoperative nerve root stimulation to confirm that the nerve root to be cut was not a motor anterior root and to identify which nerve roots were involved with knee extension. He reported impressive results and gave advice concerning selection of candidates for the procedure. He selected patients with pure spasticity and excluded those who displayed

weakness or dystonia. Despite the good results the procedure was not widely used, possibly because of the extensive deafferentation caused by sectioning the entire posterior root. Persistent sensory and proprioceptive loss may have been what made the procedure unacceptable.

In the 1960s Gros took advantage of the fact that the posterior nerve roots divide into a number of rootlets before entering the dorsal surface of the spinal cord (Gros 1979). Instead of cutting the entire posterior root he separated the rootlets and only divided four-fifths, thus sparing sufficient afferent fibers to preserve sensory functions. Unfortunately he found residual spasticity and weakness in many of his patients.

Fasano and colleagues (1978) reported that different motor responses were evoked when different nerve rootlets were stimulated. Stimulation of some rootlets produced what he termed a "normal" response, while the stimulation of others produced sustained muscular contraction that sometimes spread to muscle groups not belonging to that nerve rootlet's reflex arc. In his procedure he exposed the nerve roots at the conus of the spinal cord. He then divided those rootlets associated with an "abnormal" response but left those associated with a brief, non-spreading response intact. Fasano reported excellent reduction in spasticity and the preservation of sensation.

With an exposure of only the level of the conus of the spinal cord, however, it was difficult to identify those nerve rootlets involved with sphincter function. Consequently, Peacock exposed the cauda equina via a more extensive laminectomy (Peacock et al. 1987). This exposure allowed accurate identification of the level of the nerve roots and certainty as to whether a posterior or an anterior rootlet was being tested. Intraoperative nerve root stimulation was also used in association with electromyographic monitoring as described by Fasano and colleagues (1978).

The technique has been further modified by a number of authors with less emphasis on electrical monitoring (Cohen and Webster 1991, Steinbok et al. 1995) and those where the laminectomy has been more limited (Lazareff et al. 1990, Barolat 1991)

PATIENT SELECTION

Because cerebral palsy is a multifaceted disorder the decision as to whether a specific child is a good candidate for selective posterior rhizotomy is a complex process. Many interacting factors need to be taken into account.

First of all, the diagnosis of cerebral palsy must be confirmed based on the characteristic history and physical findings. A history of preterm birth associated with difficult delivery and intraventricular hemorrhage in the newborn period are suggestive features, with subsequent delay in motor development. During examination the following manifestations are assessed: muscle tone, posture, strength, contractures and deformities, isolated muscle control, balance and intelligence. The motivation of the child and the parents is also evaluated.

Secondly, muscle tone is assessed by testing the resistance to passive movement in both the upper and lower limbs. The presence of spasticity is confirmed by finding an increased resistance to passive movement that has a clasp-knife feel to it. With spasticity the upper limbs tend to adopt a flexed position whereas in the lower limbs extension is more characteristic. The deep-tendon reflexes are usually brisk and clonus at the ankles is often present. Dystonia, athetosis and rigidity are often confused with spasticity. Dystonia is characterized by fluctuating tone and involuntary movement. In its mildest form the involuntary movement presents with fanning of the fingers. When it is more severe and of clinical significance, rotation of the limb around its axis is noted. Brisk tendon reflexes are often not found. Rigidity manifests itself with a marked increase in resistance to passive movement that has a "lead-pipe" type of feel to it. Rigidity is often seen in children who have survived a near-drowning event or an episode of severe anoxia. Dystonia and rigidity are not muscle-spindle-dependent, but are more likely to be due to an extrapyramidal abnormality. Therefore sectioning of the posterior roots will not alter dystonia and rigidity. Rhizotomy was not found to help children with mixed spastic/dystonic cerebral palsy (Peacock et al. 1987).

In children with spastic cerebral palsy the basic lesion is damage to the upper motor neurons. There is therefore not only spasticity but also some degree of muscle weakness. Spasticity may mask this underlying weakness. It is therefore important to assess voluntary strength. This is best done by getting the child to initiate and inhibit a movement throughout its range. For example, to assess quadriceps strength, the child is asked to stand from a squatting position and to stop at various points in the ascent. In going down to a squat again attempts are made to arrest the movement at various stages When a child who is dependent on spasticity for strength is asked to stand from the squatting position the movement can only be carried out with a single thrust and similarly when going down into the squatting position the child virtually drops down when the spasticity is "turned off". Other important muscle groups to be assessed for strength are the hip-abductors and the plantarflexors.

If severe muscle contractures are present little is to be achieved by performing a selective posterior rhizotomy because the limited range of movement is mainly due to structural restrictions rather than to dynamic ones. Orthopedic procedures are more likely to be effective for the treatment of structural abnormalities.

When rhizotomy is being considered children can be placed in two groups. The first group contains those children who show reasonable functional skills, despite their spasticity, and are able to crawl and walk. The second group is composed of children who display minimal, if any, functional ability. In the first group where spasticity is the main disabling factor, following rhizotomy—when their spasticity has been reduced—function should improve.

With the second group, although functional improvement is unlikely, some important gains are possible. Comfort may be improved, and caring for the patient may be made easier. Following rhizotomy, the deforming force of spasticity is minimized so that fewer orthopedic procedures should be required. If the range of motion is improved by eliminating dynamic tightness, a less radical procedure may suffice and postoperative splinting will be reduced in duration.

An ideal candidate for rhizotomy is a child with spastic cerebral palsy aged about 4 or 5 years who has minimal contractures and is able to walk unassisted but with a crouched gait and equinus positioning of the ankles and feet (Fig. 18.6). An unsuitable candidate would display significant weakness with dystonia and poor truncal control. Severe contractures and spinal deformities would also be contraindications.

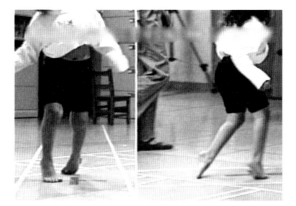

Fig. 18.6. An ideal candidate for SDR. This is the ideal patient for SDR. She was born preterm and has spastic diplegia on the basis of periventricular leukomalacia. She has dynamic spasticity with no evidence of mixed tone and/or fixed contractures. Finally, she is cognitively normal and has good selective motor control and balance. *See CD-Rom, Figures 18.6 and 18.10, for dynamic preoperative and postoperative illustrations.*

Rhizotomy only reduces spasticity. It is important to bear this in mind when assessing the child. The goal is to reduce spasticity so that the limitations in range of movement will be improved and hopefully, function will thereby be improved.

SURGICAL TECHNIQUE

A number of different operative techniques are presently used. Some surgeons place less emphasis on intraoperative monitoring (Steinbok et al. 1995), and others use minimal or no intraoperative monitoring (Cohen and Webster 1991). Others prefer to expose the nerve rootlets at the level of the conus (Barolat 1991), or the cauda equina at the L5/S1 levels (Lazareff et al. 1990). The technique described below is the one employed by the author.

Endotracheal general anesthesia is induced without the use of long-acting neuromuscular blocking agents and an indwelling urinary catheter is placed. The patient is then placed in the prone position with bolsters under the chest and pelvis to allow abdominal respiration to occur freely (Fig. 18.7). For the intraoperative electromyographic (EMG) recordings, needle electrodes are placed in five muscle groups in each leg. These are the quadriceps, the hip-adductors, the hamstrings, the gastrocnemii and tibialis anterior. Two further electrodes are placed in the anal sphincter. There is some argument as to whether intraoperative monitoring provides a valid basis for the determination of which nerve rootlets should be divided. It definitely enables the surgeon to verify accurately the level of each rootlet and to be certain that the rootlet is a posterior or an anterior (motor) rootlet. EMG is justifiable on these grounds alone. More controversial is the neurophysiological assumption that the differences in response to posterior rootlet stimulation provide a scientific basis for deciding which rootlets should be divided and which should be preserved (Cohen and Webster 1991, Steinbok et al. 1995). We have used intraoperative nerve-root stimulation and EMG monitoring for 20 years and have not found the technique to be unreliable in the determination of which nerve rootlets to divide. The number of rootlets cut has corresponded well with

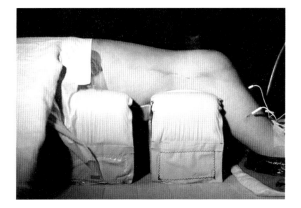

Fig. 18.7. Positioning for SDR. A child positioned for SDR before the start of the procedure. She has good chest and pelvic support without interfering with respiration. Five recording-needle electrodes have been placed on each limb for intraoperative monitoring.

the severity of the spasticity in that particular patient and there has not been a random distribution of numbers of rootlets cut as would be expected if the electrophysiological basis for the procedure was totally unfounded. The decision to divide or spare a rootlet should not be made in a rigid fashion. The clinical picture of the patient must be taken into account, and the distribution of the spasticity will also be important. If the monitoring shows few abnormal responses at the S1 level in a patient with marked equinus the surgeon should feel at liberty to cut more rootlets than strictly indicated by the monitoring to be sure that a plantigrade foot position will result.

The incision is planned by using out the bony landmarks. The intercristal plane is at the level of the L4 spinous process or at the L4/L5 interspace. By counting up and down the incision is marked out from L2 to S2. After preparing and draping the surgical area the incision is made down to the spinous processes. After separating the supraspinous ligament from the lumbodorsal fascia the paraspinal muscles are retracted laterally. The ligamentum flavum between the laminae of L5 and S1 is cleared of fat and a small window is created to expose the epidural fat on either side of the spinous process. Using a side-cutting high-speed drill with a footplate, the laminae are cut from the opening below L5, up to and including L2. This is done on both sides. The supraspinous and interspinous ligaments between L5 and S1 are cut so that the cut laminae, spinous processes and intervening ligaments can be rotated upwards, hinged on the supraspinous and interspinous ligaments between L2 and L1. This rotated segment can be secured by suturing it to the self-retaining retractor. Similarly, the laminae of S1 and S2 are cut and hinged downwards. The dura is now well exposed from the lower border of L1 to the upper border of S3. After opening the dura in the midline throughout its exposure the edges are tacked out. The cauda equina is now visible. If the arachnoid mater was not opened it should be now to provide access to the nerve roots. The nerve root of S1 is usually the largest. To verify the levels, the anterior root at this level is separated and stimulated with an increasing voltage until a motor response is seen. Normally, the response is flexion at the knee and plantarflexion. The anterior root

301

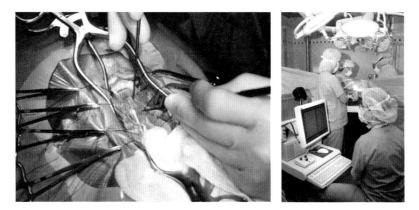

Fig. 18.8. Intraoperative stimulation of nerve rootlets. The laminae have been lifted away and the dura opened. The surgeon is stimulating a nerve rootlet while an electrophysiologist observes the results on a multichannel EMG monitor. Meanwhile a physiatrist is monitoring the response of the muscles by palpation and observation.

of S2 is now stimulated and this should produce plantarflexion and flexion of the toes with, possibly, some anal sphincter contraction. Having ascertained the level accurately, the nerve roots are counted upwards to the L2 level. At L2, the posterior root is isolated and stimulated. The voltage required to produce a response with a posterior root is about ten times greater than for an anterior root. The voltage is slowly increased until a motor response is produced. A 50 Hz train of stimuli is then applied for 1 second at approximately 75% of the threshold stimulus and the voltage increased until a motor response is recorded (Fig. 18.8). The stimulus is applied until a relatively constant EMG recording is obtained. A normal response is considered to be one where the EMG pattern is decremental, does not last longer than the 1 second of 50 Hz stimulation and there is no spread to other muscles than the ones supplied by the reflex arc of the nerve root being stimulated. An abnormal response is associated with an incremental, multiphasic or clonic response and may last longer than the 1 second of 50 Hz stimulation. An abnormal response often spreads to other muscle groups than the ones involved with the nerve root being stimulated (Fig. 18.9). Those nerve roots associated with a normal response are left intact while those associated with an abnormal response are divided with micro-neurosurgical scissors. The nerve roots from L2 to S2 on one side are dealt with and then the nerve roots on the other side are stimulated and either spared or divided in similar fashion.[1] The dura is closed in a watertight fashion and then the laminae are sutured back into their original position and the paraspinal muscles are secured to the bone. The skin is closed in layers.

---

[1] At Gillette Children's Hospital the procedure is performed from L1 to S2. We moved the operation up to L1 since both the hip-flexors and adductors take some of their innervation from that level. It is our current opinion that this change in technique has yielded better outcomes (less hip-flexor and adductor dominance and a reduction in postoperative lumbar lordosis). To date, however, we have not published a comparative study of our results.

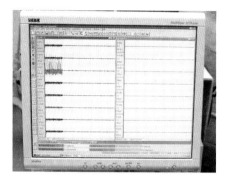

Fig. 18.9. An EMG tracing demonstrating an abnormal response to stimulation. The response to stimulation of the L5 level results in a crescendo-type signal response that spreads into other dermatome levels.

POSTOPERATIVE MANAGEMENT

The pediatric pain-management team should provide appropriate analgesia for the first 3 days. The patient is kept horizontal for 5 days and then mobilized. Physical therapy is started on the third postoperative day with gentle stretching and then, once the patient is out of bed, therapy can be continued in the physical therapy gym. At our center, the patient is usually discharged home on the eighth day to continue therapy with the familiar provider. Some institutions have kept the children for in-hospital therapy for longer periods.

The postoperative physical therapy should continue for at least 6 months before musculoskeletal surgery is contemplated. It is often difficult to determine whether the decreased range of motion is due to fixed contractures or dynamic tightness. However, once the spasticity has been reduced, 6 months of therapy may improve range of motion significantly. It is thus wise to wait as muscle-lengthening may no longer be required or, if it is, less may suffice. Maintaining length should also be easier as there is less tone to resist with casting.

RESULTS

In all post-rhizotomy series spasticity is shown to be reduced and range of motion increased (Peacock et al. 1987, Vaughan et al. 1988, Cahan et al. 1990, Steinbok et al. 1997). The majority of authors have also reported functional improvement that has persisted with long follow-up (Fasano et al. 1978, Arens et al. 1989). Assessment of function and documentation of outcome are difficult to standardize in patients with cerebral palsy because of the great variability in this particular group of patients and because of the ongoing growth and maturation. Ottfrid Foerster (1913) was the first to publish the results of rhizotomy in patients with cerebral palsy showing preoperative and postoperative photographs. More recently, standardized assessments have been used, such as the Gross Motor Function Measure (GMFM) and the Pediatric Evaluation of Disability Inventory, and most series have reported favorable results (Rosenbaum et al. 1990, Steinbok et al. 1997). Gait analysis has been used extensively (Vaughan et al. 1988, 1991, Boscarino et al. 1993) and has demonstrated improvements in hip and knee range of motion, stride length and speed of walking, with more effective joint motion and foot placement (Fig. 18.10).

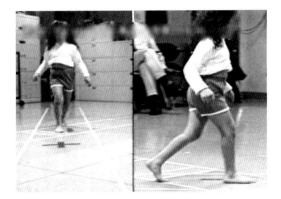

Fig. 18.10. The post-surgical result. The same child pictured in Figure 18.6, 6 months following SDR. No surgical lengthening of muscles has been done. *See CD-Rom, Figure 18.10, for a dynamic illustration.*

COMPLICATIONS

The possible complications that may occur following selective posterior rhizotomy are hemorrhage, infection and spinal fluid leakage. More specific to the procedure, problems such as increased weakness, sensory loss, bowel and bladder incontinence and sexual dysfunction may occur. In the author's recent series of 105 consecutive cases of selective posterior rhizotomy there were no serious postoperative complications such as wound infection, cerebrospinal fluid leakage, altered bowel or bladder function or sensory loss (Van de Wiele et al. 1996). The most frequently documented intraoperative were a moderate elevation of body temperature (13/105) and transient cardiac arrhythmias (8/105). The most frequent postoperative complications were fever, post-catherization cystitis and marginal oxygen saturation. Abbott (1992) reported a higher complication rate with selective posterior rhizotomy, although most were transient in nature (lower-limb dysesthesias) or related to anesthesia (bronchospasm). Transient hyperesthesias are commonly noted after rhizotomy, although it has been the observation of the author that these are seen less frequently and resolve more quickly when the percentage of rootlets sectioned is kept to a minimum. Asymptomatic, but clinically detectable, limited proprioceptive or cutaneous sensory losses are occasionally observed postoperatively, occurring in three of 51 patients in one series (Arens et al. 1989), and seven of 30 patients in a series of older children and young adults (Engsberg et al. 1998). After reduction of muscle tone by the procedure, muscle weakness may become more apparent, either unmasked or exacerbated by rhizotomy. This weakness tends to improve with postoperative physical therapy (Arens et al. 1989). Clinically significant spasticity may be noted after the procedure and this has almost always been a persistence of pre-existing spasticity rather than a delayed recurrence. This is probably due to insufficient rootlets having been cut (Lang et al. 1994, Chicoine et al. 1997). Among 51 patients undergoing multilevel laminectomy for rhizotomy 9% were found to have asymptomatic spondylolysis or spondylolisthesis (Peter et al. 1990). Interestingly, this incidence of spondylolysis is greater that of the normal population but less than the 21% found in the population of patients with spastic diplegic cerebral palsy (Harada et al. 1993).

Some patients were noted to have scoliosis, lordosis or kyphosis preoperatively, but these deformities have been reported as improving postoperatively (Harada et al. 1993). Yasuoka et al. (1982) reported a zero incidence of spinal deformity in children and young adults following multilevel lumbar laminectomies. Development of excessive lumbar lordosis has been described after rhizotomy, possibly from excessive hip-flexion in the setting of multiple laminectomies, as described by Cobb and Boop (1994), who also reported two cases of postoperative spinal stenosis several years after lumbar laminectomy. In another series of 51 patients, 6% had significant lumbar pain with out evidence of spinal instability (Arens et al. 1989). A retrospective review of 35 patients demonstrated an increased incidence of low back pain of musculoskeletal origin after minor postoperative injuries in the subgroup who underwent laminectomies, but none in the subgroup who had had replacement laminoplasties (Cobb and Boop 1994). The author has performed replacement laminoplasties routinely for many years. Greene et al. (1991) noted progression of pre-existing hip subluxation after rhizotomy in six patients with spastic quadriplegia, while other groups have noted stabilization of hip subluxation in patients after dorsal rhizotomy (Wilner and Gaebler-Spira 1989, Peter et al. 1990, Crawford et al. 1996).

CONCLUSIONS

Selective posterior rhizotomy has proven to be a safe and effective procedure for the relief of spasticity in children with spastic cerebral palsy. The candidates should be carefully selected by a competent team of experts with a thorough knowledge of all aspects of cerebral palsy as it affects children. The team should consist of a pediatric orthopaedic surgeon, one or more pediatric physical therapists and a pediatric neurosurgeon.

The procedure is most safely performed by using intraoperative nerve root stimulation and EMG with the cutting of the least number of nerve rootlets which will bring about an effective reduction of spasticity.

Intensive physical therapy is most important after the procedure to obtain the maximum benefit from the normalization of muscle tone. Stretching will increase the range of motion, but orthopaedic surgery may be necessary to overcome structural abnormalities.

Rehabilitation following spasticity reduction

There are a number of considerations in designing post-spasticity reduction rehabilitation programs for individuals with cerebral palsy. An important one is the recognition that spasticity is not the only problem associated with cerebral palsy, and most likely the individual will have significant impairments of other areas as well. The evaluation of these areas will be important as a precursor to designing the rehabilitation program. These areas of potential impairment include motor control, balance, coordination and weakness. There may be biomechanical considerations as well. Bony deformity and/or contracture may have resulted from the spasticity. People with cerebral palsy often benefit from both tone-reducing procedures and the correction of bony deformities. If tone reduction is undertaken first, the bony deformities may have an impact on the rehabilitation program and process. Also, the existence of muscle contracture will need to be addressed as well (McDonald 1991).

Another consideration in the design of a rehabilitation program is the goal of the intervention. The focus of a rehabilitation program for a child who has undergone SDR with a goal of improved ambulation and self-care will be quite different than that for a child in whom a pump has been implanted for the continuous delivery of intrathecal baclofen in order to ease care giving. It should be remembered, however, that goals of spasticity reduction do not relate to ambulation alone. The potential impact of tone reduction and rehabilitation therapy intervention on self-care, communication and fine-motor skills is important as well.

POST-SDR

When a child undergoes SDR there is an immediate, dramatic decrease in muscle tone. Often, the children initially appear to be weak, as they may have relied on their spasticity in the past to assist them with motor activities. Intensive rehabilitation after SDR is needed in order to allow them to strengthen and to relearn movement patterns without the increased tone that they had preoperatively (Guiliani 1991).

Initially there may be some activity limitations. Children are typically kept horizontal for 3–5 days after surgery to decrease the likelihood of a cerebrospinal fluid leak. Even while flat in bed, physical therapy can begin to provide gentle range of motion. At our institution, passive trunk rotation is avoided as well as passive hamstring stretching for the first 6 weeks after surgery. Active trunk rotation is allowed, as it is believed that the child will limit his/her activity if there is pain. Passive hamstring stretch is avoided to again allow for healing of the dura prior to a stretch that could be transmitted through neural bundles. Others limit this activity for 3–4 weeks (McDonald 1991). We also routinely make use of knee-immobilizers to assist with positioning and decreasing postoperative spasms. The knee-immobilizers are placed immediately after the surgical procedure, prior to reaching the nursing floor. For the first few days after surgery, they are removed only briefly for skin checks and hygiene purposes. Children often ask to have the knee-immobilizers replaced quickly for comfort, and we have generally found that, since initiating the use of knee-immobilizers, children have been more comfortable postoperatively.

We also emphasize the use of the prone position for prolonged stretch and to assist children with strengthening their neck and upper-back-extensors as well as their shoulder girdle musculature. Also, if children experience hip-flexor spasms, increasing time in prone appears to assist in decreasing them.

If a child has plantarflexion contractures, serial casting can be initiated shortly after SDR. This can be very helpful in eliminating the need for soft-tissue surgery later. Casts can be weightbearing casts so that there is minimal interference with the rehabilitation program. They do, however, preclude pool therapy until the casts are removed.

Quite frequently, the kind of orthotic device used can change after SDR. With the reduction in tone around the ankle, children can often make use of posterior leaf type ankle foot orthoses that allow ankle movement. Frequently this type of orthosis could not be used preoperatively as the amount of plantarflexor spasticity could overpower it and would not keep the foot well positioned.

Long-term the type of assistive device needed may also change. If the improvement in the base of support allows for better balance and the child is able to strengthen lower extremities, especially hip extensors and abductors, a less supportive device may be used successfully.

There is a general consensus that intensive therapy services need to continue for a period of time after SDR. This is generally thought to be 6–12 months (Oppenheim 1990, Bleck 1993, Nishida et al. 1995, Steinbok et al. 1997, McLaughlin et al. 1998, Wright et al. 1998, Olree et al. 2000). There is not, however, a consensus about the need for intensive inpatient versus outpatient intervention. Some institutions discharge patients from the hospital approximately 1 week after surgery and others continue with intensive inpatient rehabilitation programs for 4–10 weeks prior to discharging to outpatient programs (Abbott et al. 1993). Limiting movement outside of early therapy sessions is important in order to avoid old methods of movement (Abbott et al. 1989, McDonald 1991, Gormley 1999).

After SDR, physical therapy should emphasize strengthening and muscle re-education (Abbott et al. 1989). Stretching to increase range of motion, postural control and activities to increase endurance are also important (McLaughlin et al. 1994). Generally, multiple therapy methods are used including elements of neurodevelopmental therapy, proprioceptive neuromuscular facilitation and the incorporation of principles of motor control. Sometimes the use of an assistive device slows the child to allow for more specific work on the pattern of movement. It may take a significant period of time to learn more normal movement patterns with normal or nearly normal tone (Peacock et al. 1987, Wright et al. 1998).

There is general consensus that physical therapy needs to be part of the post SDR program. However, children usually benefit from other interventions as well. With tone reduction, a course of occupational therapy to work on fine-motor skills and self-care is warranted. Often upper-extremity tone is reduced as well as lower-extremity tone. This may allow for improved fine-motor skills. Also, often with tone reduction, the child has increased mobility that permits reaching his/her lower extremities more easily, so working on dressing activities is very appropriate (McDonald 1991, Nishida et al. 1995).

Buckon et al. (1995) reported on a series of 26 children who were assessed before and after rhizotomy for upper-extremity strength, range of motion, fine-motor coordination and daily-living skills, and with videotape of movement. Grasp strength improved significantly, as did manipulation patterns when assessed 1 year post-surgery. There was also a significant improvement seen in the ability to perform toileting skills, dressing and undressing. Albright and colleagues (1995) looked at upper-extremity function as impacted by SDR and continuous ITB infusion. With regard to rhizotomy, they reported that there was no significant change in range of motion; but that improvements were noted in hand function and performing daily living skills, but these changes were not quantified. Another report looked at fine-motor skills 3–5 years after SDR (Mittal et al. 2002). Their patients received a 6-week intensive inpatient rehabilitation program, including both occupational and physical therapy. After discharge from the hospital they also continued to receive both occupational and physical therapy. Their subjects showed significant improvement in fine-motor skills. The assessments showed an increase in percentile scores, not just raw scores.

There has also been a recent publication looking at the effect of intense physical therapy prior to SDR (Steinbok and McLeod 2002). This was a further examination of the two groups of patients that they had previously looked at with regard to intensive physical therapy alone, versus SDR and intensive therapy. At follow-up at least 2 years after SDR, there was no difference between the two groups using the GMFM as the assessment tool. The therapists believed that the children who received intensive therapy before SDR made more rapid gains in the early weeks after surgery.

REHABILITATION POST-INTRATHECAL BACLOFEN PUMP INSERTION

Again, the specifics of rehabilitation interventions for an individual receiving ITB need to take into consideration the goals of spasticity reduction. Also, feedback from therapists can be very helpful in the process of dose adjustment. The need for rehabilitation services arises as a result of the decreased muscle tone and the need to relearn movement patterns and to attempt to strengthen muscles to improve movement and function for those who have functional goals (Campbell et al. 1995). For those for whom the main goals are to make care-giving easier, goals are quite different and generally revolve around equipment needs and home programs. Again, one should not overlook the potential improvement in self-care activities made possible by making it easier to reach the legs and feet.

For those individuals with goals related to increasing ease of care-giving, it is imperative to reevaluate equipment that they have been using (Stempien and Tsai 2000). After ITB treatment is initiated, spasms are likely to be eliminated. For some with total body involvement cerebral palsy, muscle spasms may have served as automatic weight shifts and pressure-relief assists. We have found that re-evaluating the seating systems including cushions is necessary. Straps may also need to be padded or repositioned to avoid pressure over the pump site. If individuals had anti-thrust seat modifications prior to the implant, these are likely to no longer be necessary. A small percentage of individuals appear to develop significant difficulty with trunk control. Additional trunk support may be needed.

It is also important to re-evaluate orthoses. If contractures had been dynamic rather than true muscle shortening, different orthoses may now be tolerated. It may be possible to use orthoses that can assist with increasing range of motion over time such as turnbuckle splints.

Bed positioning is another consideration in the individual with total body involvement. Again, periodic spasms might have helped with pressure relief prior to pump implantation. The use of extensor tone may also have been used to assist with rolling and repositioning. These are likely to be decreased with ITB treatment. Pressure-relief mattresses could be required to decrease the likelihood of ischemic ulcer formation. Different adaptations may be necessary to assist the individual to be able to reposition him/herself.

With significantly lower tone, the individual with total body involvement cerebral palsy will tolerate range of motion better. This is an excellent time to review range of motion techniques with those who provide care on an ongoing basis. The individual is also likely to tolerate stretch better, including positioning for effective stretching, so those techniques need to be reviewed as well.

One negative effect of ITB in the individual with total body involvement could be a decreased ability to bear weight for transfers. It is important to evaluate transfers after pump implantation. Even for some who have been lifted or who have used a mechanical lift, the reduction in tone may affect the transfer. Some have required longer slings for mechanical lifts in order to provide support for the head and neck.

Another potentially negative effect can be excessive weight gain. For some individuals with total body involvement cerebral palsy, their spasticity is a major energy-user. With the reduction of tone, they may actually require fewer calories. Careful monitoring of weight following pump implantation is warranted.

For those with some volitional movement and the ability to use switches and augmentative communication or environmental control devices, it is important to re-evaluate the placement of the devices. Evaluation for the possible use of adaptive equipment to increase ADL independence is important as well, as unexpected functional improvements may be possible. For example, one individual in whom a pump was implanted at our center with the goals of increasing comfort and easing care-giving was able to learn to feed herself with adaptive equipment and set up.

For those individuals with functional goals, rehabilitation should focus on strengthening, increasing range of motion and improving specific functional activities. Just as with SDR, the individual must relearn how to move with lower tone and learn to make use of individual muscle strength rather than tone and movement patterns. Goals can include walking, wheelchair ambulation, transfers, increasing ADL independence and improving communication, both verbally and with an augmentative communication device. Again, therapist feedback is very important in assisting with dose titration.

Questions arise concerning the best time to increase therapies and in what setting. It can take 6–9 months to reach a stable dose of ITB, and certainly takes weeks until tone reduction is sufficiently titrated to allow for optimal therapy involvement. Does one wait weeks or months after implant to begin an intensive therapy program? Some needs are immediate, such as the evaluation of weightbearing ability and equipment. There is no consensus about the timing of therapies, but intensive intervention would most logically wait until there has been some opportunity for dose titration.

Nor is there consensus about whether rehabilitation therapies should be in an inpatient or an outpatient setting. Most centers opt for outpatient therapies, but some have reported success with brief courses of inpatient therapies addressing very specific goals (Scheinberg et al. 2001). Scheinberg and colleagues also reported a small improvement in functional skills with an increase in outpatient physical therapy for 1–3 months after pump implantation. Conversely, however, inpatient rehabilitation is stated to be important to allow individuals to have optimal benefit from both the reduction in tone and apparent increase in motor control seen after implantation of a pump for the continuous delivery of ITB (Meythaler et al. 2001). The frequency of therapy can also vary depending on the goal of tone reduction (Albright 1996).

CONCLUSIONS

Rehabilitation programs need to be individualized for the specific goals, strengths and weaknesses of the person receiving the intervention. Before undertaking any spasticity-reduction procedure, it is important to discuss and evaluate all available information about the various potential deficits associated with cerebral palsy in addition to tonal abnormalities. These include problems with motor control, coordination, weakness and balance. A discussion of potential secondary impairments, such as bony abnormalities and contractures, and their possible implications is important as well. This discussion will assist in the formulation of realistic goals.

Rehabilitation services are seen as important to the ultimate success of tone-reducing procedures. Anecdotes can be shared illustrating a lack of change in movement patterns seen in children who underwent SDR without an intensive rehabilitation program. It would be helpful to prospectively study therapy intensity and ascertain the optimal amount of therapy to be recommended after these procedures.

REFERENCES

Abbott R. (1992) Complications with selective posterior rhizotomy. *Pediatr Neurosurg* **18:** 43–47.

Abbott R, Forem SL, Johann M. (1989) Selective posterior rhizotomy for the treatment of spasticity: a review. *Childs Nerv Syst* **5:** 337–346.

Abbott R, Johann-Murphy M, Siminski-Maher T, Quartermain D, Forem SL, Gold JT, Epstein FJ. (1993) Selective dorsal rhizotomy: outcome and complications in treating spastic cerebral palsy. *Neurosurgery* **33:** 851–857.

Albright AL. (1996) Intrathecal baclofen in cerebral palsy movement disorders. *J Child Neurol* **11** (suppl. 1): S29–S35.

Albright AL. (1999) Implantation of pumps for treatment of dystonia. In: Krauss JK, Jankovic J, Grossman RG, editors. *Movement Disorders Surgery.* Philadelphia: Lippincott, Williams and Wilkins. p 316–322.

Albright AL, Shultz BL. (1999) Plasma baclofen levels in children receiving continuous intrathecal baclofen infusion. *J Child Neurol* **14:** 408–409.

Albright AL, Barry M, Fasick MP, Janosky J. (1995) Effects of continuous intrathecal baclofen infusion and selective posterior rhizotomy on upper extremity spasticity. *Pediatr Neurosurg* **23:** 82–85.

Albright AL, Barry MJ, Shafton DH, Ferson SS. (2001) Intrathecal baclofen for generalized dystonia. *Dev Med Child Neurol* **43:** 652–657.

Almeida GL, Campbell SK, Girolami GL, Penn RD, Corcos DM. (1997) Multidimensional assessment of motor function in a child with cerebral palsy following intrathecal administration of baclofen. *Phys Ther* **77:** 751–764.

Arens LJ, Peacock WJ, Peter J. (1989) Selective posterior rhizotomy: a long-term follow-up study. *Childs Nerv Syst* **5:** 148–152.

Ashby P, Mailis A, Hunter J. (1987) The evaluation of "spasticity". *Can J Neurol Sci* **14:** 497–500.

Barolat G. (1991) Dorsal selective rhizotomy through a limited exposure of the cauda equina at L-1. Technical note. *J Neurosurg* **75:** 804–807.

Barry MJ, VanSwearington J, Albright AL. (1999) Reliability and responsiveness of the Barry–Albright Dystonia Scale. *Dev Med Child Neurol* **41:** 404–411.

Bleck E. (1993) Posterior rootlet rhizotomy in cerebral palsy. *Arch Dis Child* **68:** 717–719.

Boscarino LF, Õunpuu S, Davis RB 3rd, Gage JR, DeLuca PA. (1993) Effects of selective dorsal rhizotomy on gait in children with cerebral palsy. *J Pediatr Orthop* **13:** 174–179.

Buckon CE, SienkoThomas S, Aiona MD, Piatt JH. (1995) Assessment of upper-extremity function in children with spastic diplegia before and after selective dorsal rhizotomy. *Dev Med Child Neurol* **38:** 967–975.

Butler C, Campbell S. (2000) Evidence of the effects of intrathecal baclofen for spastic and dystonic cerebral palsy. AACPDM Treatment Outcomes Committee Review Panel. *Dev Med Child Neurol* **42:** 634–645.

Cahan LD, Adams JM, Perry J, Beeler LM. (1990) Instrumented gait analysis after selective dorsal rhizotomy. *Dev Med Child Neurol* **32:** 1037–1043.

Campbell SK, Almeida GL, Penn RD, Corcos DM. (1995) The effects of intrathecally administered baclofen on function in patients with spasticity. *Phys Ther* **75:** 352–362.

Chicoine MR, Park TS, Kaufman BA. (1997) Selective dorsal rhizotomy and rates of orthopedic surgery in children with spastic cerebral palsy. *J Neurosurg* **86:** 34–39.

Cobb MA, Boop FA. (1994) Replacement laminoplasty in selective dorsal rhizotomy: possible protection against the development of musculoskeletal pain. *Pediatr Neurosurg* **21:** 237–242.

Coffey RJ, Edgar TS, Francisco GE, Graziani V, Meythaler JM, Ridgely PM, Sadiq SA, Turner MS. (2002) Abrupt withdrawal from intrathecal baclofen: recognition and management of a potentially life-threatening syndrome. *Arch Phys Med Rehabil* **83**: 735–741.

Cohen AR, Webster HC. (1991) How selective is selective posterior rhizotomy? *Surg Neurol* **35**: 267–272.

Corcos DM, Gottlieb GL, Penn RD, Myklebust B, Agarwal GC. (1986) Movement deficits caused by hyperexcitable stretch reflexes in spastic humans. *Brain* **109**: 1043–1058.

Crawford K, Karol LA, Herring JA. (1996) Severe lumbar lordosis after dorsal rhizotomy. *J Pediatr Orthop* **16**: 336–339.

Engsberg JR, Olree KS, Ross SA, Park TS. (1998) Spasticity and strength changes as a function of selective dorsal rhizotomy. *J Neurosurg* **88**: 1020–1026.

Evans P, Elliott M, Alberman E, Evans S. (1985) Prevalence and disabilities in 4 to 8 year olds with cerebral palsy. *Arch Dis Child* **60**: 940–945.

Faigle JW, Keberle H. (1972) The chemistry and kinetics of lioresal. *Postgrad Med J* **Oct**: 9–13.

Fasano VA, Broggi G, Barolat-Romana G, Sguazzi A. (1978) Surgical treatment of spasticity in cerebral palsy. *Childs Brain* **4**: 289–305.

Foerster O. (1913) On the indications and results of the excision of posterior spinal nerve roots in man. *Surg Gynecol Obstet* **16**: 463–474.

Galloway A, Falope FZ. (2000) Pseudomonas aeruginosa infection in an intrathecal baclofen pump: successful treatment with adjunct intra-reservoir gentamicin. *Spinal Cord* **38**: 126–128.

Gerstzen PC, Albright AL, Johnstone GF. (1998) Intrathecal baclofen infusion and subsequent orthopedic surgery in patients with spastic cerebral palsy. *J Neurosurg* **88**: 1009–1013.

Gilmartin R, Bruce D, Storrs BB, Abbott R, Krach L, Ward J, Bloom K, Brooks WH, Johnson DL, Madsen JR, McLaughlin JF, Nadell J. (2000) Intrathecal baclofen for management of spastic cerebral palsy: multicenter trial. *J Child Neurol* **15**: 71–77.

Gormley ME. (1999) The treatment of cerebral origin spasticity in children. *NeuroRehabilitation* **12**: 93–103.

Grabb PA, Guin-Renfroe S, Meythaler JM. (1999) Midthoracic catheter tip placement for intrathecal baclofen administration in children with quadriparetic spasticity. *Neurosurgery* **45**: 833–837.

Greene WB, Dietz FR, Goldberg MJ, Gross RH, Miller F, Sussman MD. (1991) Rapid progression of hip subluxation in cerebral palsy after selective posterior rhizotomy. *J Pediatr Orthop* **11**: 494–497.

Gros C. (1979) Spasticity: clinical classification and surgical treatment. *Adv Tech Stand Neurosurg* **6**: 55–97.

Guiliani CA. (1991) Dorsal rhizotomy for children with cerebral palsy: support for concepts of motor control. *Phys Ther* **71**: 248–259.

Harada T, Ebara S, Anwar MM, Kajiura I, Oshita S, Hiroshima K, Ono K. (1993) The lumbar spine in spastic diplegia. A radiographic study. *J Bone Joint Surg Br* **75**: 534–537.

Knutsson E, Martensson A. (1980) Dynamic motor capacity in spastic paresis and its relation to prime mover dysfunction, spastic reflexes and antagonist co-activation. *Scand J Rehabil Med* **12**: 93–106.

Kopell BH, Sala D, Doyle WK. (2001) Subfascial placement of intrathecal baclofen pumps in children: technical note. *Neurosurgery* **49**: 753–757.

Lance JW. (1980) *Disordered Motor Control*. Philadelphia: Lippincott.

Lang FF, Deletis V, Cohen HW, Velasquez L, Abbott R. (1994) Inclusion of the S2 dorsal rootlets in functional posterior rhizotomy for spasticity in children with cerebral palsy. *Neurosurgery*. **34**: 847–853.

Lazareff JA, Mata-Acosta AM, Garcia-Mendez MA. (1990) Limited selective posterior rhizotomy for the treatment of spasticity secondary to infantile cerebral palsy: a preliminary report. *Neurosurgery*. **27**: 535–538.

Lee WA, Boughton A, Rymer WZ. (1987) Absence of stretch reflex gain enhancement in voluntarily activated spastic muscle. *Exp Neurol* **98**: 317–335.

Lundberg A. (1975) Mechanical efficiency in bicycle ergometer work of young adults with cerebral palsy. *Dev Med Child Neurol* **17**: 434–439.

McDonald CM. (1991) Selective dorsal rhizotomy: a critical review. *Phys Med Rehabil Clin N Am* **2**: 891–915.

McLaughlin JF, Bjornson KF, Astley SJ, Hays RM, Hoffinger SA, Armantrout EA, Roberts TS. (1994) The role of selective dorsal rhizotomy in cerebral palsy: critical evaluation of a prospective clinical series. *Dev Med Child Neurol* **36**: 755–769.

McLaughlin JF, Bjornson KF, Astley SJ, Graubert C, Hays RM, Roberts TS, Price R, Temkin N. (1998) Selective dorsal rhizotomy: efficacy and safety in an investigator-masked randomized clinical trial. *Dev Med Child Neurol* **40**: 220–232.

McLaughlin J, Bjornson K, Temkin N, Steinbok P, Wright V, Reiner A, Roberts T, Drake J, O'Donnell M, Rosenbaum P, Barber J, Ferrel A. (2002) Selective dorsal rhizotomy: meta-analysis of three randomized controlled trials. *Dev Med Child Neurol* **44**: 17–25.

311

Meythaler JM, Guin-Renfroe S, Law C, Grabb P, Hadley MN. (2001) Continuously infused intrathecal baclofen over 12 months for spastic hypertonia in adolescents and adults with cerebral palsy. *Arch Phys Med Rehabil* **82**: 155–161.

Mittal S, Farmer J-P, Al-Atassi B, Montpetit K, Gervais N, Poulin C, Cantin M-A, Benaroch TE. (2002) Impact of selective posterior rhizotomy on fine motor skills: long-term results using a validated evaluative measure. *Pediatr Neurosurg* **36**: 133–141.

Moto F, Buonaguro V, Carletti T. (2001) Intrathecal baclofen therapy (ITBT) in children affected by spastic diplegia. A comparison of results among gait analysis, functional and subjective patient evaluations. (abstract). *Dev Med Child Neurol* **43**: 17.

Müller H, Zierski J, Dralle D, Kraub D, Mart-Schler E (1988) Pharmacokinetics of intrathecal baclofen. In: Müller H, Zierski J, Penn RD, editors. *Local Spinal Therapy of Spasticity.* Berlin: Springer. p 155–214.

Nishida T, Thatcher SW, Marty GR. (1995) Selective posterior rhizotomy for children with cerebral palsy: a 7-year experience. *Childs Nerv Syst* **11**: 374–380.

Olree KS, Engsberg JR, Ross SA, Park TS. (2000) Changes in synergistic movement patterns after selective dorsal rhizotomy. *Dev Med Child Neurol* **42**: 297–303.

Oppenheim WL. (1990) Selective posterior rhizotomy for spastic cerebral palsy. *Clin Orthop* **253**: 20–29.

Peacock WJ, Arens LJ, Berman B. (1987) Cerebral palsy spasticity. Selective posterior rhizotomy. *Pediatr Neurosci* **13**: 61–66.

Peter JC, Hoffman EB, Arens LJ, Peacock WJ. (1990) Incidence of spinal deformity in children after multiple level laminectomy for selective posterior rhizotomy. *Childs Nerv Syst* **6**: 30–32.

Rosenbaum PL, Russell DJ, Cadman DT. (1990) Issues in measuring changes in motor function in children with cerebral palsy. *J Phys Ther* **70**: 125–131.

Sallerin-Caute B, Lazorthes Y, Monsarrat B, Cros J, Bastide RCS. (1991) baclofen levels after intrathecal administration in severe spasticity. *Eur J Clin Pharmacol* **40**: 363–365.

Samilson RL. (1975) *Orthopaedic Aspects of Cerebral Palsy.* Philadelphia: Lippincott.

Scheinberg A, O'Flaherty S, Chaseling R, Dexter M. (2001) Continuous intrathecal baclofen infusion for children with cerebral palsy: a pilot study. *J Paediatr Child Health* **37**: 283–288.

Sherrington CS. (1898) Decerebrate rigidity and reflex coordination of movement. *J Physiol (London)* **22**: 319–337.

Stanley FJ. (1979) An epidemiological study of cerebral palsy in Western Australia, 1956–1975. I: Changes in total incidence of cerebral palsy and associated factors. *Dev Med Child Neurol* **21**: 701–713.

Steinbok P, McLeod K. (2002) Comparison of motor outcomes after selective dorsal rhizotomy with and without preoperative intensified physiotherapy in children with spastic diplegic cerebral palsy. *Pediatr Neurosurg* **36**: 142–147.

Steinbok P, Gustavsson B, Kestle JR, Reiner A, Cochrane DD. (1995) Relationship of intraoperative electrophysiological criteria to outcome after selective functional posterior rhizotomy. *J Neurosurg* **83**: 18–26.

Steinbok P, Reiner AM, Beauchamp R, Armstrong RW, Cochrane DD, Kestle J. (1997) A randomized clinical trial to compare selective posterior rhizotomy plus physiotherapy with physiotherapy alone in children with spastic diplegic cerebral palsy. *Dev Med Child Neurol* **39**: 178–184.

Stempien L, Tsai T. (2000) Intrathecal baclofen pump use for spasticity: a clinical survey. *Am J Phys Med Rehabil* **79**: 536–541.

Stout JL, Gage JR, Koop SE. (1993) A comparison of metabolic energy expenditure after surgery or selective dorsal rhizotomy. *Proceedings of the Eighth Annual East Coast Gait Laboratories Conference*, 101. (Abstract.)

Tabary JC, Tardieu C, Tardieu G, Tabary C. (1981) Experimental rapid sarcomere loss with concomitant hypoextensibility. *Muscle Nerve* **4**: 198–203.

Tardieu G, Tardieu C. (1987) Cerebral palsy. Mechanical evaluation and conservative correction of limb joint contractures. *Clin Orthop* 63–69.

Van de Wiele BM, Staudt LA, Rubinstein EH, Nuwer M, Peacock WJ. (1996) Perioperative complications in children undergoing selective posterior rhizotomy: a review of 105 cases. *Paediatr Anaesth* **6**: 479–486.

Vaughan CL, Berman B, Staudt LA, Peacock WJ. (1988) Gait analysis of cerebral palsy children before and after rhizotomy. *Pediatr Neurosci* **14**: 297–300.

Vaughan CL, Berman B, Peacock WJ. (1991) Cerebral palsy and rhizotomy. A 3-year follow-up evaluation with gait analysis. *J Neurosurg* **74**: 178–184.

Waters RL, Hislop HJ, Perry J, Antonelli D. (1978) Energetics: application to the study and management of locomotor disabilities. Energy cost of normal and pathologic gait. *Orthop Clin N Am* **9**: 351–366.

312

Wilner L, Gaebler-Spira DJ. (1989) Growth parameters of cerebral palsy children: status post selective dorsal rhizotomy. *Arch Phys Med Rehabil* **70:** A45–A46.

Wright FV, Sheil EMH, Drake JM, Wedge JH, Naumann S. (1998) Evaluation of selective dorsal rhizotomy for the reduction of spasticity in cerebral palsy: a randomized controlled trial. *Dev Med Child Neurol* **40:** 239–247.

Yasuoka S, Peterson HA, MacCarty CS. (1982) Incidence of spinal column deformity after multilevel laminectomy in children and adults. *J Neurosurg* **57:** 441–445.

19
HEMIPLEGIA: PATHOLOGY AND TREATMENT

Jean Stout, James R. Gage and Ann E. Van Heest

Etiology

The term hemiplegia connotes involvement of only one side. When gait analysis is done, however, these children often have some motor involvement on the contralateral side as well, particularly in those cases with the more severe types of hemiparesis (subtypes III and IV) (Winters et al. 1987). Etiologies of hemiplegia include *periventricular hemorrhagic infarction* (PVHI), which commonly occurs in the preterm infant or in the term infant, *focal arterio-occlusive injury or stroke*. The former condition affects pathways to the arms, legs and even the face, producing the typical form of hemiparesis seen in surviving preterm infants. In the latter condition, the long-term sequelae depend on the particular arteries involved. As was discussed in Chapter 2, the acute presentation of an infant stroke is often with focal neonatal seizures in the first days of life (Clancy et al. 1985, Levy et al. 1985). The motor deficits may be subtle, however, and may not be detected for 6 months or more. Right hemiparesis is more common than left, since strokes most commonly involve the left middle cerebral artery (Volpe 2001). Unlike the hemiparesis that follows PVHI in the preterm infant, hemiparesis in the term infant tends to affect the arm and face more than the lower extremity. Hemiparesis can also arise from parasagittal vascular injury (see Figs 2.6, 2.7). In this case the upper-extremity weakness is predominantly proximal, whereas in focal stroke the distal upper extremities are the more impaired. Hemiparesis is virtually assured when occlusion of the proximal middle cerebral artery segment causes injury of the entire territory including the basal ganglia, white matter, posterior limb of the internal capsule and cortex (de Vries et al. 1997). Other causes of hemiparesis include intradural or subdural hemorrhage, which is often secondary to birth injury, or head trauma occurring prior to the age of 2 years. Computer-augmented tomography or magnetic resonance imaging will frequently demonstrate porencephalic cysts in the affected hemisphere.

Finally, as Dr du Plessis pointed out in Chapter 2, "*Parasagittal cerebral injury* resulting from watershed ischemia between the anterior and middle cerebral arteries affects the motor cortex, particularly regions innervating the upper extremities (especially proximal muscles) and trunk (Figs 2.6, 2.7, left side), usually with lesser involvement of areas representing the pelvic girdle and leg muscles. This topography of injury results in a characteristic type of spastic quadriparesis involving the arms more than the legs, i.e. the reverse of spastic diparesis in the preterm infant. . . . The *gradient* of weakness (i.e. arm more than leg), which resembles that in hemiplegia following middle cerebral artery stroke, has led to the use of the term 'bilateral hemiplegia', which is a confusing and inappropriate way of referring to the motor deficits after parasagittal injury. Because the parasagittal watershed area is particularly broad in the important association areas of the parietal cortex, *cognitive/intellectual deficits* are common after this form of injury, as are distinct learning disabilities (Yokochi 1998). *Visual function* following parasagittal cerebral injury in infants is not well described. However, in adults watershed injury in this area causes visual neglect, disordered tracking and difficulties interpreting complex diagrams (Balint's syndrome). Because of the cortical involvement, epilepsy is particularly common following this form of brain injury."

Clinical presentation

MUSCLE TONE

Depending on the location of the brain lesion, the tone can be spastic, athetoid or mixed. However, spasticity is the predominant presentation. Although mixed tone can occur in hemiplegia, particularly with occlusion of the proximal middle cerebal artery that involves the territory of the basal ganglia, in the discussion of surgical treatment of the motor lesions that follow *spastic hemiplegia* will be presumed.

COGNITIVE AND VISUAL DISORDERS

In children with hemiplegia, attention deficit disorder with or without compartmentalized learning disabilities such as dysnomia or dyslexia are much more common than mental retardation. In addition, many may be emotionally labile, perseverative and/or impulsive (Silver 1986). According to Rang and colleagues (1986), more than half of these children have an IQ within the normal range. In our personal experience mental retardation is relatively infrequent, whereas attention deficit disorders are fairly common. In addition, roughly one-third of these children have seizures. Seizures and compartmentalized learning disorders are in accordance with the pathology of localized brain damage, since the neural loss tends to be focal and the scar that results from such damage can result in a seizure locus. Strabismus may also be present and may require surgical correction or patching. If the visual cortex is involved, hemianopsia can occur. If this is the case and the child happens to be sitting on the wrong side of the classroom, s/he may miss a great deal of visual information. Accordingly, all children with hemiplegia should have an adequate visual examination at an early age. Our pediatric ophthalmologists prefer to see them as soon as possible after the diagnosis of cerebral palsy is made.

MOTOR PROBLEMS

Children with hemiplegia have much less difficulty with overall body balance; almost all of them are able to walk, and many of them can ride a bicycle without much difficulty. This is because in hemiplegia, as opposed to diplegia, there is a relatively intact unilateral sensory and motor system. Given the background of the neuropathology presented in Chapter 2, the reasons for this should now be clear. As a general rule, the upper extremity is more severely involved than the lower, and the individual typically walks with the upper extremity postured in internal rotation at the shoulder and flexion at the elbow. The hand is frequently clenched, with the thumb in the palm, and the wrist is usually ulnarly deviated and flexed.

In the past, hemiplegia has been considered to be a homogeneous condition. As such, lower-extremity management has traditionally focused on the ankle equinus deformity that is frequently present. However, with modern gait analysis it has been shown that there is a spectrum of involvement in the lower extremities (Becky et al. 1977, Perry et al. 1978, Winters et al. 1987). Consequently, if treatment is to be optimized it must be tailored to the patient's particular pattern of involvement. Although Perry's work was mainly with adult stroke patients, she did recognize that these individuals had varying patterns of involvement. Perry et al. (1978) emphasized that following a neurologic injury, recovery of function proceeds from proximal to distal. They described three forms of incomplete locomotor pattern independence. (1) Voluntary control of the hip has recovered and thus the hip has escaped the fixed-limb synergy. The individual is now able to maintain the hip in flexion even though the knee is in extension with a corresponding increase in step length. However, ankle control continues to be tied to the knee. (2) Selective control is possible at all three joints on command, but during patterned activities such as walking control reverts to one of locomotor pattern action. (3) Selective motor control is possible only when the limb is in a facilitatory posture, e.g. voluntary plantarflexion of the ankle is possible when the knee is extended, but not when the knee is flexed. During walking, however, muscle action may be accomplished entirely through locomotor patterns. Perry feels that this last pattern is the one seen most often in patients with spastic hemiplegia.

Lower extremity
PATTERNS OF MOTOR INVOLVEMENT

Previous work with modern gait analysis has described four basic patterns of involvement (types I–IV) in spastic hemiplegia, which depend on Perry's premise that recovery proceeds from the proximal to distal end of the limb (Winters et al. 1987):

Type I

The principle finding in this group is equinus in swing secondary to a relative dominance of the triceps surae compared to the anterior tibial musculature. As such initial contact is either foot flat or on toe, and first rocker is absent. Second rocker begins at initial contact, but is otherwise normal. There is no limitation of dorsiflexion in stance. Compensatory gait deviations in this subtype of hemiplegia are (1) increased knee flexion at terminal swing, initial contact and loading response, (2) hyperflexion of the hip in swing, and (3) increased pelvic lordosis. (Fig. 19.1) This pattern may be characteristic of individuals who have voluntary control of the hip and knee, but not the ankle.

Treatment of the type I pattern consists of restoring proper pre-positioning of the foot in swing. The easiest way to accomplish this is with a leaf-spring type ankle–foot orthosis (AFO). Some of these individuals recruit their extensor hallicis longus (EHL) to assist in dorsiflexion in swing. If so, transfer of the EHL to the first or second metatarsal in conjunction with fusion of the first interphalangeal (IP) joint as described by Jones (1916) may be useful. Since the flexor hallicis longus (FHL) is also spastic, however, when this transfer is done it is necessary to combine it with an intramuscular lengthening of the FHL to avoid

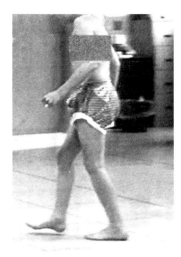

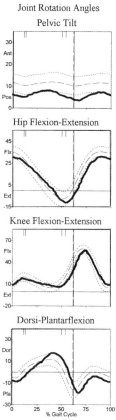

Joint Rotation Angles

Fig. 19.1. Child with type I hemiplegia (left), and the sagittal-plane kinematics of his gait (right). Since selective control extends down only as far as the knee, the foot and ankle must be controlled through "automatic" or "habitual" locomotor patterns. As such, ankle plantarflexion is tied to knee extension. Consequently, the foot drops into equinus in terminal swing and first rocker does not occur. Second and third rockers are normal, and the only major abnormality noted on kinematics is an equinus deformity that persists from toe-off to initial contact. In these children the peroneal and anterior tibial muscles (tibialis anterior and long toe extensors) are weak and poorly controlled, and the biarticular gastrocnemius is spastic and hyperactive. The result is a problem with priority III of normal gait: foot position at initial contact (see Chapter 4 for a discussion of gait priorities). *See CD-Rom, Figure 19.1, for a dynamic illustration.*

overpull of the antagonist. Anterior transfer of the long toe-flexors as described by Hiroshima et al. (1988) can also be used to augment dorsiflexion. The authors claim improved gait in up to two-thirds of the cases. Hiroshima et al. describe transfer of both flexor digitorum longus and flexor hallucis longus. This is a logical approach since the long toe-flexors are often spastic and begin action prematurely in late swing. However, since we feel the flexor hallucis is important in stabilizing the foot in terminal stance and pre-swing, in selected cases we have used a variation of this procedure in which only the flexor digitorum longus is transferred to the dorsum of the foot. In addition to augmenting dorsiflexion, this transfer also has the benefit of correcting claw toes if present (although toe-clawing is unusual in hemiplegic cerebral palsy). We have not specifically studied the postoperative outcomes of this procedure, but it is our clinical impression that the flexor digitorum longus transfer usually will not eliminate the foot-drop in swing sufficiently to obviate the need for a leaf-spring orthosis.

Type II

The cardinal feature in this group is that in addition to a drop foot in swing, there is restricted

317

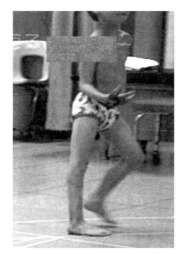

Joint Rotation Angles

Pelvic Tilt

Hip Flexion-Extension

Knee Flexion-Extension

Dorsi-Plantarflexion

Fig. 19.2. Child with type II hemiplegia (left), and the sagittal-plane kinematics of his gait (right). Selective motor control is still intact to the knee. However, because of greater spasticity and/or fixed contractures of the posterior calf musculature, second rocker is also restricted. This restriction in ankle dorsiflexion produces an excessive plantarflexion/knee-extension couple with resultant knee hyperextension on the hemiplegic side in late stance. These children frequently have overactivity/contracture of the tibialis posterior as well, which results in a varus hindfoot in stance. Sagittal-plane kinematics are identical to type I except that now there is true equinus of the ankle in stance, which in turn produces knee hyperextension in late stance. Type II hemiplegics have a problem with priority I of normal gait: stability in stance. *See CD-Rom, Figure 19.2, for a dynamic illustration.*

ankle dorsiflexion in stance. Unlike the type I subjects who have normal functional length of the posterior calf muscles, type II individuals have static or dynamic contracture of the triceps surae, tibialis posterior, and/or the long toe-flexors. As such, second rocker is arrested prematurely with resultant hyperextension of the knee and hip in stance (Fig. 19.2). Type II individuals may just be a more severe variant of type I with similar or identical neuromuscular control patterns. They also have a slower walking velocity than those individuals with type I involvement (Stout et al. 1994).

Treatment of the type II pattern of involvement consists of restoring appropriate dorsiflexion in stance as well as insuring proper pre-positioning of the foot in swing. Gait analysis reveals that the two muscles most commonly involved are the gastrocnemius and the tibialis posterior. Therefore, at our hospital, the usual surgical correction consists of intramuscular lengthening of the tibialis posterior (Majestro et al. 1971), split posterior tibial tendon transfer (Kling et al. 1985) and a Baker-type lengthening of the gastrocsoleus fascia (Baker 1956). In hemiplegic cerebral palsy, usually both the gastrocnemius and the soleus are contracted, whereas in diplegia the soleus is usually of normal length. However, even if both muscles are contracted, they will not be contracted to the same degree (Delp

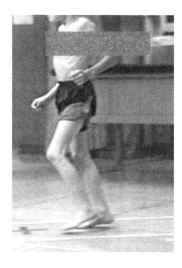

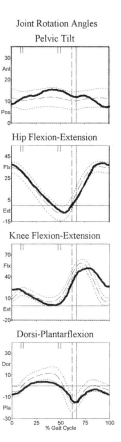

Joint Rotation Angles

Pelvic Tilt

Hip Flexion-Extension

Knee Flexion-Extension

Dorsi-Plantarflexion

Fig. 19.3. Type III hemiplegia. Left: child with type III hemiplegia. Right: the sagittal-plane kinematics of his gait. In type III hemiplegia, the biarticular muscles crossing the knee (rectus femoris and hamstrings) are also involved. The co-spasticity of these muscles results in limited knee flexion in swing, which in turn leads to a problem with priority 2 of normal gait: foot clearance in swing phase. Femoral anteversion commonly occurs with this pattern of involvement, which results in internal rotation of the lower extremity in the coronal plane. *See CD-Rom, Figure 19.3, for a dynamic illustration.*

et al. 1995). Since the Baker tendoachilles lengthening has the advantage of lengthening the fascias of both muscles at a point where they are still independent of each other, it will allow proportionate lengthening of both muscle groups. Once the posterior calf contractures are corrected, one still needs to manage the foot drop in swing as has been described in the type I pattern.

Type III

In addition to the gait anomalies of the type II patients, this group demonstrates limited knee flexion in the swing phase of gait. This limited knee motion will cause additional problems with foot clearance in swing. A young child will usually compensate for this by vaulting on the contralateral side. With the onset of the adolescent growth spurt, however, body mass makes this too energy-inefficient, so the older individual tends to circumduct the hip on the hemiplegic side. The sagittal-plane ankle kinematics of type III involvement are similar to those with type II, but the knee kinematics are now affected as well (Fig. 19.3). This pattern probably represents a group of individuals who have voluntary control of the hip, but not the knee and ankle. For reasons pointed out in Chapter 12, biarticular muscles are more involved in cerebral palsy than those that are monoarticular. Thus the principal biarticular muscles that are involved in the type III pattern are the hamstrings, rectus femoris and gastrocnemius.

Treatment of the type III pattern consists of restoring knee flexion in swing as well as knee extension in stance. To accomplish the latter, one must correct the type II abnormalities of the ankle and foot. At the ankle, the surgical principles would be identical to those outlined for type II involvement. At the knee, hamstring lengthening is often required. Unfortunately, because of the co-spasticity with the rectus femoris, hamstring lengthening alone usually further restricts knee flexion in swing (Baumann et al. 1980, Gage et al. 1987, Fabry et al. 1999).

Restoring knee flexion in swing is more complicated. Duncan (1955), and later Sutherland and colleagues (1975), recommended proximal rectus femoris release, but this leaves the unwanted action of the muscle as an extensor of the knee, and deprives the hip of a necessary flexor. In individuals who have lost normal selective motor control, Eccles and Lundberg (1958) found that the rectus femoris reacted with either the hip flexors (iliacus and sartorius) or the knee extensors (vasti). Neurologically, therefore, it would seem that the muscle is part of two primitive synergies or patterns. Using dynamic electromyography (EMG), Perry demonstrated that the muscle usually aligns itself with the hip-flexors and is active in swing (Waters et al. 1979, Perry 1987). Frequently, however, it may continue to fire throughout the entire period of swing. Since the walking speed of a child with cerebral palsy is usually slower than normal, deceleration of knee flexion is unnecessary and in fact disadvantageous. In addition the plantarflexion force, which drives the knee into flexion, is greatly diminished because of the poor distal selective motor control. Thus, in an individual with spastic cerebral palsy affecting the knee, coactivation of the rectus femoris and hamstrings is present in mid-swing (a time when neither muscle should be active). Transfer of the distal end of the rectus femoris back to the sartorius or one of the hamstrings will augment knee flexion in swing rather than inhibit it (Gage et al. 1987, Perry 1987, Sutherland et al. 1990), and is a better solution.

Type IV
This group has all the features of type III, but the neurological involvement has progressed proximally to the hip such that the psoas and adductors are also involved. Subjects with type IV involvement demonstrate ankle plantarflexion in swing and stance, restricted sagittal-plane motion of the knee, and flexion and adduction contracture of the hip. They compensate for the limited hip motion through the use of increased lumbar lordosis in terminal stance. (Fig. 19.4) This is the most severe pattern of involvement in which affected individuals ambulate by reciprocating primitive flexion and extension patterns. As in the type III subjects, most of the involved muscles in this pattern are biarticular (psoas, hamstrings, rectus femoris and gastrocnemius). Individuals with more severe type IV involvement usually have an adductor longus contracture at the hip as well. Femoral anteversion, secondary to persistent fetal alignment, is frequently present in types III and IV. It is interesting to note that the individuals with femoral anteversion frequently have an external tibial torsion on the non-hemiplegic side. The reasons for this will be discussed when we come to the case example.

320

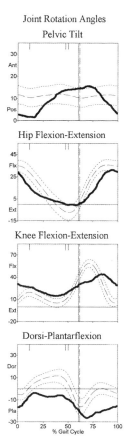

Pelvic Tilt

Hip Flexion-Extension

Knee Flexion-Extension

Dorsi-Plantarflexion

% Gait Cycle

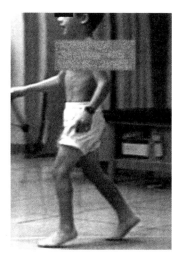

Fig. 19.4. Child with type IV hemiplegia (left), and the sagittal-plane kinematics of his gait (right). In this pattern, spasticity and loss of selective motor control go all the way up to the hip with involvement, at a minimum, of the biarticular muscles that cross these joints (gastrocnemius, hamstrings, rectus femoris and psoas). As such, this pattern of involvement features ankle equinus and restricted sagittal-plane motion of the knee and hip. Loss of knee flexion produces difficulties with foot clearance in swing, whereas limited hip-extension forces the pelvis to tip forward (anterior pelvic tilt). Excessive trunk lordosis is then necessary to keep the mass of the trunk back over the base of support in late stance. Internal hip rotation secondary to femoral anteversion plus hip adduction secondary to spasticity/contracture of the hip-adductors are often present in type IV hemiplegia as well. *See CD-Rom, Figure 19.4, for a dynamic illustration.*

Treatment of type IV involvement requires correction of the deformities that are common to the type III pattern plus correction of the psoas contracture. For reasons discussed previously, the psoas, which is biarticular, is usually spastic whereas the monoarticular iliacus is not. Therefore we reduce the spasticity of the psoas with simple intramuscular tenotomy, as originally described by Salter (1966), without disturbing the iliacus. This is analogous to the lengthening of the biarticular gastrocnemius without disturbing the soleus. Novacheck et al. (2002) have shown that this does not produce weakening of the hip-flexors.

In the coronal plane these children may have pelvic obliquity and an adduction contracture, and in the transverse plane they often have internal rotation of the hip secondary to femoral anteversion. If these deformities are present, they need to be corrected as well.

SUMMARY OF PATTERN TYPES

In summary, with the aid of kinematics we defined a spectrum of involvement of spastic hemiplegia that can be differentiated into four principal subtypes of involvement with type I being the least and type IV the most severely involved (Winters et al. 1987). More recently, using kinetics in a larger series of patients, we were able to break types III and IV into two

321

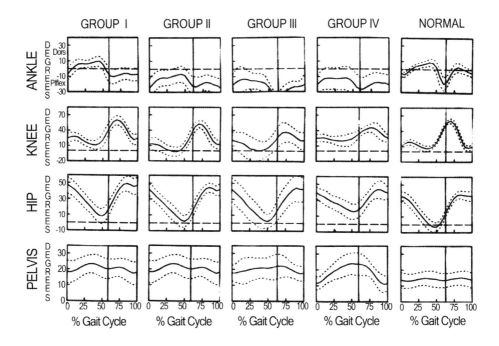

Fig. 19.5. Kinematics of the sagittal plane in each of the four subtypes of hemiplegia. The solid line on each of the graphs indicates the mean value for the group, and the dotted lines indicate 1 S.D. The right-hand column illustrates the normal sagittal-plane motions of the ankle, knee, hip and pelvis. Delineating subtypes of hemiplegia, allows the development of specific treatment protocols.

subtypes each (Stout et al. 1994). In the milder type III pattern, the hamstrings are only minimally involved and in the milder type IV pattern, the adductors are minimally involved. In the new classification there would now be two types of involvement at the ankle (A1-2), knee (K1-2), and hip (H1-2) respectively. Consequently, type I of the older classification becomes A1 and type II becomes A2. Once again, anteversion is commonly associated with the knee and hip types. Regardless of which system is used, breaking spastic hemiplegia into subtypes allows the development of treatment protocols (Fig. 19.5). With appropriate orthopaedic treatment, the gait of a patient with the more severe subtypes of involvement can be significantly improved, so that his/her gait approaches that of a patient with type I involvement. This is illustrated by the following case example.

Lower-extremity treatment with gait analysis: case study
R.S. is a 9 ½-year-old boy with left spastic hemiplegia cerebral palsy. He was born approximately 6 weeks preterm with a birthweight of 4 lb 8 oz. Difficulties following birth included jaundice, respiratory distress, and apnea but no known intracranial hemorrhage. A diagnosis of cerebral palsy was made at 18 months of age. R.S. has no history of orthopaedic intervention or Botox treatment. Functionally it has become increasingly difficult for him to keep pace with peers when running, jumping, and participating in

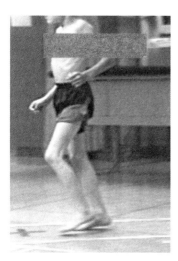

Fig. 19.6. R.S. walking without braces prior to surgery. *See CD-Rom, Figure 19.6, for a dynamic illustration.*

sporting activities.

R.S. walks with apparent bilateral internal femoral rotation, an external foot-progression angle on the right and an internal foot-progression angle on the left. Initial contact on the right is with the heel, whereas there is a foot-flat initial contact on the left. Increased knee flexion on the left is noted at initial contact as well. As he progresses into stance phase, gastrocnemius tightness produces an early heel rise and drives the leg posteriorly so that the knee reaches nearly full extension in terminal stance. In swing, knee flexion is decreased and a foot drop is apparent (Fig. 19.6). As such, R.S. utilizes a vault over the right extremity plus circumduction on the left to achieve left foot clearance in swing. The asymmetry of initial contact patterns, the stiff left knee, and the vaulting in swing produces a visual "limp".

Physical exam findings on the left include evidence of internal femoral torsion, posterior tibialis spasticity, and gastrocnemius contracture and spasticity with a positive Silfverskiöld sign. The Duncan–Ely stretch test (an indication of rectus femoris spasticity) is positive on the left side as well. On the left (hemiplegic) side, R.S. has partially isolated movement selectivity at the knee and ankle with grade 4–5 strength by manual muscle testing throughout the lower extremity. With the exception of an external tibial torsion, the right lower extremity is normal.

Kinematic assessment of the coronal plane demonstrates a mild pelvic obliquity (right side high and left side low) in the absence of leg-length discrepancy or adductor tightness. Transverse-plane data demonstrate a pelvic retraction on the left with internal rotation of the hips bilaterally. The foot-progression angle on the left is more internal than would be expected for the pelvis and hip positions. By contrast, the foot-progression angle on the right is more external than expected for the pelvis and hip positions. Sagittal-plane kinematics and ankle kinetics of the both the right (non-hemiplegic) and left (hemiplegic) sides are shown with a normal comparison (Fig. 19.7). Note that modulation (the pattern of movement) of the left ankle is normal, despite the tightness present on clinical exam. The modulation

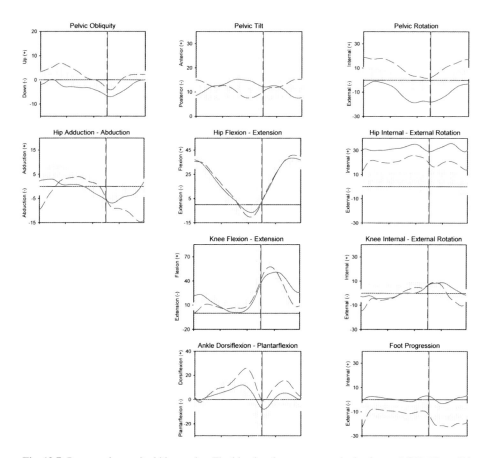

Fig. 19.7. Preoperative sagittal kinematics. The blue band represents typical values ± 1 S.D. The solid line indicates the left (hemiplegic) side and the dashed line the right (non-hemiplegic) side (see Chapter 7 for a review of the interpretation of kinematics). In the coronal plane (left column, first row), there is a mild pelvic obliquity. In the sagittal plane (middle column, third row), the left knee is mildly hyperextended in late stance with diminished and delayed knee flexion in swing. The left knee remains in about 20° of flexion at terminal swing and initial contact. In the transverse plane (right column) the pelvis is retracted on the left, and protracted on the right. Both hips are internally rotated referable to the pelvis (left > right). If one calculates the rotations, starting from the pelvis down, it can be seen that the right foot progression is in external rotation referable to the segment above. This represents a compensatory external rotation of the non-hemiplegic side and, in order to bring the pelvis into appropriate alignment in the rotational plane the external torsion (non-hemiplegic side) it needs to be corrected along with the internal femoral torsion on the hemiplegic side.

of the right ankle is abnormal, which is consistent with a vault. The left knee graph exhibits abnormality in swing phase. The kinematics of the hip are normal. The pelvis demonstrates mildly increased lordosis.

Dynamic electromyograms (not illustrated) demonstrate excessive activity of the rectus femoris in swing; prolonged activity of the hamstrings in stance; and early activity of the triceps surae (activity starting in late swing rather than midstance).

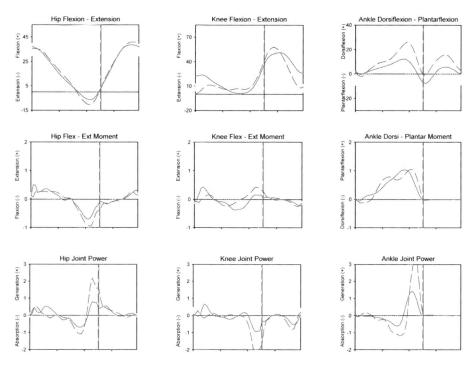

Hip Flexion - Extension	Knee Flexion - Extension	Ankle Dorsiflexion - Plantarflexion
Hip Flex - Ext Moment	Knee Flex - Ext Moment	Ankle Dorsi - Plantar Moment
Hip Joint Power	Knee Joint Power	Ankle Joint Power

Fig. 19.8. Preoperative sagittal kinetics. The blue band represents typical values ± 1 S.D. The solid line indicates the left (hemiplegic) side and the dashed line the right (non-hemiplegic) side. The top row of graphs actually represents the kinematics; the middle row moments; and the bottom row power about the hip, knee and ankle respectively (see Chapter 8 for a review of the interpretation of kinetics). Note that most of the power for walking comes from the normal right side. The difference is particularly striking at the ankle.

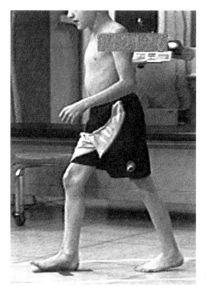

Fig. 19.9. R.S. walking without braces after recovery from surgery. *See CD-Rom, Figure 19.6, for dynamic illustration.*

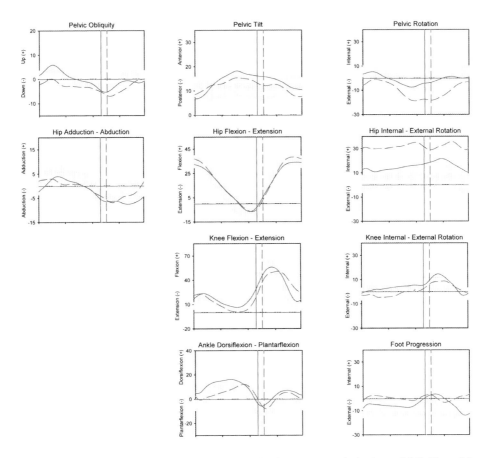

Fig. 19.10. Postoperative sagittal kinematics. The blue band represents typical values ± 1 S.D. The solid line indicates the left side postoperatively and the dashed line the same side before surgery. Note that the graphs have normalized in all three planes. In particular, the sagittal plane (middle column) is now within normal limits.

Kinetics of the ankle indicate diminished terminal stance-phase power production. The contrast between right and left sides is quite striking (Fig. 19.8).

On the basis of the clinical examination and the gait analysis, the patient's abnormalities of gait can be summarized as follows. (1) Left contracture of the triceps surae (gastrocnemius > soleus) with a positive Silfverskiöld test (see Fig. 5.2) on clinical exam and premature firing of the triceps surae on dynamic EMG. (2) Left posterior tibialis spasticity (spasticity noted on clinical exam and the foot progression angle was more internal than expected for pelvis/hip positions). (3) Left rectus femoris spasticity: positive Duncan–Ely sign (see Fig. 5.3) on clinical exam, inappropriate EMG activity in mid-swing, and decreased swing-phase knee motion on kinematics. (4) Left internal femoral torsion (possible right internal femoral torsion) as demonstrated by the findings of femoral anteversion on clinical exam and excessive internal hip rotation on kinematics. (5) Right external tibial torsion (excessive

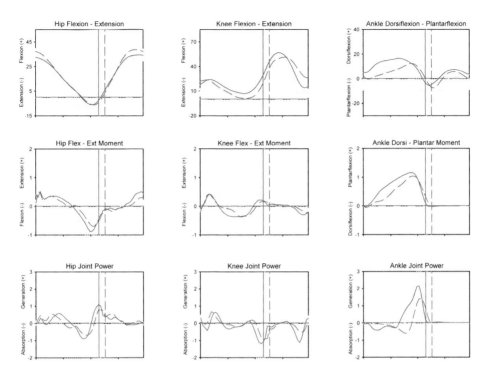

Fig. 19.11. Postoperative sagittal kinetics. The blue band represents typical values ± 1 S.D. The solid line indicates the left side after surgery and the dashed line the same side before surgery. As in Figure 19.8, the top row is kinematics, the middle is moments, and the bottom is powers. Note that almost all of the graphs have normalized compared with the position before surgery. Again, the difference is particularly striking at the ankle.

thigh foot and bimalleolar axis measurements on clinical exam and greater than expected external foot progression angle based on pelvis and hip positions on kinematics).

These findings are consistent with a type III pattern of left hemiplegia with associated left femoral internal torsion and right external tibial torsion. In the alternate classification system of hemiplegia (Stout et al. 1994) this would represent a K-1 pattern in which rectus femoris spasticity is present without hamstring tightness. The presence of the external tibial torsion on the less affected right side may seem unusual, but often develops as a secondary deformity over time. Probably the pelvic retraction of the affected side necessitates pelvic protraction on the less affected side, which in turn creates an abnormal internal foot progression angle. Consequently, to maintain foot progression neutral to the direction of progression while walking, the child places an external torque on the tibia. Eventually this produces a true bony torsion.

Based on this analysis, the following procedures were performed during the course of a single surgery: (1) Strayer-type gastrocnemius recession (left); (2) intramuscular lengthening of the posterior tibialis (left); (3) distal transfer of the rectus femoris to gracilis intramuscular tendon (left); (4) intertrochanteric femoral derotation osteotomy (left); (5) supramalleolar tibial derotation osteotomy (right); and (6) pin placement to assess internal torsion on right.

Ten months post-surgery, the clinical appearance of his gait is much better (Fig. 19.9). Functionally his parents report he is able to run better, bike-riding is easier, and he has increased walking endurance. Gait analysis was repeated following recovery from surgery and compared to the preoperative analysis. The kinematics of the knee and ankle in the sagittal plane and the hip-rotation and foot-progression angle in the transverse plane have been restored to within normal limits (Fig. 19.10). The asymmetric pelvic rotation is also reduced suggesting that much of the asymmetry was a compensation for the previous internal femoral torsion. The vault noted in the ankle kinematics and kinetics on the right side has disappeared, since with improved knee and ankle motion during swing on the left side the compensation is no longer necessary (Fig. 19.11). In this case, gait analysis has provided objective evidence of improvement.

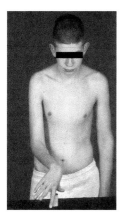

Fig. 19.12. Typical upper-limb deformity in spastic hemiplegia. In spastic hemiplegia due to cerebral palsy, the most common peripheral manifestations in the upper limb are shoulder internal rotation, elbow flexion, forearm pronation, wrist flexion/ulnar deviation, finger-clenching or swan-necking, and thumb-in-palm deformity.

Upper extremity

In the past, most evaluations and treatments of cerebral palsy were centered on the lower extremities and the patient's ability to walk. In the 21st century, however, with improved motorized wheelchair controls and public access for the disabled, and with increased opportunities for individuals to access computers and assistive communication devices, treatment now emphasizes maximizing functional use of the upper extremities as well.

In spastic hemiplegia due to cerebral palsy, the most common peripheral manifestations in the upper limb are shoulder internal rotation, elbow flexion, forearm pronation, wrist-flexion/ulnar deviation, finger-clenching or swan-necking, and thumb-in-palm deformity (Fig. 19.12). Increased muscle spasticity causes muscle imbalance across joints, which leads to impaired function acutely, and joint contractures with skeletal deformation chronically. This portion of the chapter will deal with the evaluation of the upper extremity in spastic hemiplegia, followed by an outline of treatment options and surgical results.

PATIENT EVALUATION

Patient evaluation begins with an interviewing the parents, regarding use of the affected limb. Most commonly children with spastic hemiplegia will show premature hand dominance

TABLE 19.1
Classification of upper-extremity functional use

Class	Designation	Activity level
0	Does Not Use	Does not use
1	Poor Passive Assist	Uses as stabilizing weight only
2	Fair Passive Assist	Can hold and object placed in hand
3	Good Passive Assist	Can hold onto object placed in hand and stabilize it for use by other hand
4	Poor Active Assist	Can actively grasp object and hold it weakly
5	Fair Active Assist	Can actively grasp object and stabilize it well
6	Good Active Assist	Can actively grasp object and then manipulate it against other hand
7	Partial Spontaneous	Use Can perform bimanual skills easily and occasionally uses the hand spontaneously
8	Full Spontaneous Use	Uses hand completely independently without reference to the other hand

Reprinted from Van Heest AE, House JH, Cariello C. (1999) Upper extremity surgical treatment of cerebral palsy. *J Hand Surg Am* **24**: 324, by permission.

favoring the unaffected side even as young as 6 months of age, and may be the presenting complaint leading to the diagnosis. Delay of normal pinch and grasp function patterning at 1 year of age is evident. Generalized patterns of upper-extremity use for activities of daily living, commensurate with the child's age, are discussed with the parents and child. In addition, we evaluate the child's ability to do bimanual skills such as zippers, buttons, cutting food and tying shoes. The child's *functional use* of the hand can be quantified using House's Classification of Upper-Extremity Functional Use (Van Heest et al. 1999a) (Table 19.1). In this 9-level classification, functional use is assessed as "does not use", "passive assist" (poor, fair, good), "active assist" (poor, fair, good), and "spontaneous use" (partial, complete). This provides a baseline that can be used to help the physician communicate the functional goals of treatment with the parents. Agreement with the parents on the child's present overall level of limb function lays the groundwork against which outcome of subsequent treatments can be compared.

In the early stages of spastic hemiplegia, the joints and muscles will be supple, with full passive range of motion. With skeletal growth, the muscle imbalance across joints over time leads to muscle-tendon unit shortening and joint contractures, eventually leading to skeletal deformity. Physical examination begins with evaluation for *static deformity* by examining the limb for passive range of motion of the shoulder, elbow, forearm, wrist and hand. In addition, the examiner evaluates joint contractures and shortening of the muscle-tendon units. Passive range of motion needs to be done slowly to overcome muscle tone. Note that the finger- and thumb-flexor muscles are biarticular muscles meaning they cross both the wrist and finger joints. Wrist-joint contractures can be checked first with the fingers flexed, to assess if contractures exists in the joint itself; then with fingers extended, to assess if the finger and thumb-flexor muscles are contracted. Zancolli (1968) classified the degree of muscle-tendon contractures (Fig. 19.13). If there is full passive mobility of each joint and muscle, no static deformity exists, and assessment proceeds to dynamic deformities by looking at motor function.

Dynamic deformity is assessed by observation of joint position during active use of the

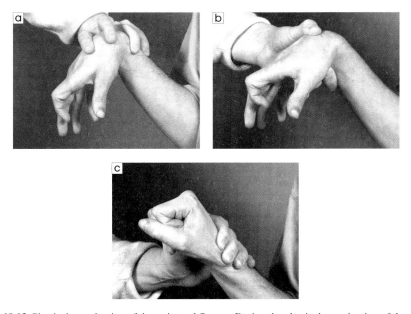

Fig. 19.13. Physical examination of the wrist and fingers. During the physical examination of the wrist and fingers, the fingers are held in maximum extension, and the wrist is extended until the fingers begin to flex. In the patient shown in (a), when the wrist is maximally flexed, full digital extension is possible. As the wrist is brought into extension (b), with wrist extension of -60°, the fingers start to flex due to contracture of the finger-flexor muscles. When the wrist is fully extended (c), the fingers fully flex due to muscle contracture of the flexor digitorum muscles.

arm and assessing for cortical control of positioning the arm in space for grasp, release and pinch function. Videotaping is a useful adjunct for physical examination as it allows assessment of the spasticity encountered during routine activities of daily living and eliminates the stress of performance on demand in the physician's office. Identification of the specific spastic muscle can be determined by the joint position; for example, excessive dynamic wrist flexion with ulnar deviation identifies the flexor carpi ulnaris as the spastic deforming force. Palpation of specific spastic muscles also localizes the source of the dynamic imbalance. The examiner needs to assess the extent of voluntary muscle control in the limb. Additionally, spasticity (increased muscle tone) versus dystonia (lack of central nervous system control with position of dynamic deformity varying with time) should be noted. In the higher functioning child, the Pediatric Jebsen Taylor standardized test (Jebsen et al. 1969) can be used both as a baseline from which to measure the effect of subsequent treatment, but also as a screen of which subtest functions have the greatest impairment (e.g. pinching small objects versus grasping large cans).

Dynamic EMG is another diagnostic tool that has been used to help assess motor tone and phasic control of specific muscles (Hoffer 1993, Hoffer et al. 1990). In major centers that have motion labs for gait analysis, the same technology can be used for upper-extremity assessment. For example, Kozin and Keenan (1993) have shown that either biceps and/or

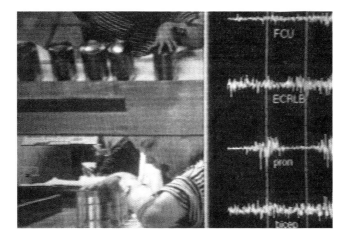

Fig. 19.14. The Pediatric Jebsen Taylor Test of Hand Function. The two video-frames on the left show a front and side view of the child lifting cans, one of several items on the test. Looking at the two angles simultaneously allows assessment of the deformity in both the sagittal and coronal planes. For example, this child can be seen to demonstrate a wrist flexion and ulnar deviation deformity. The EMG data on the right shows 3 seconds of EMG activity of four muscles: biceps brachii, pronator teres, flexor carpi ulnaris and extensor carpi radialis longus/brevis. Needle electrodes are used for the pronator teres and the flexor carpi ulnaris. Surface electrodes are used for the biceps brachii and the radial wrist-extensor muscles. The box encompassing the central one-third of the EMG data highlights the 1 second of activity that is simultaneously shown on the video-frames on the left. The EMG recording evidences continuous firing activity of the flexor carpi ulnaris, indicating poor motor control. Despite this it also demonstrates that this child is able to actively control some muscles for functional use (such as the pronator teres, which in the child shows good phasic control).

brachialis spasticity can lead to elbow flexion deformity; preoperative dynamic EMG can assess spastic tone and phase control of each muscle in order to direct treatment to the specific offending muscle(s). Differences in phasic control of muscles versus continuous spastic activation can be assessed, as well as determination of central control of muscles as children are viewed carrying out functional tasks. Use of the motion lab in assessment of upper-extremity activities is demonstrated in Figure 19.14.

In addition to assessment of the efferent ability of the brain to control upper-limb function, the afferent sensory ability of the brain needs to be evaluated as well. *Sensation* can be evaluated by stereognosis, two-point discrimination, and proprioception. In our review of 40 children with spastic hemiplegia (Van Heest et al. 1993), we have found that stereognosis is the most sensitive discriminator of degree of sensibility impairment. We found that 97% had a stereognosis impairment using the 12 objects shown in Table 19.2. The six objects listed on the left discriminate gross-motor function, and the six objects listed on the right discriminate fine motor function. These children demonstrated 12/12 object recognition on the unaffected side, verifying understanding of the test. Furthermore, we found that those children with severe sensibility impairment had a significant size-discrepancy when compared to the unaffected side. The shortened limb can be a useful clue to underlying sensibility deficiency, particularly in the child too young or too mentally impaired to reliably

TABLE 19.2
Objects for assessment of stereognosis function

12 common objects	
Cube	Button
Key	Safety-pin
Pencil	Pill
Rubber-band	Penny
Spoon	Marble
String	Paper-clip

perform a sensibility assessment. Children with sensibility deficiencies need to be coached to use the eyes rather than their touch for afferent feedback. Several studies have indicated that poor sensation is *not* a contraindication for surgery (Van Heest et al. 1999a). In fact, one study has reported an improvement in sensibility function after surgical intervention (Dahlin et al. 1998), presumably associated with increased postoperative functional use.

In summation of the evaluative process, the physician needs to integrate the results of the assessment of overall patterns of functional use (Table 19.1), static contractures, dynamic deformities of motor imbalance for multiple levels of involvement (shoulder, elbow, wrist and hand), as well as sensory deficiencies. This information is combined with a general assessment of the child's mentation, motivation, and generalized medical condition. An overall treatment plan is synthesized, taking into account the child's capabilities, disabilities, and potential, in the context of the child's age. Discussion with the parents and the child is imperative in formulating the individualized treatment plan and its expected outcome.

NON-OPERATIVE TREATMENT OPTIONS
Occupational therapy has includes use of splints, stretching/strengthening programs, and active functional use activities. Two types of splints can be used: night-time serial static splinting is used for treatment of muscle or joint contractures; and daytime splints are used for pre-positioning the hand to improve active function. The indication for *night-time splinting* is the existence of contractures; if no contractures of the muscles or joints exist, night-time splinting is not necessary and is a waste of time and money for the child and family. If contractures *do* exist at the elbow, serial static splints can be employed. If contractures exist at the wrist or fingers/thumb, a night-time forearm-based wrist–hand orthosis may be helpful. Pronation contractures are difficult to splint and are usually treated with passive stretching. *Daytime splints* are usually used to pre-position the wrist in a neutral to slight "cock-up" position to help improve grasp; and to pre-position the thumb out of the palm to help improve pinch. If the splint is bulky or cumbersome, it will interfere rather than enhance function, defeating its purpose. Care should be given to ensure proper fit of the splint so that its purpose can be achieved. Stretching and strengthening programs, along with active functional use activities, are both carried out by therapist as well as instructed to the parents and child as a home program. The efficacy of these treatments has been documented in limited studies but no controlled studies have been done.

For patients with more focal muscle tone imbalance, botulinum toxin type-A injections (Botox™, Allergan Pharmaceuticals, Irvine, CA) has been shown to be effective in reducing spasticity in the muscles injected and in improving hand function (Wall et al. 1993, Van Heest 1997, Autti-Ramo et al. 2000, Fehlings et al. 2000). Botox locally blocks the release of acetylcholine at the neuromuscular junction with a reversible action typically lasting 3–4 months. (See Chapter 16, page 259, for a full discussion of botulinum toxin and its actions.) During this period, assessment of the antagonist muscles can be made, possible surgical benefits can be assessed. In addition, during this time, antagonist muscles can be strengthened and spastic muscles can be stretched with the benefits lasting beyond the direct effects of the medication. For the mildly involved child, treatment with Botox injections may obviate the need for surgical intervention.

Optimal surgical candidates are patients at least 7 years of age (or mature enough to comply with postoperative regimens), with a joint positioning deformity interfering with active functional use of the arm. After children are diagnosed with cerebral palsy, there exists a period of about 7 years before children would even be considered surgical candidates. In the meantime, non-operative treatment of these children is the norm. Most of the non-operative regimen revolves around parent and child education in active functional use of the affected arm to the extent that the child is able to perform.

Yearly or twice-yearly monitoring by the physician is important to assess for development of contractures and overall developmental progress regarding age appropriate use of the arm. For example, babies are assessed for their ability to bear weight on the arm for sitting and crawling; young children are assessed for bimanual gross-motor skills such as dressing and ball catching; school age children are assessed for fine-motor skills such as buttoning and shoe-tying; all children are assessed for development of contractures with growth. If failure to meet developmental milestones is encountered, a specific therapy protocol is instituted to help keep the child as close to "on target" as their physical disabilities will allow. Therapists are in a unique position to develop a relationship with the family and child in patient education regarding use patterns and adaptive patterns, and their services can be an integral part of delivering medical attention to these children.

SURGICAL OPTIONS, INDICATIONS AND OUTCOMES
Surgical principles
The surgical principles for treatment of spastic deformities in cerebral palsy are as follows: (1) release or lengthen the spastic or contracted muscle(s), (2) augment (tendon transfers into) the weak or flaccid antagonist muscle(s), and (3) stabilize the joint for severe joint instability or severe fixed contractures.

The major goal in surgical reconstruction is *balance* across the affected joint(s). Surgical treatment targets joint imbalance in order to prevent fixed deformity and to improve functional use. Ideally, joint balance can be achieved through appropriate releases or lengthening of the spastic muscles, with tendon transfers to augment the weak antagonist muscles, as necessary. If severe fixed deformity is already present, joint-stabilization procedures may be necessary.

The surgeon is required to carefully assess the type of deformity and its treatment at each joint separately, and then synthesize them together to organize a comprehensive surgical reconstructive plan. Adequate shoulder, elbow, and forearm function is necessary for the patient to be able to appropriately position the limb in space; adequate wrist, finger, and thumb function is necessary for the patient to appropriate grasp, pinch and release. Surgical treatment options for each joint deformity are listed in Table 19.3. As in the lower extremity, surgical intervention is reserved primarily for the spastic limb, as surgical treatment in the athetoid patient has been unpredictable.

Shoulder

In spastic hemiplegia, the most *common* deformity at the shoulder is internal rotation and adduction, which usually is not very symptomatic as this positions the arm effectively by the side. The most *symptomatic* deformity at the shoulder is external rotation and abduction. This is particularly troublesome during ambulation when the arm flies out from the body and interferes with normal balance. If conservative measures fail, a slide of the deltoid insertion for abduction deformity or an internal humeral derotational osteotomy for external rotation deformity can be performed.

Elbow

The most common deformity at the elbow is flexion. The primary muscles contributing to this deformity are the biceps and brachialis. The secondary offenders are the brachioradialis and flexor pronator wad muscles as these muscles cross the elbow joint as well.

   The primary procedure used to treat elbow-flexion deformity is z-lengthening of the biceps tendon with fractional lengthening of the brachialis muscle. With severe contractures, the brachioradialis may need to be released off its origin as well. A flexor pronator slide, as treatment for a wrist- and finger-flexion deformity, will have a secondary effect of lessening the elbow-flexion deformity.

   Elbow-flexion deformities of less than 45° rarely functionally impair use of the limb and are usually treated non-operatively with serial static splints or a turnbuckle splint. Elbow-flexion deformities of greater than 90° should be approached with caution as the neurovascular bundle may be shortened and will limit the amount of surgical correction possible. Improvement of 40° has been reported as an average result after biceps and brachialis lengthening (Mital and Sakellarides 1981).

Forearm

The most common deformity of the forearm is pronation, which can severely limit the child's ability to position the arm in space for grasping objects or for bringing the palms of the hands together for two-handed activities. The offending muscle is primarily the pronator teres, and secondarily the pronator quadratus.

   The two surgical options for lessening forearm pronation are pronator teres release and pronator teres re-routing. The pronator teres release works primarily through release of a deforming spastic muscle and relies on the biceps and/or supinator to provide active supination. This operation is indicated if the child exhibits a severely spastic pronator teres with little control of its activity. The pronator teres is released from its insertion on the middle

TABLE 19.3
TABLE 19.3
Surgical treatment options in the spastic upper extremity

Procedures		Deformity			
	Elbow flexion	Forearm pronation	Wrist flexion/UD	Finger deformity	Thumb-in-palm
Soft-tissue releases	Biceps lengthenings (Mital 1979)	PT releases (Strecker et al. 1988)	FCR lengthenings (Zancolli 1968)	FDS lengthenings (Zancolli 1968)	Adductor and/or 1st DI releases (Matev 1963)
	Brachialis lengthenings (Mital 1979)	Biceps aponeurosis Releases	Flexor pronator slides (Inglis and Cooper 1966, White 1972)	First web z-plastics	
		PQ release	FCU lengthenings (Zancolli 1968)		FPL lengthenings
Tendon transfers		PT re-routing (Sakellarides et al. 1981)	BR to ECRB/L (House and Gwathmey 1978, McCue et al. 1970)	FCU to EDC	FCR to APL
			ECU to ECRB/L	BR to EDC	PL to APL (House et al. 1981)
			FCU to ECRB/L	FDS tenodesis (Swanson 1960)	PL to EPB
			FCR to ECRB/L (Green 1942, Green and Banks 1962)	Lateral band re-routings (Tonkin et al. 1992)	BR to APL
			PT to ECRL	SORL (Littler, 1967)	BR to EPB
Bone/joint stabilization		Rotational osteotomies	Wrist fusion with PRC	Palmar plate Capsulodesis	PL to EPL
			PRC (Omer and Capen 1976)	PIP fusions	EPL re-routings
				DIP fusions	BR to EPL
					FCR to EPB
					Accessory muscle of APL to EPB
					MCP fusions (Goldner et al. 1990)
					MCP capsulodesis (Filler et al. 1976)
					IP fusions

APL, abductor pollicis longus; BR, brachioradialis; DI, dorsal interosseous; DIP, distal interphalangeal joint; ECRB/L, extensor carpi radialis brevis and/or longus; ECU, extensor carpi ulnaris; EDC, extensor digitorum communis; EPB, extensor pollicis brevis; EPL, extensor pollicis longus; FCR, flexor carpi radialis; FCU, flexor carpi ulnaris; FDS, flexor digitorum superficialis; FPL, flexor pollicis longus; IP, interphalangeal joint; MCP, metacarpophalangeal joint; PIP, proximal interphalangeal joint; PL, palmaris longus; PQ, pronator quadratus; PRC, proximal row carpectomy; PT, pronator teres; SORL, spiral oblique retinacular ligament reconstruction; UD, ulnar deviation.

Reprinted from Van Heest AE, House JH, Cariello C. (1999) Upper extremity surgical treatment of cerebral palsy. *J Hand Surg Am* **24**: 325, by permission.

one-third of the radius. The pronator rerouting procedure, by transferring the pronator back on to the radius in the opposite direction so that it works as a supinator, releases the pronator teres as a deforming pronation force. This operation provides greater correction than the pronator teres release, as it both diminishes the agonist (pronation) force and augments the antagonist (supination) force. However, care needs to be taken that the pronator teres is not too spastic, as this will lead to overcorrection.

Studies of results of these two procedures report similar results: 35°–40° of supination were the most common expected outcome. (Sakellarides et al. 1981, Strecker et al. 1988, Gschwind and Tonkin 1992).

Several procedures provide forearm supination as a secondary effect. The flexor pronator slide, diminishes the strength of the pronator teres by releasing it off its origin. Release of the pronator quadratus has been described as well for a milder deformity (Gschwind and Tonkin 1992). Transfer of the flexor carpi ulnaris (FCU) to the extensor carpi radialis longus or brevis provides a supination moment arm as it wraps around the ulna onto the dorsum of the wrist, which is greatest if the FCU is released two-thirds the length of the forearm (Van Heest et al. 1999b). Conversely, transfer of the flexor carpi radialis or pronator teres for wrist extension provides a pronation moment arm as the transferred muscle wraps on the radial side of the wrist; these transfers exacerbates the forearm pronation deformity and should be avoided as a wrist-tendon transfer in this population.

Wrist
The most common deformity of the wrist is flexion, often with ulnar deviation as well. This is the most functionally disabling deformity in hemiplegia as it significantly interferes with grasp and release function. Several different surgical options exist, with the choice dependent on the degree of deformity and the extent of volitional control of each muscle involved. Application of the surgical principles listed above is necessary and part of the art of designing a successful reconstructive plan: release or lengthen the deforming spastic muscles (FCU, FCR); transfer tendons to augment the weak wrist extension; and stabilize the joint only for the severe, fixed, non-functioning wrist (wrist fusion).

If the wrist-flexion deformity is mild, and wrist-extensor control exists, weakening the wrist-flexor(s) through fractional lengthening may be sufficient. If the mild wrist-flexion deformity exhibits concomitant wrist-ulnar deviation, the FCU would be lengthened. If the mild wrist-flexion deformity exhibits concomitant finger flexion and pronator spasticity, the entire flexor pronator mass can be lengthened using a flexor pronator slide (Inglis and Cooper 1966, White 1972).

If the wrist-flexor deformity is more severe, and wrist-extensors are not functional, then tendon-transfer surgery to augment wrist extension may be necessary. Muscles that can be transferred into wrist extensors include the brachioradialis (BR), the extensor carpi ulnaris (ECU), or the FCU. Using the BR or the ECU as the donor tendon has the advantage of leaving both flexor tendons intact, thus avoiding overcorrection; yet the disadvantage of not achieving balance unless the wrist-flexors are lengthened if their spasticity is significant. Using the ECU tendon has the advantage of correction of the ulnar deviation deformity, although this may require FCU-lengthening concomitantly; yet the disadvantage of not providing significantly more wrist-extension force than is already present. Using the FCU tendon has the advantage of removing its force as a spastic wrist-flexor/ulnar-deviator, while transferring its forces into wrist extension; yet the disadvantage is the possibility of over-correction if the deformity is not severe or if the transfer is tensioned too tight. This is particularly likely to occur in the younger child.

In all cases of transfer into the wrist-extensors, the finger function must be assessed preoperatively with the wrist in neutral, the desired postoperative position. If the finger-flexors are too tight when the wrist is brought into neutral, then a finger-flexor lengthening will be necessary as part of the procedure. If the patient does not have finger-extensor control to allow for release of grasped objects, then a transfer into the finger extensors (EDC) may be indicated. If the patient has such severe wrist-joint contracture that functional use of the hand is reduced to that of a paperweight, consideration should be given to either a proximal-row carpectomy (PRC) to shorten the skeletal column across the wrist joint, or to a wrist fusion to hold the wrist in a fixed, more functional position. The PRC is used in combination with tendon transfers and releases in those cases when passive mobility of the wrist cannot be achieved into extension. Passive mobility of the wrist is a necessary prerequisite to tendon-transfer surgery, which aspires to improve active mobility as well.

Wrist fusion predictably maintains the wrist in fixed position and is usually indicated only for improved cosmesis and use of the hand as a paperweight, in the skeletally mature individual. The proximal carpal row can be removed as part of the wrist fusion to facilitate positioning of the wrist into slight extension. Wrist fusion is contraindicated in the individual who uses wrist flexion tenodesis for release function, as this function would be lost if the wrist were to be fixed in a single position.

The greatest functional benefit in upper-extremity surgery has been reported with correction of the wrist-flexion deformity, regardless of the transfer used. As a representative example of the correction achieved, Beach and colleagues (1991) reported a postoperative arc of motion of almost 50°, centered around the neutral axis at greater than 5-year follow-up. Significant aesthetic improvement was noted as well in 90% of patients.

Fingers

The most common finger deformities are spastic flexion deformity and swan-neck deformity. Spastic flexion deformities are addressed in the above section on wrist deformities, as these muscles are biarticular muscles, crossing both the wrist and finger joints. Thus they need to be lengthened in concert with the wrist-flexion deformity correction, either as part of the flexor pronator slide or with selective fascial lengthenings. For the most severe clenched-fist deformity, which causes hygiene problems in a child with little active functional use of the fingers, a superficialis to profundus (STP) transfer would be indicated.

Swan-neck deformity of the fingers is due to dynamic imbalance of the muscles acting on the proximal interphalangeal (PIP) joint. Swan-neck finger deformity is characterized by PIP joint hyperextension with distal interphalangeal (DIP) joint flexion, due to intrinsic muscle spasticity. Additionally, many patients with cerebral palsy have better volitional control of their extrinsic finger extensors than they have of their wrist-extensors and will attempt to extend their wrists through overactivity of their extrinsic finger-extensors, further

337

exacerbating finger swan-necking.

Furthermore, excessive lengthening, or surgical release of the flexor digitorum superficialis (FDS), such as employed in the STP transfer, will often unmask intrinsic spasticity resulting in significant swan-neck deformities.

Surgical correction of swan-neck deformities is indicated if locking swan-neck deformities (usually greater than 40°) are not responsive to splinting and are found to be interfering with function, in the generalized assessment of upper-limb function. For the patient with significant wrist-flexion deformities and only mild swan-necking, surgical correction of wrist position alone may be adequate for treatment. For the patient with severe swan-necking (>40°), rebalancing of the muscle forces at the PIP joint will be necessary. Surgical options include lateral-band re-routing, lateral-band tenodesis, spiral oblique ligament reconstruction, intrinsic muscle slide, a resection of the ulnar-nerve motor branch in Guyon's canal, or superficialis tenodesis. The author's preferred method is lateral band re-routing procedure because it requires less extensive dissection and rebalances both the intrinsic and extrinsic tendons as deforming forces.

Thumb

The most common deformity for the thumb is in the palm. Thumb-in-palm deformity is also the most complex and challenging muscle imbalance to correct. Treatment requires a thorough understanding of the actions of the nine muscles that act on the thumb, and how these can be surgically rebalanced to provide pinch function.

Many different surgical combinations exist, with the choice dependent on the degree of deformity and the extent of volitional control of each muscle involved. Application of the surgical principles listed above is a necessary component in the design of a successful reconstructive plan: (1) release or lengthen the spastic muscles causing thumb flexion and adduction, i.e. release or lengthen the adductor pollicis, flexor pollicis brevis (FPB), and/or the flexor pollicis longus; (2) transfer tendons to augment the weak thumb extension and abduction; and (3) stabilize the joint for instability (metacarpophalangeal [MCP] joint capsulodesis or fusion).

Four types of thumb-in-palm deformity have been described, which help the surgeon to identify which spastic muscles need to be released or lengthened. In all types, the thumb adductor is a spastic deforming force. In the *type I thumb-in-palm deformity*, spasticity in the adductor pollicis causes significant adduction of the first metacarpal, narrowing the first web and limiting grasp. The adductor pollicis is the primary deforming force. In the type I deformity, two options exist for decreasing the spastic forces of the adductor pollicis muscle as shown in (Fig. 19.15): the Matev (1963) adductor slide or the partial adductor myotomy.

In the *type II thumb-in-palm deformity* (Fig. 19.16), not only does adductor pollicis spasticity cause significant adduction of the first metacarpal, but also flexor pollicis brevis spasticity causes significant thumb MCP joint-flexion deformity. In the type II deformity, the adductor is released as in the type I deformity, and the flexor brevis is released as well.

In the *type III thumb-in-palm deformity* (Fig. 19.17), prolonged adductor pollicis spasticity with metacarpal adduction leads to secondary, the thumb extension and abduction

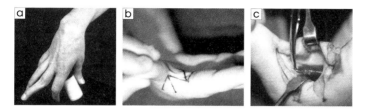

Fig. 19.15. The type I thumb-in-palm deformity. (a) Spasticity in the adductor pollicis causes significant adduction of the first metacarpal, narrowing the first web and limited grasp. The adductor pollicis is the primary deforming force. The thumb is pulled across the palm of the hand by the adductor pollicis, without significant deformity of the MCP or IP joints. Treatment of the type I thumb-in-palm includes a release of the adductor pollicis muscle, which can be performed through a first web z-plasty incision (b). The four-part z-plasty is used to increase the width of the first web skin for grasp function, and allows release of the transverse head of the adductor pollicis near its insertion as shown in (c). The oblique head of the adductor pollicis is left to preserve pinch function.

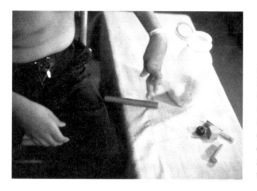

Fig. 19.16. The type II thumb-in-palm deformity. In addition to the thumb metacarpal adduction deformity from the adductor pollicis muscle spasticity, the type II thumb-in-palm deformity additionally has thumb MCP joint-flexion deformity due to FPB spasticity. Surgical correction would include release of the FPB in addition to the thumb adductor as described in type I.

through the MCP joint; this leads to secondary MCP joint instability, subluxation, and dislocation. The MCP becomes dorsally unstable with an incompetent volar plate. In the type III deformity, the adductor is released as in the type I deformity. Additionally, the thumb MCP joint is stabilized through a radial mid-lateral incision using a capsulodesis technique (Filler et al. 1976) or fusion (Goldner et al. 1990).

In the *type IV thumb-in-palm deformity* (Fig. 19.18), in addition to the thumb metacarpal adduction deformity due to adductor pollicis spasticity, and the MCP flexion due to FPB spasticity, the IP joint has a flexion deformity due to flexor pollicis longus spasticity. In the type IV deformity, the adductor and FPB are released as described for the type II thumb, but the FPL is also lengthened in the forearm.

For the milder deformities, when antagonist control is present, a release or lengthening of the spastic muscles is indicated without additional procedures. For more severe deformities without sufficient antagonist control, tendon transfers into the abductor pollicus longus (APL) or extensor pollicus brevis (EPB) is indicated. The exception is that transfers into the extensor pollicis brevis is not indicated for the type III thumb-in-palm deformity, unless the joint is fused, as a strong MCP extensor will exacerbate the MCP extension instability.

Tendon transfers to augment extension and abduction of the thumb include transfers into

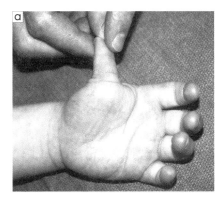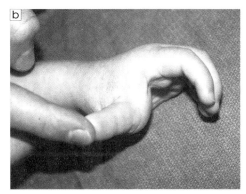

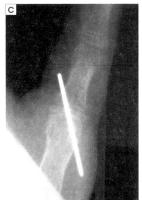

Fig. 19.17. The type III thumb-in-palm deformity. With prolonged adductor pollicis spasticity, the thumb will extend and abduct through the MCP joint with eventual secondary MCP joint instability, subluxation, and dislocation. The MCP becomes dorsally unstable with an incompetent volar plate as shown in (a) and (b). In addition to correction of the thumb-adduction deformity, the MCP joint is surgically stabilized by capsulodesis or fusion (c).

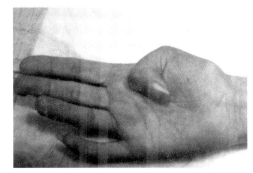

Fig. 19.18. The type IV thumb-in-palm deformity. In addition to the thumb metacarpal adduction deformity due to adductor pollicis spasticity and the MCP flexion due to flexor pollicis brevis spasticity, the type IV thumb-in-palm deformity also has IP joint-flexion deformity due to flexor pollicis longus spasticity. This is best corrected by a myotendinous lengthening in the forearm.

the APL or EPB, or re-routing of the EPL into the first dorsal compartment. Donor tendons for transfer include flexor carpi radialis (if the FCU is not transferred as part of the wrist correction); the brachioradialis, and the palmaris longus. If satisfactory tendon donors are not available, tenodeses can be carried out in the lower functioning hand. Re-routing of the EPL from the third dorsal compartment, where it acts as a secondary thumb-adductor, into the first dorsal compartment, will convert it into a thumb extensor–abductor (Manske 1985).

POSTPERATIVE MANAGEMENT

I advocate multiple simultaneous upper-extremity procedures for multilevel correction of the spastic limb in cerebral palsy. Postoperatively, a well-padded cast that will allow for swelling, but maintain intraoperative positioning is applied. The cast is removed 4 weeks later and the patient is fitted with a custom orthoplast splint. The splint is worn full-time for 4 weeks, removing it for active range of motion, light at-table activities, and hygiene. After 4 weeks of full-time wear, if the patient is maintaining the position of joint correction and learning active range of motion, then the patient is progressed to part-time use (at night, and for protection at school or in sports) and is started on strengthening exercises with gentle passive range of motion if needed for mobility. After this 3-month postoperative program, we recommend a long-term upper-extremity functional-use protocol, encouraging long-term bimanual skills.

COMPLICATIONS

All surgical procedures carry risk, which must be weighed against the potential benefits that most commonly are achieved. *Preoperatively*, patients must be screened for anesthetic complications: a bleeding screen for patients on long-term Depakote anti-seizure medications; screening for bladder and lung infections, particularly for patients with poor urinary or pulmonary control; and nutritional status (height and weight percentiles for age). *Intraoperative* attention to wound care is imperative to avoid wound-healing problems, particularly in z-plasty approaches. Large wounds should be treated with a postoperative drain to prevent hematoma formation. Nerve and artery injury due to overzealous correction of joint position is to be avoided. *Postoperatively*, the splint or cast should be adequate to allow for postoperative swelling and should be split if excessively swelling is encountered. Many children with spasticity do not have a normal preoperative sensory or motor exam, and may not have normal mentation, so normal parameters cannot be used to monitor for compartment syndrome. Premature removal of the cast or splint, as well as overzealous patient activities, can lead to tendon rupture or attenuation. Excessive immobilization can lead to excessive adhesion formation diminishing the eventual functional use.

Long-term problems most commonly center on loss of the balance achieved at the time of the surgery. Many children have tendon transfers as young as 7 years old and, due to their continued skeletal growth, may have recurrent deformity. Overcorrection can also occur with the "opposite" deformity occurring. Additionally, further "fine-tuning" surgery may be necessary to address complications that develop after correction of the original deformity.

Several principles will help prevent these complications: (1) do not overcorrect deformity, particularly in the younger child; (2) leave options to reverse the surgical correction if necessary; (3) keep functional grasp and release as your highest priority in your surgical planning; and (4) avoid wrist arthrodesis as this precludes the tenodesis effect of the wrist for finger use.

OUTCOMES

A review of the literature indicates an overall functional improvement in children with spastic hemiplegia after operative treatment (Eliasson et al. 1998, Van Heest et al. 1999a,

Nylanders et al. 1999). Nylanders and colleagues (1999) documented that functional improvement was achieved by 6 months postoperatively and was maintained at 4½-year follow-up in 24 children. Eliasson et al. (1998) reported on 32 children treated with tendon transfers and muscle releases and showed functional improvement in all children regardless of the degree of preoperative impairment. They noted that the extent of improvement based on preoperative functional level. We reported on 134 patients treated with soft-tissue release, tendon transfer and joint stabilization procedures (Van Heest et al. 1999a). Most commonly, all deformities were corrected during one operation, with an average of four procedures performed per surgery. Surgical results showed an average improvement of 2.6 levels using the House Classification of Upper Extremity Functional Use (Table 19.1). This functional improvement was not affected by level of mentation, 2-point discrimination, stereognosis function or type of cerebral palsy. (Note that only three athetoid patients were treated surgically over 25 years.) Patients with poor motor control did have less improvement in functional use. Most patients treated surgically were highly motivated.

Surgical procedures and outcomes should be discussed fully with your patient and their parents to prevent unrealistic expectations. In general, using the functional use scale in Table 19.1, an average of 2½ functional levels of improvement can be achieved with surgical intervention. Most commonly, this would mean that a child who presents with a severely flexed wrist with a thumb-in-palm deformity that limits him/her to use of the limb as a good passive assist could be improved to a fair-to-good active assist with better wrist and thumb positioning.

As surgeons, we must remember that we are treating only the secondary peripheral manifestations of a primary central nervous system dysfunction that persists. However, do not underestimate the importance of correcting upper-limb dysfunction in the hemiplegic patient. With careful preoperative assessment, judicious surgical planning, and appropriate surgical planning, your patient can exclaim: "It looks like a real arm!"

REFERENCES

Autti-Ramo I, Larsen A, Peltonen J, Taimo A, von Wendt L. (2000) Botulinum toxin injection as an adjunct when planning hand surgery in children with spastic hemiplegia. *Neuropediatrics* **31:** 4–8.
Baker LD. (1956) A rational approach to the surgical needs of the cerebral palsy patient. *J Bone Joint Surg Am* **38:** 313–323.
Baumann JU, Ruetsch H, Schurmann K. (1980) Distal hamstring lengthening in cerebral palsy. An evaluation by gait analysis. *Int Orthop* **3:** 305–309.
Beach WR, Strecker WB, Coe J, Manske PR, Schoenecker PL, Dailey L. (1991) Use of the Green transfer in treatment of patients with spastic cerebral palsy: 17 year experience. *J Pediatr Orthop* **11:** 731–736.
Becky GA, Chang CW, Perry J, Hoffer MM. (1977) Pattern recognition of multiple EMG signals applied to the description of human gait. *Proceedings of IEEE* **65:** 674–681.
Clancy R, Malin S, Laraque D, Baumgart S, Younkin D. (1985) Focal motor seizures heralding stroke in full-term neonates. *Am J Dis Child* **139:** 601–606.
Dahlin LB, Komoto-Tufvesson Y, Salgeback S. (1998) Surgery of the spastic hand in cerebral palsy. Improvement in stereognosis and hand function after surgery. *J Hand Surg Br* **23:** 334–339.
Delp SL, Statler K, Carroll NC. (1995) Preserving plantar flexion strength after surgical treatment for contracture of the triceps surae: a computer simulation study. *J Orthop Res* **13:** 96–104.
de Vries LS, Groenendaal F, Eken P, van Haastert IC, Rademaker KJ, Meiners LC. (1997) Infarcts in the

vascular distribution of the middle cerebral artery in preterm and fullterm infants. *Neuropediatrics* **28:** 88–96.

Duncan WR. (1955) Release of the rectus femoris in spastic paralysis. *J Bone Joint Surg Am* **37:** 634. (Abstract.)

Eccles RN, Lundberg A. (1958) Integrative patterns of Ia synaptic actions on motoneurons of hip and knee muscles. *J Physiol* **144:** 271–298.

Eliasson AC, Ekholm C, Carlstedt T. (1998) Hand function in children with cerebral palsy after upper-limb tendon transfer and muscle release. *Dev Med Child Neurol* **40:** 612–621.

Fabry G, Liu XC, Molenaers G. (1999) Gait pattern in patients with spastic diplegic cerebral palsy who underwent staged operations. *J Pediatr Orthop B* **8:** 33–38.

Fehlings D, Rang M, Glazier J, Steele C. (2000) An evaluation of botulinum-A toxin injections to improve upper extremity function in children with hemiplegic cerebral palsy. *J Pediatr* **137:** 300–303, 331–337.

Filler BC, Stark HH, Boyes JH. (1976) Capsulodesis of the metacarpophalangeal joint of the thumb in children with cerebral palsy. *J Bone Joint Surg Am* **58:** 667–670.

Gage JR, Perry J, Hicks RR, Koop S, Werntz JR. (1987) Rectus femoris transfer to improve knee function of children with cerebral palsy. *Dev Med Child Neurol* **29:** 159–166.

Goldner JL, Koman LA, Gelberman R, Levin S, Goldner RD. (1990) Arthrodesis of the metacarpophalangeal joint of the thumb in children and adults: adjunctive treatment of thumb-in-palm deformity in cerebral palsy. *Clin Orthop* **253:** 75–89.

Green WT. (1942) Tendon transplantation of the flexor carpi ulnaris for pronation-flexion deformity of the wrist. *Surg Gynecol Obstet* **75:** 337–342.

Green WT, Banks HH. (1962) Flexor carpi ulnaris transplant and its use in cerebral palsy. *J Bone Joint Surg Am* **44:** 1343–1352.

Gschwind C, Tonkin M. (1992) Surgery for cerebral palsy: part 1. Classification and operative procedures for pronation deformity. *J Hand Surg Br* **17:** 391–395.

Hiroshima K, Hamada S, Shimizu N, Ohshita S, Ono K. (1988) Anterior transfer of the long toe flexors for the treatment of spastic equinovarus and equinus foot in cerebral palsy. *J Pediatr Orthop* **8:** 164–168.

Hoffer MM. (1993) The use of the pathokinesiology laboratory to select muscles for tendon transfers in the cerebral palsy hand. *Clin Orthop Rel Res* **288:** 135–138.

Hoffer MM, Perry J, Melkonian G. (1990) Postoperative electromyographic function of tendon transfers in patients with cerebral palsy. *Dev Med Child Neurol* **32:** 789–791.

House JH, Gwathmey FW. (1978) Flexor carpi ulnaris and the brachioradialis as a wrist extension transfer in cerebral palsy. *Minn Med* **61:** 481-484.

House J, Gwathmey F, Fidler M. (1981) A dynamic approach to the thumb-in-palm deformity in cerebral palsy. *J Bone Joint Surg Am* **63:** 216–225.

Inglis AE, Cooper W. (1966) Release of the flexor-pronator origin for flexion deformities of the hand and wrist in spastic paralysis. *J Bone Joint Surg Am* **48:** 847–857.

Jebsen RH, Taylor N, Trieschmann RB, Trotter MJ, Howard LA. (1969) An objective and standardized test of hand function. *Arch Phys Med Rehabil* **50:** 311–319.

Jones R. (1916) The soldier's foot and the treatment of common deformities of the foot: part II. Claw-foot. *Br Med J* **1:** 749.

Kling TF, Kaufer H, Hensinger RN. (1985) Split posterior tibial tendon transfers in children with cerebral spastic paralysis and equinovarus deformity. *J Bone Joint Surg Am* **67:** 186–194.

Kozin SH, Keenan MH. (1993) Using dynamic electromyography to guide surgical treatment of the spastic upper extremity in the brain-injured patient. *Clin Orthop* **288:** 109–117.

Levy SR, Abroms IF, Marshall PC, Rosquete EE. (1985) Seizures and cerebral infarction in the full-term newborn. *Ann Neurol* **17:** 366–370.

Littler JW. (1967) The finger extensor mechanism. *Surg Clin North Am* **47**: 415–432.

Majestro MD, Ruda MD, Frost MD. (1971) Intramuscular lengthening of the posterior tibialis muscle. *Clinical Orthopaedics and Related Research* **79:** 59–60.

Manske PR. (1985) Redirection of extensor pollicis longus in the treatment of spastic thumb-in-palm deformity. *J Hand Surg Am* **10:** 553–560.

Matev I. (1963) Surgical treatment of spastic "thumb-in-palm" deformity. *J Bone Joint Surg Br* **45:** 703–708.

McCue FC, Honner R, Chapman WC. (1970) Transfer of the brachioradialis for hands deformed by cerebral palsy. *J Bone Joint Surg Am* **52:**1171–1180.

Mital MA. (1979) Lengthening of the elbow flexors in cerebral palsy. *J Bone Joint Surg Am* **61:** 515–522.

Mital MA, Sakellarides HT. (1981) Surgery of the upper extremity in the retarded individual with spastic cerebral palsy. *Orthop Clin N Am* **12**: 127–141.

Novacheck TF, Trost JP, Schwartz MH. (2002) Intramuscular psoas lengthening improves dynamic hip function in children with cerebral palsy. *J Pediatr Orthop* **22**: 158–164.

Nylanders G, Carlstrom C, Adolfsson L. (1999) 4.5 years follow-up after surgical correction of upper extremity deformities in spastic cerebral palsy. *J Hand Surg Br* **24**: 719–723.

Omer GE. Capen DA. (1976) Proximal row carpectomy with muscle transfers for spastic paralysis. *J Hand Surg Am* **1**: 197–204.

Perry J. (1987) Distal rectus femoris transfer. *Dev Med Child Neurol* **29**: 153–158.

Perry J, Giovan P, Harris LJ, Montgomery J, Azaria M. (1978) The determinants of muscle action in the hemiparetic lower extremity (and their effect on the examination procedure). *Clin Orthop* 71–89.

Rang M, Silver R, de la Garza J. (1986) Cerebral palsy. In: Winter R, editor. *Pediatric Orthopaedics,* 2nd edn. Philadelphia: J.B. Lippincott. p 385–395.

Sakellarides HT, Mital MA, Lenzi WD. (1981) Treatment of pronation contractures of the forearm in cerebral palsy by changing the insertion of the pronator radii teres. *J Bone Joint Surg Am* **63**: 645–652.

Salter RB. (1966) Role of inominate osteotomy in the treatment of congenital dislocation and subluxation of the hip in the older child. *J Bone Joint Surg Am* **48**: 1432–1439.

Silver LB. (1986) Controversial approaches to treating learning disabilities and attention deficit disorders. *Am J Dis Child* **140**: 1045–1052.

Stout JL, Gage JR, Bruce R. (1994) Joint kinetic patterns in spastic hemiplegia [abstract]. *Dev Med Child Neurol* **70** (suppl.): 8–9.

Strecker WB, Emanuel JP, Dailey L, Manske PR. (1988) Comparison of pronator tenotomy and pronator rerouting in children with spastic cerebral palsy. *J Hand Surg Am* **13**: 540–543.

Sutherland DH, Larsen LJ, Mann R. (1975) Rectus femoris release in selected patients with cerebral palsy: a preliminary report. *Dev Med Child Neurol* **17**: 26–34.

Sutherland DH, Santi M, Abel MF. (1990) Treatment of stiff-knee gait in cerebral palsy: a comparison by gait analysis of distal rectus femoris transfer versus proximal rectus release. *J Pediatr Orthop* **10**: 433–441.

Swanson AB. (1960) Surgery of the hand in cerebral palsy and the swan neck deformity. *J Bone Joint Surg Am* **42**: 951–964.

Tonkin MA, Hughes J, Smith KL. (1992) Lateral band translocation for swan-neck deformity. *J Hand Surg Am* **17**: 260–267.

Van Heest AE. (1997) Applications of Botulinum toxin in orthopaedics and upper extremity surgery. *Tech Hand Upper Extrem Surg* **1**: 27–34.

Van Heest AE, House J, Putnam M. (1993) Sensibility deficiencies in the hands of children with spastic hemiplegia. *J Hand Surg Am* **18**: 278–281.

Van Heest AE, House JH, Cariello C. (1999a) Upper extremity surgical treatment of cerebral palsy. *J Hand Surg Am* **24**: 323–330.

Van Heest AE, Murthy NS, Sathy MR, Wentorf FA. (1999b) The supination effect of tendon transfer of the flexor carpi ulnaris to the extensor carpi radialis brevis or longus: a cadaveric study. *J Hand Surg Am* **24**: 1091–1096.

Volpe JJ. (2001) *Neurology of the Newborn*. Philadelphia: W. B. Saunders. p 217–276.

Wall SA, Chait LA, Temlett JA, Perkins B, Hillen G, Becker P. (1993) Botulinum A chemodenervation: a new modality in cerebral palsied hands. *Br J Plast Surg* **46**: 703–706.

Waters RL, Garland DE, Perry J, Habig T, Slabaugh P. (1979) Stiff-legged gait in hemiplegia: surgical correction. *J Bone Joint Surg Am* **61**: 927–933.

White WF. (1972) Flexor muscle slide in the spastic hand: the Max page operation. *J Bone Joint Surg Br* **54**: 453–459.

Winters TF Jr, Gage JR, Hicks R. (1987) Gait patterns in spastic hemiplegia in children and young adults. *J Bone Joint Surg Am* **69**: 437–441.

Yokochi K. (1998) Clinical profiles of subjects with subcortical leukomalacia and border-zone infarction revealed by MR. *Acta Paediatr* **87**: 879–883.

Zancolli EA. (1968) *Structural and Dynamic Bases of Hand Surgery*. Philadelphia: Lippincott.

20
DIPLEGIA AND QUADRIPLEGIA: PATHOLOGY AND TREATMENT

Tom F. Novacheck

The general pathology of cerebral palsy as it pertains to walking was covered in Chapter 12. Specific lower-extremity abnormalities of the hips, knees and ankles were covered in Chapter 13. The genesis of spasticity as a primary abnormality was discussed in Chapter 3. In addition, abnormal muscle tone and its consequences were touched upon in Chapters 5, 12, 14 and 15. Nonoperative treatment of abnormal tone was discussed in Chapter 16, and Chapter 18 was devoted exclusively to the surgical correction of abnormal tone. The purpose of this chapter is to demonstrate how these methods can be used to improve ambulation in children with diplegia and quadriplegia. To accomplish this, it will attempt to integrate the treatment principles that have been presented. Accordingly, this chapter will focus on the specifics of interpreting gait analysis, and provide further insights into the role of gait analysis in the management of these patients. Finally, we discuss the means by which the specific orthopaedic anomalies that are common in these children can be corrected.

Since the focus of this book is on the correction of problems with gait, most of the management principles discussed in this chapter will apply not only to children with spastic diplegia, in which walking is the norm, but also to those with quadriplegia who are ambulatory. The former group tends to have better balance and selective motor control, whereas the latter tends to have poorer selective motor control, balance difficulties that often require walking aids (crutches or walkers), and more difficulties with abnormal muscle tone, which is frequently mixed due to a combination of spasticity plus basal ganglia injury. In reality, diplegia and quadriplegia are not separate conditions, but blend into each other. Consequently it is not possible to draw a distinct line between them. For example, how much, if any, upper-extremity involvement can one have and still be considered diplegic? As such, the individual with quadriplegia should be seen as representing the more severe end of the pathology spectrum. The two ends of the spectrum are clear; the middle is fuzzy. In addition, children with more severe involvement potentially have other issues as well, which may include seizures, perceptual problems and learning disability.

Goal assessment
It is important that the treating physician/surgeon and the patient/family communicate optimally. That is, the goals and expectations of treatment both present and future must be clear to both parties. Short-term goals might include improving walking speed, maintaining or increasing walking distance, reducing fatigue, improving stability to reduce the frequency of falling, and/or improving the child's ability to keep up with peers. Improving the

appearance of gait and/or decreasing gait asymmetries may be a concern to some patients and their families, whereas for other individuals with more severe involvement, treatment may need to focus on reducing pain or making a limb more braceable. When considering orthopaedic interventions the physician/surgeon should also look towards long-term goals such as avoiding joint degeneration and the pain that accompanies it, and preventing the decrease in walking ability that commonly occurs in young adults with cerebral palsy (Murphy et al. 1995, Bottos et al. 2001). For the more involved child, long-term goals may need to focus on maintaining or improving ability to stand for transfers, improving the child's ability to transfer from bed to chair, and/or improving independence for toileting or other activities of daily living. Because the severity of the condition varies so widely, functional abilities can be extremely different. With more severe involvement, the patient, family and caregiver need to recognize that the preferred means of mobility in the community will be accomplished via a wheelchair rather than walking. In that case, gait preservation will not be the primary goal, although limited ambulation may still be necessary for transfers and mobility within the home, particularly if the individual is to live independently as an adult. In instances such as these, it is important to focus more on the primary goals of communication, activities of daily living and mobility enumerated by Bleck (1987). Early and appropriate recognition of this situation will enable the team to direct time and energy towards realistic, obtainable goals and to prevent unrealistic family expectations.

In order to work through these complex issues, clear lines of communication are necessary. One of the roles of the motion analysis laboratory is to help promote this communication by documenting the severity of involvement. As an example, both walking speed and oxygen consumption provide useful insight into the severity of the child's involvement. In addition, the Functional Assessment Questionnaire, which is administered prior to any treatment intervention, includes specific questions about the family's goals of treatment, and the post-intervention questionnaire includes questions directed towards patient/family satisfaction with the treatment outcome. In addition the post-intervention questionnaire offers the opportunity to assess and set new goals. The use of such a tool has proved to be an invaluable asset in the management of the complex problems of these individuals.

Role of gait analysis
Gait analysis provides clear insight into the safety and efficacy of surgical intervention. The practitioner's knowledge, which is based on the patient's current gait analysis and physical examination plus his/her experience with previous patients, helps to provide a clear direction for counseling new patients whose families are considering surgical intervention. Experience gained through preoperative and postoperative assessment of patients in the motion analysis laboratory provides the surgeon with insight into the safety and efficacy of a potential intervention for any particular patient. Furthermore, the knowledge gained through the critical analysis of previous patients endows the practitioner with the ability to recognize the specific problems of the new patient and to develop a problem list. Once that problem list is formulated, it can then become the basis of communication. Working from the list, the patient, family, and surgeon can discuss which portions of the

pathology can be corrected surgically and which cannot. The problems that remain on the list can then be examined to determine whether additional treatment modalities, such as orthotics, medications and therapy might be used to control or minimize them. Here the reader may recognize the principles of the well-known "Serenity prayer" (see Chapter 12).

As mentioned previously, it is essential for all concerned to recognize that solutions must be tied not only to short-term but also to long-term goals. General principles of surgical management include (1) the reduction of spasticity, (2) the restoration of normal bony lever-arms, (3) the preservation of power generators, (4) the correction of contractures, and (5) the simplification of the control system.

Obviously the orthopaedist does not directly perform spasticity reducing procedures such as implantation of an intrathecal baclofen pump or selective dorsal rhizotomy (SDR). However, s/he needs to recognize the appropriateness of spasticity reduction and the indications for the procedures when they are present. At our institution, even though the orthopaedist in question might be a contributing member of the spasticity evaluation clinic, in order to get the benefit of the team's experience, s/he would still refer the patient for assessment.

Gait analysis for spasticity evaluation
Gait analysis provides valuable information as to the appropriateness of selection for SDR. As was discussed in Chapter 18, these criteria include (1) significant spasticity, (2) appropriate etiology, (3) good selective motor control, (4) the presence of pure spasticity (exclude rigidity, athetosis and/or other evidence of mixed tone patterns), (5) appropriate age (ideally between 4 and 8 years), and (6) adequate underlying muscle strength.

The child's spasticity must be severe enough to warrant a major permanent intervention such as SDR. In the spectrum of children with cerebral palsy, in some cases the spasticity will be too mild to consider a procedure of this magnitude. For these children, attention can better be directed to other aspects of gait dysfunction. In other children, neurological impairment will be so severe that their spasticity is overwhelming and/or motor control and muscle strength would be inadequate to maintain antigravity support of body weight if the spasticity were to be eliminated. For example, in some cases children rely on their spasticity for standing function or transfers. In this circumstance, rhizotomy may lead to loss of function and is contraindicated.

The motion analysis laboratory helps to delineate spastic movement patterns from those driven by "primitive reflexes". In Figure 20.1, for example, the hip, knee and ankle kinematics in the sagittal plane are consistent with spastic movement, and the overall joint excursions are decreased due to the stiffness associated with that spasticity. In this example there is a lack of hip extension in terminal stance, which may well be due to psoas spasticity. When this occurs there may or may not be an anterior pelvic tilt (usually with an associated "double-bump pattern" of pelvic motion in the sagittal plane). Hamstring spasticity frequently limits knee extension in terminal swing, which in turn leads to excessive knee flexion at initial contact and during loading response. Spasticity of the gastrocnemius can produce an amplification of the plantarflexion/knee-extension (PF/KE) couple, such that despite hamstring spasticity, there may be normal or near-normal extension of the knee in mid-

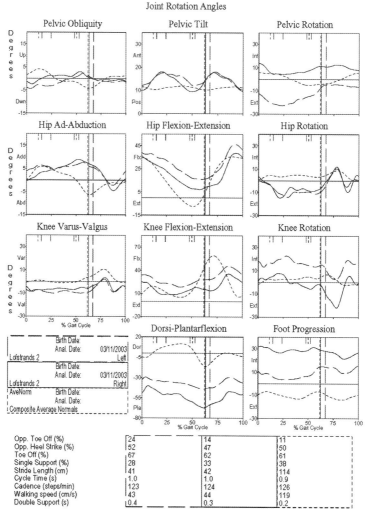

GILLETTE CHILDREN'S SPECIALTY HEALTHCARE GAIT LABORATORY
Joint Rotation Angles

Fig. 20.1. Sagittal-plane kinematics of a child with severe spasticity. The hip, knee and ankle kinematics in the sagittal plane are consistent with spastic movement, and the overall joint excursions are decreased due to the stiffness associated with that spasticity

stance. Since the biarticular gastrocnemius crosses both the knee and the ankle, however, spasticity of this muscle can also contribute to insufficient knee extension in terminal swing, at initial contact and during loading response. Gastrocnemius spasticity also can limit the duration of second rocker, producing premature plantarflexion with inappropriate power generation in mid-stance. Since the body is directly over the foot at that time, the power burst produces upward displacement of the trunk (the so-called "bounce gait") as opposed to useful forward propulsion. Finally, rectus femoris spasticity usually causes decreased and delayed knee flexion in swing. The reader should note that, as discussed in Chapter

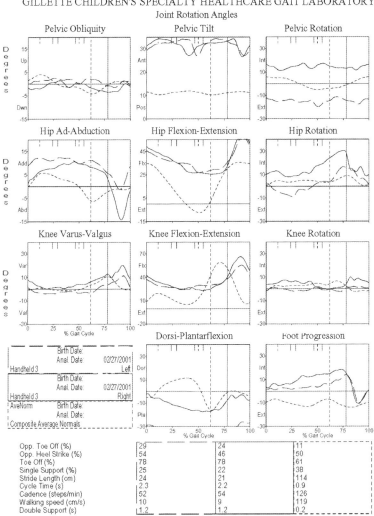

GILLETTE CHILDREN'S SPECIALTY HEALTHCARE GAIT LABORATORY

Joint Rotation Angles

Opp. Toe Off (%)	29	24	11
Opp. Heel Strike (%)	54	46	50
Toe Off (%)	78	78	61
Single Support (%)	25	22	38
Stride Length (cm)	24	21	114
Cycle Time (s)	2.3	2.2	0.9
Cadence (steps/min)	52	54	126
Walking speed (cm/s)	10	9	119
Double Support (s)	1.2	1.2	0.2

Fig. 20.2. Sagittal-plane kinematics of a child with poor selective motor control. Movement is characterized by a pattern in which the individual is reciprocating two primitive reflexes: mass flexion in swing for limb advancement and mass extension in stance for support.

12, the principal muscles that are producing these problems (psoas, hamstrings, gastrocnemius and rectus femoris) are all biarticular. The spasticity-reducing effect of SDR may be an appropriate recommendation in this circumstance as the gait pattern is dominated by spasticity.

In Figure 20.2, on the other hand, movement is characterized by a pattern in which the individual is reciprocating two primitive reflexes (mass flexion and mass extension). This is apparent because in swing phase, hip and knee flexion and ankle dorsiflexion occur simultaneously. In the same way during stance phase, all joints are extending at the same

349

time. SDR in this case would not be appropriate as the primary movement pattern is dictated by reflexive movement, rather than spasticity.

Assessment of oxygen consumption helps to identify patients in whom spasticity is a major contributing factor to gait pathology. Patients with oxygen consumption 1.8–2.2 times normal may have the best potential to benefit from SDR. Assuming they have the other findings consistent with multilevel spasticity, SDR will probably improve gait efficiency and decrease oxygen consumption (see Chapter 23). Children, in whom spasticity is not severe enough to warrant SDR, typically have oxygen consumption levels that are only slightly increased (up to 1.6/1.7 times normal, or about 20% outside of normal range). Patients with energy consumptions that are extremely high might also benefit from SDR. As a rule, however, these children have additional problems that relate to selective motor control and balance, which also adversely affect their function. Consequently, although patients in this category may improve with SDR, the benefits are less apparent because of their other problems with motor control and balance.

If optimal results with spasticity reduction are to be achieved, the spasticity evaluation team also must be certain that the diagnosis is correct. In order to accomplish this they need to determine which central nervous system studies have been done to document the diagnosis, and whether other central nervous system problems such as hydrocephalus, congenital brain malformations, and Arnold–Chiari malformation have been ruled out. In addition to demonstrating absence of mixed tone, adequate balance and sufficient selective motor control, the ideal patient for spasticity reduction via SDR is the product of preterm birth with evidence that his/her CNS lesion is secondary to periventricular leukomalacia.

Gait analysis should include an assessment of selective motor control. This author is not familiar with validated scales that are documented to be reliable. In our laboratory, we currently use a relatively simple scale:

0   Selective motor control is absent
1   Movement is not completely selective and is tied to associated movements at other joints, e.g. the Strümpel Confusion Test
2   The individual is able to isolate the desired muscular activity selectively, without other associated movements.

Selective motor control is rated at each joint. When considering SDR, the ability to selectively isolate and control movement about the hips and knees is an important criterion. As was discussed in Chapter 12, cerebral palsy causes the greatest difficulties with selectivity and motor control at the distal end of the limb, i.e. the foot and ankle. When motor control is poor, there is greater dependence on patterns of movement (the so-called "primitive movement patterns" that do not emanate from the cerebral cortex). Some individuals who demonstrate an inability to selectively control movements of the foot and ankle may still be appropriate rhizotomy candidates. In more severe cases, the child's underlying selective motor control can be overshadowed by his/her spasticity. If the physician remains mindful that one of the prerequisites for rhizotomy is a consistent gait pattern characterized by restricted joint movement, SDR can still be an appropriate recommendation in a case such as this.

Through the use of electromyography (EMG) and kinematics, the motion analysis

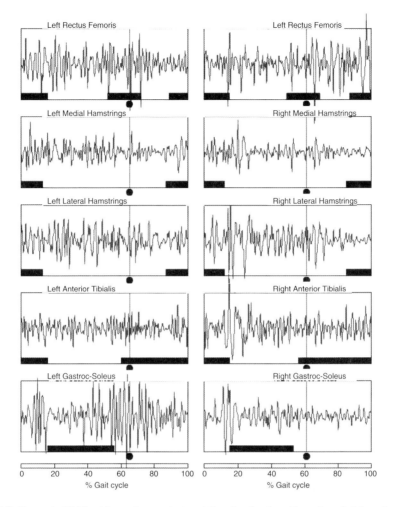

Fig. 20.3. Dynamic EMG with nearly constant multilevel activation. Even though this patient has multilevel spasticity, the nearly constant activity in multiple muscle groups suggests that he/she may be a less ideal candidate for SDR. In the absence of any distinct "off" times, the patient may be relying on multilevel spasticity to maintain an upright, antigravity position.

laboratory can provide further insight into tone type and motor control. Dynamic EMG, for example, which demonstrates constant activity in multiple muscle groups without any distinct "off" times, is less ideal for SDR (Fig. 20.3). In the patient data depicted in Figure 20.4, on the other hand, multilevel prolonged activation of dynamic EMG can be seen in association with distinct "off" times. Such a patient would fulfil the criteria for multilevel spasticity and have a high likelihood for improvement with SDR. The rhizotomy can reduce co-spasticity between agonist and antagonist muscles allowing the child's underlying coordinated muscular activity to emerge.

One of the orthopaedist's principal roles in the spasticity evaluation team is to identify

Trial Number 03   bf 1

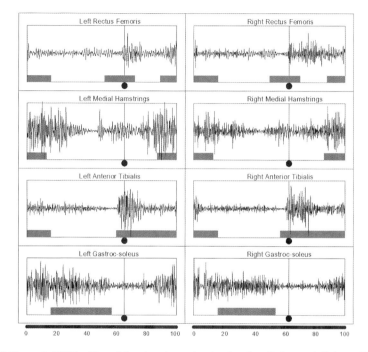

Fig. 20.4. Dynamic EMG with multilevel prolonged activation, but distinct on/off times. This patient would typically be considered a better candidate for SDR. There is prolonged and simultaneous activation of antagonistic muscle groups compared to normal (compared to normal activation bars). The "off times" suggest that he/she is able to rely on other muscle groups to maintain postural alignment rather than co-spastic activation.

and point out lever-arm dysfunction (LAD) accurately. To accomplish this, radiographs (including an anteroposterior pelvis, weightbearing x-rays of the feet, and mortise x-rays of the ankles) are typically necessary. Physical examination for LAD (femoral anteversion, hip subluxation, tibial torsion and/or foot deformity) falls within his/her expertise. The orthopaedist also must be able to confirm the presence and severity of torsional problems that were identified on gait analysis. It is important for the orthopaedist on the spasticity evaluation team to identify joint- and lever-arm dysfunction that might adversely affect rehabilitation following SDR. Finally, because these issues are complex, it is imperative that the spasticity team communicates the findings of the evaluation with the family and patient in language and terms they can understand. To achieve maximum benefit, most of the children who require spasticity reduction will also need correction of LAD, so the orthopaedist needs to participate actively in future planning. In fact, at times the child's LAD is so severe as to produce hip subluxation and/or interfere with rehabilitation following

352

rhizotomy. In a case such as this, correction of LAD should be the first procedure. At the completion of the evaluation, each team member must be available to answer the family's follow-up questions, so the participation of an experienced nurse coordinator is essential.

Gait interpretation session

The mechanics of the gait interpretation session will depend upon the experience of the reviewers. The therapist who performed the gait analysis and the physician interpreter (typically a pediatric orthopaedist) will interpret the data jointly. If the patient's past medical history, level of disability and prior treatment are not known to the physician interpreter, the therapist will typically review that material with him/her while the patient's videotape is playing. Next the patient's and/or family's stated goals of intervention are reviewed. This important information was gathered earlier when the gait analysis was done. If the interpreter suggests an intervention, s/he must be sure that the treatment addresses the patient's and family's concerns. The orthopaedist also should be alert to short- and long-term goals suggested by the family that are unlikely to be achieved.

During the review of the videotape and the motion analysis data, the interpreter should consider the five prerequisites of normal gait: (1) stability in stance, (2) clearance in swing, (3) appropriate pre-positioning of the foot for initial contact, (4) adequate step length, and (5) energy conservation (see Chapter 4). This helps both to organize one's thinking and to link problems identified on gait analysis with their adverse impact on function.

By separating the abnormal findings demonstrated by the gait analysis into primary, secondary, and tertiary gait problems (see Chapter 12), the relative impact on function of spasticity (a primary problem) versus LAD (a secondary/growth problem) can be assessed. It also is essential that the interpreter is able to recognize that some of the abnormalities in gait data (kinematics, kinetics and EMG) are compensations (tertiary problems) employed by the patient to maximize efficiency or avoid other difficulties created by the primary and secondary abnormalities of gait. This approach will help the interpreter to avoid the mistake of recommending treatment for gait compensations. One of the most obvious examples is to recognize vaulting as a compensation to avoid problems with foot clearance in swing phase. The video will reveal an early heel-rise. Kinematics confirm premature plantarflexion in mid-stance. Kinetics shows an abnormally increased ankle plantarflexion moment in mid-stance. EMG in this case, however, should show that the triceps surae is appropriately quiet in swing and immediately following initial contact during first rocker. If the problem that requires the compensation is corrected, the compensation will disappear spontaneously. Many iatrogenic problems have occurred because gait compensations were operated upon rather than being recognized for what they were.

Next, the physical examination is reviewed to identify torsional deformities (femoral anteversion and tibial torsion) as well as joint deformities. In particular, contractures that are inconsistent with a normal gait pattern should be noted. For example, to achieve normal gait the knee must come to within 5° of full extension. Consequently, a knee-flexion contracture of 15° precludes a normal walking pattern. Attention also must be paid to muscle strength, muscle imbalance and abnormalities of motor control. To continue with the example of the knee begun above, quadriceps insufficiency (e.g. muscle strength less

353

than or equal to 3/5) is inconsistent with the knee's normal response to load during the first 20% of the gait cycle. Therefore, absence of knee flexion during the loading response portion of stance phase (greater than normal knee extension) would be a necessary gait compensation for this muscular insufficiency.

Muscular imbalance in the joint's functional position during walking should also be assessed. Until recently, the impact of a knee-extension lag (due to knee-extensor insufficiency) has been underappreciated. To attain normal knee extension in mid- and terminal stance, an individual must not only have adequate joint flexibility, but also quadriceps-extension strength adequate to stabilize the knee in a position of extension (see Chapter 21).

Currently, an adequate assessment of foot deformities cannot be obtained using only kinematic and kinetic data. The need for weightbearing X-rays of the foot has already been emphasized. In addition, however, the physical evaluation of foot deformities can be supplemented with close-up videotape views of the foot during walking (anterior, posterior, and medial/lateral). Moreover, static close-up videotape views of the feet in quiet standing (single and double leg), as well as videotape documentation of the Root sign (see Chapter 5) are extremely helpful. If the therapist notes significant coronal-plane foot deformities, close-up videotape views with the placement of medial or lateral forefoot wedges in appropriate locations can help distinguish hindfoot from forefoot deformity. The Coleman block test is an example of this (see Chapter 5).

Gait analysis always is performed within the context of other clinical information. Ideally, in order to complete the generation of the problem list, appropriate radiographs should be present at the time of the gait interpretation session. These might include an anteroposterior pelvis, lateral X-ray of both knees in maximum extension (to assess joint contracture and/or patella alta), weightbearing X-rays of both feet and mortise X-rays of both ankles (see Chapter 5). Radiographs provide further insight into many deformities that are fairly common in cerebral palsy. These include lever-arm dysfunction such as hip joint subluxation, coxa valga, acetabular dysplasia, patella alta, fixed knee contractures, ankle valgus, an abnormal orientation between the ankle joint and forefoot and instability of the midfoot.

Some of the other items from the physical examination that also need to be considered during motion analysis interpretation include (1) the extent of spasticity, (2) the degree of motor control, (3) right/left side asymmetry, and (4) leg-length discrepancy.

When three-dimensional joint kinematics and kinetics are reviewed, gait consistency should be ensured by comparing at least three cycles of data for both the right and left sides. If the consistency data shows significant variability from one cycle to the next, information from a single gait cycle must be interpreted with caution. Fortunately, in most cases, the gait is consistent. An inconsistent gait pattern may be due to a number of factors, including gait immaturity, poor balance, cerebellar dysfunction and basal ganglia dysfunction (often referred to as extrapyramidal involvement).

Details of the identification of specific gait deviation patterns are provided in Chapter 14. The current state of interpretation of muscle length plots is early in its clinical implementation (Fig. 20.5). Muscle-length data are determined by modeling the origin to insertion distance for the muscle in question based on the patient's kinematic data. It has great potential for use in the assessment of two-joint (biarticular) muscles. When compared

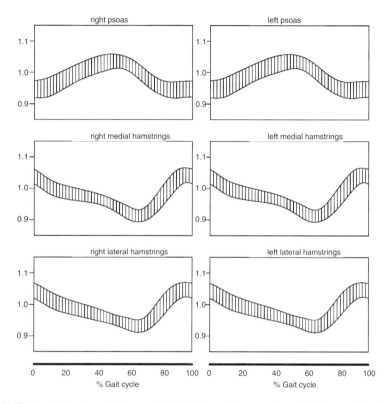

Gillette Children's Specialty Healthcare Gait Laboratory

Muscle lengths

* Muscle lengths are normalized to the anatomical position origin to insertion length

Fig. 20.5. Muscle-length graphs (normal). Muscle-length data are determined by modeling the origin to insertion distance for the muscle in question based on the patient's kinematic data. Not only does it provide needed information about the length of a biarticular muscle group, it also provides information regarding the excursion (flexibility) and modulation (pattern of motion) of those muscles.

to normalized gait data, we find it particularly useful to assess both hamstring and psoas length and spasticity. That is, the graphs not only provide information about the length of the muscles in question, they also provide needed information about the muscle's modulation (or lack of it) during the gait cycle. As an example, since spasticity tends to be worse distally, we often note that the hamstrings are virtually isometric throughout the gait cycle, whereas the psoas, although frequently short, tends to modulate fairly normally (Fig. 20.6). If spasticity is reduced by means of SDR, hamstring modulation usually improves significantly on the post-rhizotomy gait analysis. Again, this cannot be used as stand-alone information, e.g. hamstrings that measure longer than normal during the gait cycle, for a patient in crouch

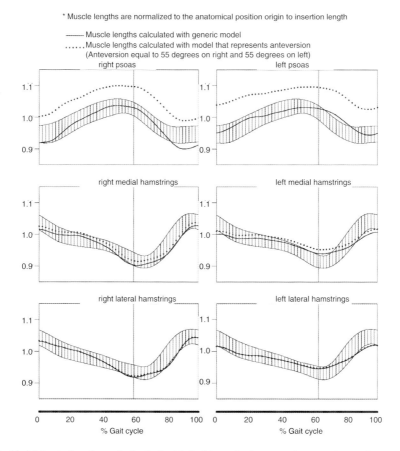

Gillette Children's Specialty Healthcare Gait Laboratory

Muscle lengths

* Muscle lengths are normalized to the anatomical position origin to insertion length

—— Muscle lengths calculated with generic model
····· Muscle lengths calculated with model that represents anteversion
(Anteversion equal to 55 degrees on right and 55 degrees on left)

Fig. 20.6. Muscle-length graphs (pathologic). In this particular example one notes nearly normal range, excursion, and modulation of the psoas whereas the left hamstrings are at length, but nearly isometric in action. This is a fairly common pattern, since spasticity and selective motor control both tend to worsen as one moves distally in the limb.

gait, may still require some surgical lengthening. Perhaps the development of muscle-length data has raised as many questions as it answers. However, it has greatly increased our understanding of crouch gait (Hoffinger et al. 1993, Delp et al. 1996, Schutte et al. 1997, Thompson et al. 1998, Schmidt et al. 1999). If the patient is in crouch and has longer-than-normal measured hamstring length, there must be an increased anterior pelvic tilt. In this situation, treatment must focus on reducing pelvic tilt. This might include elimination of femoral anteversion via femoral derotational osteotomy and/or psoas lengthening at the pelvic brim in conjunction with a therapy program aimed at strengthening the abdominals and hip extensors. Botulinum toxin injection to the hamstrings also may be used at the time of surgical intervention to facilitate the stretching program. If successful, the existing hamstring length may be sufficient to allow adequate knee excursion without resorting to surgical lengthening.

At the conclusion of the gait interpretation session, a problem list is generated. Occasionally, there are conflicting pieces of information that may require further review by physical exam, supplemental radiographs, and/or rarely by repeat gait analysis. At a subsequent clinic appointment, the problem list is reviewed with the family. If adequate X-rays had not been done earlier, these can be done at that time. In addition conflicting or questionable physical exam data usually can be clarified at the time of this gait analysis review session.

Ultimately, final treatment decisions must be made in conjunction with the family. An informed decision about treatment cannot be made without an adequate and complete problem list. As a result of this step-wise progression, it should be apparent to the reader that there are three steps in clinical gait analysis. In the first step, objective information (physical exam, X-rays, kinematics, kinetics, EMG, muscle lengths, oxygen consumption) is gathered. The second step is to develop a problem list based on that data. If you stop to consider it, data interpretation really is just a subjective extrapolation of the objective information gathered from the various pieces of the examination. Finally, the third step, involves the formulation of a "solution list" that addresses the problem list (step 2). The development of a problem list is relatively consistent from one experienced interpreter to another and/or between institutions, whereas the formulation of the solution list is much less uniform because it depends so heavily on the experience and background of the individual (Skaggs et al. 2000, Noonan et al. 2003, Gage 2003). When we performed an informal study comparing three experienced pediatric orthopaedic physician interpreters with similar background and experience, we found this to be the case even within our own institution. While at first this seems to be a cause for concern, in many aspects of medical care it is not without precedent. Take, for example, a child with talipes equinovarus. In all likelihood there would be little disagreement among pediatric orthopaedists that the child has talipes equinovarus, but treatment recommendations would be likely to vary substantially from one surgeon to the next. Treatment decision-making in Legg-Calve-Perthes disease is another good example. Pediatric orthopaedic surgeons will have little difficulty agreeing with the diagnosis, but commonly will recommend different care pathways, each of which may meet with varying degrees of success. As Cervantes wrote in *Don Quixote*, "The proof of the pudding is in the eating!" Fortunately, however, postoperative gait analysis now also provides us with an objective assessment of the treatment outcome, which over time should allow us to compare the relative merits of various treatment protocols (see *Functional Assessment*, Chapter 23).

Orthopaedic surgical treatment

To a large extent, success with the multiple lower-extremity procedure (MLEP) depends on obtaining rigid fixation of osteotomized bone segments to allow for early healing, comfort, and rapid remobilization. As will be discussed in Chapter 22, the period of non-

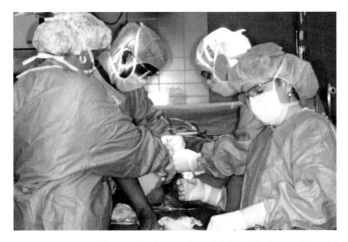

Fig. 20.7. The "two-team approach" to surgical correction of deformities in a patient with diplegia. The two surgeons are working simultaneously but independently on each lower extremity.

weightbearing is minimized (usually to no more than 3–4 weeks). Weightbearing is allowed prior to radiographic evidence of bone-healing. Prolonged immobility delays and extends rehabilitation, limits potential improvement, and potentially could even cause treatment failure. As a result, success depends on a close working relationship with the other members of the team involved in the care of the patient, which includes nursing, cast-room services, physical therapy and orthotics. The first and second follow-up appointments following discharge from the hospital after MLEP are typically lengthy. It takes several hours for all of the steps (cast removal, X-ray, physician appointment, molding for new braces, potential recasting, and a physical therapy session) to be performed.

Proper postoperative pain management is crucial. Again this requires a multidisciplinary approach with involvement of the inpatient nursing staff and the pain management team (anesthesia) for monitoring and dosing of epidural catheters or patient controlled analgesia (PCA). All of this will be discussed in greater detail in Chapter 22.

Botulinum toxin may be injected at the time of surgery in order to help with pain management due to spasticity (Barwood et al. 2000), to facilitate rehabilitation during the first three or four months following surgery, and to limit the amount of surgical lengthening of musculotendinous units (Thompson et al. 1998, Sutherland et al. 1999, Zurcher et al. 2001).

With experience the surgeon gains confidence in the speed and efficacy with which surgery can be done. As a result, the reliability of attaining the goals of the intervention increases and the risk of surgical complications decreases. All of these factors are important in order to have the confidence to recommend and carry out the multiple interventions. For extensive bilateral cases, two surgical teams working simultaneously on both lower extremities shortens the surgical time and avoids surgeon fatigue (Fig. 20.7). The reader is referred to prior publications for details of the particular surgeries that we commonly perform (Gage et al. 1987, Gage 1990, Novacheck 1996, Gage and Novacheck 2001, Novacheck et al. 2002).

This discussion will therefore focus on the lessons learned, nuances of treatment, and surgical "pearls".

HIP-FLEXION DEFORMITY

It is extremely difficult to identify who needs surgery to improve hip-extension flexibility. However, the use of the multivariate statistic, hip-flexor index (HFI) is helpful (Schwartz et al. 2000). We do not believe that the decision can be made based merely on the presence or absence of a hip-flexion contracture on physical exam. The Thomas test is inaccurate and variable. Additionally, spasticity, which greatly affects the test, varies greatly depending on the position and emotional state of the patient. Lastly, one should recognize that normal gait requires hip extension beyond 0°. Consequently, extension of the hip to neutral (0°) is not sufficient to achieve this goal.

There has been significant reluctance to perform psoas-lengthening surgery due to the concern that the hip-flexors, which are an important source of power for movement, would be weakened. The details of the intramuscular psoas lengthening technique have been published (Novacheck et al. 2002). If one uses this technique, the procedure can be done in 20–30 minutes. Intramuscular psoas lengthening at the pelvic brim has been shown to be effective (Novacheck et al. 2002) while other surgeries such as recession of the psoas off the trochanter to the capsule as described by Bleck (1971) excessively weaken hip flexion. If one starts to think about why this is true, it becomes apparent that the triceps surae and the iliopsoas are anatomically similar (in both cases a monoarticular and a biarticular muscle come together on a common tendon. As such, recession of the psoas tendon from the lesser trochanter to the hip capsule is analogous to tendo-Achilles lengthening in that both tendo-Achilles lengthening and recession of iliopsoas tendon to the hip capsule effectively lengthen both the mono- and biarticular elements of their respective muscles (the soleus and gastrocnemius in the former and the iliacus and the psoas in the latter). Furthermore, it is now known that in children with spastic diplegia the biarticular muscles are prone to develop contractures whereas the monoarticular muscles rarely do (see Chapter 12). Therefore, in carrying our reasoning further, both procedures are very likely to produce iatrogenic weakening of muscles that are critically important to gait. With rare exception, in children with cerebral palsy, proximal rectus femoris release has also been proven to do little more than produce iatrogenic weakening of hip flexion. Perry has presented arguments as to why this might be true and Sutherland has shown that distal transfer of the rectus femoris is more effective than proximal release (Perry 1987, Sutherland et al. 1990, McMulkin et al. 2001). By exposing the psoas tendon in the interval between the iliacus and the ileum (under the iliacus muscle belly), the surgery can be done safely, although the surgeon is very close to the femoral nerve (Skaggs et al. 1997). Accordingly, the reader should be aware that, although there are no publications to document these, we are aware of several malpractice cases that have been filed in the USA as a result of damage to the femoral nerve and/or artery. Because of this concern, Sutherland and colleagues (1997) have recommended dissection medial to the psoas/iliacus muscle mass with direct visualization of the femoral neurovascular bundle.

In our study, we showed no weakening of hip-flexion function following intramuscular psoas lengthening. However, if the patient demonstrated significant hip-flexor weakness preoperatively, rather than surgically lengthening the psoas, we frequently choose to inject the psoas with botulinum toxin injection and then use appropriate therapy to stretch the hip-flexors and strengthen the hip-extensors and abdominal muscles. In these cases, we reserve psoas lengthening for failure of the more conservative approach. In some cases, the hip-flexion deformity is largely dynamic and, as a result, may respond well to botulinum toxin injection. We use a transcutaneous technique through the abdominal wall under general anesthesia to inject botulinum toxin into the psoas that Molenaers has described in a personal communication, but has not published.

TALIPES EQUINOVALGUS

The equinovalgus foot is an inadequate lever. It is not only maloriented, but the midfoot instability prevents normal progression of the center of pressure path along the length of the foot during stance phase. The presentation of the calcaneal lengthening procedure by Mosca at the POSNA meeting in 1993, led to the rebirth of the procedure that was initially popularized by Evans (1975). This led to an immediate change in the nature of our management of this foot deformity (Mosca 1995, 1996, 1998). The instability and hypermobility of the foot are directly treated. We think of this procedure as a stiffener of the excessively flexible midfoot in this extremely common foot deformity. The procedure helps to block the excessive eversion range of motion. Oeffinger and colleagues (2000) have shown dynamic improvement in foot function using plantar pressure measurements.

In our experience, the os calcis lengthening procedure alone is often not sufficient to restore adequate lever-arm function. For example, associated external tibial torsion is frequently present and if this is the case, the tibial torsion must also be corrected in order to fully correct the lever-arm dysfunction that is interfering with the PF/KE couple. Usually the gastrocnemius is contracted as well. If so, it will act to restrict ankle dorsiflexion during second rocker and the resultant restriction of motion at the tibial–talar joint will generate additional motion and strain on the midfoot. To correct this problem it is almost always necessary to perform these bony procedures in conjunction with gastrocnemius lengthening or recession, as once dorsiflexion flexibility of the tibial–talar joint is restored, the hypermobility and stress on the midfoot is decreased (Strayer 1958, Saraph et al. 2000). Finally, the soft-tissue structures on the medial side of the foot (talar–navicular capsule and spring ligament) have usually stretched out over time. If this is the case, reefing of the talonavicular capsule (occasionally in conjunction with advancement of the posterior tibialis tendon) is performed as well. To date the efficacy of this additional soft-tissue surgery on the medial side of the foot has not been scientifically evaluated. Based on our clinical impression, however, it is beneficial.

With long-standing and/or more severe deformities, significant subtalar joint deformity is frequently present as well. Correction of this problem requires the use of the subtalar arthrodesis as described by Dennyson and Fulford (1976) in conjunction with the os calcis lengthening procedure (Fig. 20.8). The quadriplegic patient, who has poorer motor control and strength, will require the use of ankle–foot orthoses (AFOs) or, if there is no foot-drop in swing phase, appropriate foot orthotics. The orthotics protect the adjacent joints from

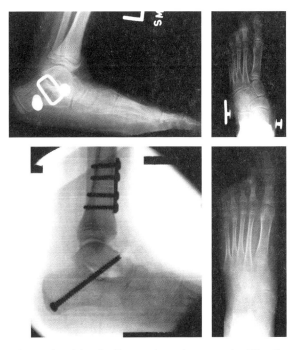

Fig. 20.8. Correction of severe foot deformity. Preoperative and postoperative AP and lateral roentgenograms demonstrating the results of surgical correction of a severe planovalgus foot with associated external tibial torsion. In order to maximize lever arm deformity correction (restore foot-to-knee alignment), we combined os calcis lengthening with subtalar arthrodesis and derotational tibial osteotomy.

the increased stresses that are generated by the loss of subtalar motion. These children have higher-energy consumptions and slower walking velocities, which act to limit their walking distance as well. All of these factors mitigate concern that premature osteoarthritis may develop in the joints adjacent to the subtalar fusion.

As stated earlier, the current state of motion analysis does not permit an adequate evaluation of complex foot deformities. For that reason, many laboratories (including ours) are trying to develop improved methods of foot modeling and assessment. Because of this inadequacy, precise determination of severity of the deformity, detection of associated deformities and evaluation of outcome of the foot are inaccurate. Consequently, to identify the presence of other deformities, the surgeon still must rely on physical and videotape examination plus roentgenograms. Two deformities, however, are commonly associated with the equinovalgus foot. The first is forefoot varus deformity. Some refer to this as supination of the forefoot on the hindfoot. Regardless of the fact that there is a lack of consensus regarding terminology, as pressure advances to the mid and forefoot in second rocker, excessive subtalar eversion occurs before the medial side of the forefoot can contact the floor and become stable enough to accept weight. A plantar, closing-wedge osteotomy of the first cuneiform can correct this deformity (Mosca 1995). The second associated deformity is valgus of the ankle mortise. This deformity produces the appearance of a hindfoot valgus during weightbearing. A mortise view X-ray of the ankle joint is diagnostic. Because this deformity is so commonly associated with planovalgus foot deformity, this view should be part of the routine preoperative X-ray evaluation of any patient who is at or near skeletal maturity. If there is sufficient distal tibial growth remaining, ankle valgus can be treated with a screw across the medial aspect of the distal tibial epiphysis (Davids et al. 1997). After maturity a distal tibial varus osteotomy is necessary. The correction of the valgus deformity can be done in conjunction with derotation of the tibia as there is often an associated external tibial torsion, which if present, will need to be corrected as well.

PATELLA ALTA

Until recently, the adverse effects of patella alta and quadriceps insufficiency with which it is associated have been under appreciated. In the last 4–5 years, however, we have focused much more attention to its detection and assessment. Patellar subluxation, patellofemoral pain and pain due to inferior pole sleeve avulsion fracture, are all recognized consequences of this condition (Kaye and Freiberger 1971, Insall et al. 1972, Lotman 1976, Rosenthal & Levine 1977, Lloyd-Roberts et al. 1985, Villani et al. 1988, Feldkamp 1990, Pietu and Hauet 1995, Topoleski et al. 2000). We investigate the genesis and etiology of this condition further in Chapter 21.

During the physical examination, we look for patella alta by assessing the patellar position relative to the knee. If the length of the patellar tendon is longer than the length of the patella, patella alta is present. In order to relax the hamstrings and isolate quadriceps action to the greatest degree possible, we assess extension lag in the supine position. The difference between maximum passive and active knee extension is then measured and is recorded as the knee-extensor lag. It is also important to assess strength in that position. Most of these children also have contracture of the posterior knee capsule with an associated fixed knee-flexion contracture.

Numerous methods to measure patella alta have been described (Insall and Salvati 1971, Blackburne and Peel 1977, Soejbjerg et al. 1986, Koshino and Sugimoto 1989, Walker et al. 1998, Seil et al. 2000). Of these, the Koshino index is probably the most applicable to children with open epiphyses. In assessing patella alta roentgenographically, we prefer to have the child tension his/her quadriceps and then take a lateral x-ray of the knee in maximum extension. In a normal child the superior pole of the patella will lie at or near the distal femoral physis (Fig. 20.9). When we correct this problem surgically, with the knee in full extension, we again rely on the position of the inferior pole of the patella relative to the joint line and/or the position of the superior pole of the patella relative to the distal femoral growth plate to gauge the appropriateness of our correction (Gage et al. 2002). This will be discussed in greater detail in the next chapter.

FEMORAL DEROTATIONAL OSTEOTOMY

Abduction capacity is markedly diminished by lever-arm dysfunction produced by femoral anteversion. Even with a normal neck-shaft angle, femoral anteversion decreases the abduction moment arm nearly 40% (Arnold et al. 1997). Excessive hip flexion and adverse rotational moments at the knee can also be introduced with femoral anteversion (Delp et

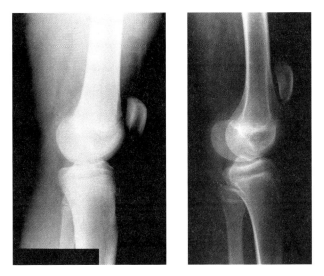

Fig. 20.9. Patella alta. On a normal lateral knee X-ray, the superior pole of the patella lies at or just above the distal femoral physis (left). A child with cerebral palsy typically has patella alta (right). Clinically, this is frequently associated with a knee-extensor (quadriceps) lag and crouch gait. This problem will be discussed in more detail in the next chapter.

al. 1999, Arnold and Delp 2001). When one understands the adverse effects of lever-arm dysfunction on gait (described in Chapter 13), which have been confirmed by modern gait modeling, the importance of correction of femoral torsion becomes apparent.

Because of persistent abnormal motor control and muscle imbalance, the goal at the time of surgery is slight overcorrection of femoral anteversion. In our experience, in diplegia and quadriplegia slight overcorrection never causes adverse effects. In the vast majority of cases, we have been pleased with the results of femoral derotation. However, even when femoral anteversion has been surgically corrected, poor motor control and persistent muscle imbalance can lead to persistent internal hip rotation. Occasionally this can be the cause of postoperative dissatisfaction with the results of femoral derotation. At the time of surgery, our goal is to correct anteversion to between 5° and 10° with maximum internal hip rotation restricted to 20°. In our experience, undercorrection of femoral anteversion leads to persistent internal rotation gait. Typically the amount of overcorrection just described results in proper alignment. In our experience, this has produced good results. It rarely if ever has resulted in excessive external hip rotation positioning in diplegia and quadriplegia. The reader should be aware that despite femoral derotation in hemiplegia, pelvic malrotation due to poor motor control may persist. In hemiplegia, therefore, slight undercorrection of anteversion is preferred to prevent an externally rotated knee and external foot progression.

TIBIAL TORSION

Tibial torsion is notoriously difficult to detect and measure accurately. In our experience, the classic physical exam methods, including thigh-foot angle and bimalleolar axis angle, have relatively high inter- and intra-observer error. This difficulty is compounded by the fact that even relatively small tibial torsions ($\geq 15°$) can have significant adverse effects on proper lever-arm alignment for ankle plantarflexor function (Schwartz and Lakin 2003). Since tibial torsion is a transverse-plane deformity, and transverse-plane rotation is limited at the knee or ankle, the patient is unable to compensate. On the other hand, a child with good underlying motor control can compensate for relatively small degrees of excessive anteversion by externally rotating the hip joint without major adverse consequences on lever-arm position (Arnold et al. 1997). In diplegia and quadriplegia, most tibial torsions are external. Occasionally, a young child will have persistence of infantile internal tibial torsion that can be equally adverse in its effect. In addition, internal malalignment can cause problems with clearance and tripping. Unless it is severe, however, most internal tibial torsions will remodel spontaneously and surgical correction is rarely necessary. External tibial torsion, on the other hand, does not resolve spontaneously, and in fact tends to worsen over time. Therefore surgical correction is usually required.

We have adopted a third physical exam measure for torsion that we refer to as the second-toe test (see Fig. 20.10). The subject in the figure has an external tibial torsion of $20°$. Figure 20.10a shows that at rest (prior to moving the leg of the patient) the foot is externally rotated relative to vertical. In Figure 20.10b, the hip has been internally rotated to direct the second toe perpendicular towards the floor (heel bisector/second metatarsal head line vertical). The thigh is then held rigidly in this position (preventing internal or external hip rotation) as the knee is flexed to $90°$ (Fig. 20.10c). The angular difference between the vertical and the axis of the tibia indicates the degree of tibial torsion (in this case $20°$ off vertical, external). It should be noted that for an individual with internal tibial torsion, external rotation of the hip would be required to bring the second toe vertical. Knee flexion would then result in medial orientation of the tibia (as opposed to lateral orientation as in this case).

At our institution, correction of malrotations of the foot, tibia and femur are done with the child in the prone position. Correction of the foot (usually pes planovalgus deformity) is done first, as tibial torsion is very difficult to assess in the presence of foot deformity. However, once the foot has been corrected, the second-toe test is very accurate, particularly under general anesthesia. Because of the extra confidence gained in the physical exam measurement with this test plus recognition of the fact that even small tibial torsions can adversely affect function, tibial torsions as small as $15°$ are now commonly corrected at our institution. In order to avoid delayed or non-union, in the skeletally mature individual one should be careful to avoid overheating of the tibia while cutting the bone and/or excessive stripping of the periosteum.

HAMSTRING SURGERY

In light of recent information suggesting that there is normal-to-long hamstring functional length in crouch gait, less hamstring-lengthening surgery is done now than in the past (Hoffinger et al. 1993, Delp et al. 1996, Schutte et al. 1997). In addition, rhizotomy has markedly decreased the need for hamstring surgery (Schwartz et al. 2003). It is not uncommon that botulinum toxin injection of the hamstrings is carried out at the time of lower-extremity surgery. In severe cases, botulinum toxin is injected in conjunction with hamstring lengthening

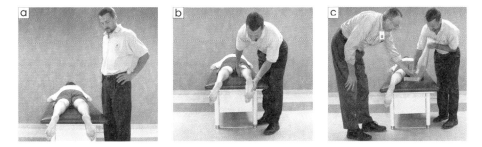

Fig. 20.10. The second-toe test. At rest in the prone position in the case of an external tibial torsion, the foot is externally rotated relative to vertical (a). It is necessary to internally rotate the hip (b) to direct the second toe perpendicular towards the floor (heel bisector/second metatarsal head line vertical). The thigh is then held rigidly in this position (preventing internal or external hip rotation) as the knee is flexed to 90° (c). The angular difference between the vertical and the axis of the tibia indicates the degree of tibial torsion (in this case 20° off vertical, external). This subject has an external tibial torsion of 20°. *See CD-Rom, Figure 20.10, for a dynamic illustration.*

in an effort to minimize the amount of lengthening done and to decrease postoperative pain and spasm. Medial and lateral hamstring lengthening is seldom performed, and proximal hamstring release is never done in an ambulatory patient. The surgeon must keep in mind that the hamstrings function not only as knee-flexors but also as important hip-extensors (Waters et al. 1974). Because anterior pelvic tilt is a common problem, proximal or combined medial and lateral lengthening of the hamstrings, will exacerbate the anterior tilt of the pelvis and the resultant lumbar hyperlordosis may increase lumbar strain.

With increased crouch, the moment arm for the hamstrings becomes longer at the knee and shorter at the hip (see Fig. 12.15 and explanatory text). Because of this, as crouch increases the hamstrings become less efficient as hip-extensors and more efficient as knee-flexors. Therefore crouch tends to lead to more crouch. As such, strategies that might lead to decreased anterior pelvic tilt, for example, intramuscular psoas lengthening or spasticity reduction, may allow the already normal or longer than normal hamstrings to function well without hamstring-lengthening surgery.

In the ambulatory diplegic and quadriplegic patients at our center, medial and lateral hamstring lengthening with posterior capsulotomy has been eliminated from the treatment algorithm for fixed knee-flexion contractures. Distal femoral extension osteotomy is preferred. If this is to be effective, this procedure must be combined with patellar advancement (Gage et al. 2002). In this case, because of the bone-shortening effect of the extension osteotomy, minimal lengthening and/or Botox injection of the hamstrings may be all that is necessary.

On occasion, we see patients referred with "overlengthened hamstrings" and associated genu recurvatum. While this might represent a true overlengthening, it may in fact be more representative of an inappropriate lengthening performed in a patient who had one or more of the following associated problems: (1) equinus contracture, (2) ligamentous laxity, (3) pre-existing anterior pelvic tilt, a condition in which hamstrings are frequently longer than normal (Hoffinger et al. 1993, Delp et al. 1996, Schutte et al. 1997), (4) psoas contracture,

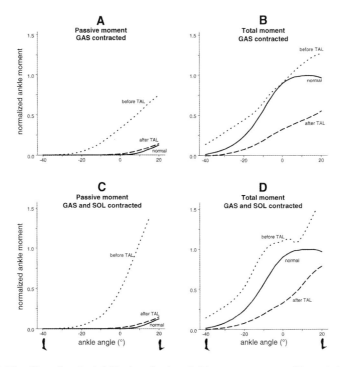

Fig. 20.11. The effect of tendo-Achilles lengthening. Ankle moment versus ankle angle before and after simulated tendo-Achilles lengthening (TAL) with isolated gastrocnemius (GAS) contracture (A, B) and with contracture of both the gastrocnemius and the soleus (SOL) (C, D). After tendo-Achilles lengthening, the passive moment developed by the triceps surae is restored to approximately normal (A, C); however, the total moment is substantially less than normal (B, D). The data suggests that Achilles tendon lengthening should not be used to treat isolated gastrocnemius contracture because doing so may decrease the strength of the plantarflexors greatly (from Delp et al. 1995).

and/or (5) hamstring lengthening that was done without regard to coexistent rectus femoris spasticity. Any or all of these can lead to genu recurvatum and the finding of "overlengthened hamstrings".

GASTROCSOLEUS

Muscle-length models indicate that the soleus is extremely sensitive to lengthening (Delp et al. 1995). It has been shown by these models that a 1 cm lengthening of the soleus will lead to a 50% loss of the force-generating capacity of the muscle (Fig. 20.11). It should be recognized by the orthopaedic surgeon that a lengthening of the tendon distal to the muscle belly of the soleus leads to a more horizontal orientation of the muscle fibers of the bipennate soleus. Contraction of the muscle fibers in their new line of action is inefficient in generating force along the length of the tendon. In addition, muscles with short muscle-fiber lengths are much more sensitive to lengthening than those with long fiber lengths due to the fact that the percentage change in resting muscle-fiber length is much greater. This should lead one to the reasonable conclusion that lengthening of the heel-cord in the ambulatory patient should be avoided, because in almost all cases the pathological shortening occurs in the gastrocnemius alone. This two-joint muscle is much more subject to spasticity than the soleus and because of crouch gait and/or foot deformity, the gastrocnemius cannot be stretched adequately to allow its normal growth during the course of daily functional activities. At our institution, the most common treatment for gastrosoleus contracture is an isolated Strayer recession or Baumann procedure (Strayer 1958, Saraph et al. 2000). Occasionally, it is necessary to obtain some further length of the soleus musculotendinous unit. In that case, typically the soleus fascia is lengthened underneath the reflected gastrocnemius prior to repair of the gastrocnemius fascia to the underlying soleus fascia.

A second option for obtaining greater length of the soleus is a Baker lengthening (Baker 1956). This procedure represents a lengthening of the combined fascias of the gastrocnemius and soleus. It is performed at a higher level than most of the muscle fibers of the soleus and therefore technically should help preserve soleus force-generating capacity better than lengthening of the heelcord itself. The goal of operative intervention is 10° of ankle dorsiflexion under anesthesia with the knee in extension. Botox to the soleus at the time of MLEP in conjunction with postoperative casting, which is necessary in any event, can oftentimes eliminate the need for surgical lengthening of the soleus.

The gastrocnemius and soleus have distinctly different functions during gait. The gastrocnemius muscle is a fast-twitch, precisely timed muscle that is responsible for the coordinated movement of the ankle and knee, particularly in terminal stance and pre-swing. The soleus is a slow-twitch, stance-phase eccentric stabilizer that is primarily responsible for maintaining the integrity of the normal PF/KE couple during mid-stance. The PF/KE couple, which generates an extension moment on the knee during second rocker, provides knee stability in the second half of stance without the need for quadriceps action (see Chapter 4). It also provides about half of the total support needed for upright posture (Winter 1991). Thus it is not surprising that crouch gait is a frequent sequela of heelcord lengthening.

Case studies

PATIENT EXAMPLE NO.1 (Fig. 20.12)
This 10-year-old with spastic diplegic cerebral palsy is an independent community ambulator without the use of assistive devices or orthoses. At 1 year of age, he underwent bilateral tendo-Achilles lengthening and plantar fascia release.

Gait by observation shows toe–toe initial contact bilaterally, worse on the right. There is bilateral knee hyperextension in mid-stance and bilateral internal foot-progression angles.

Physical examination shows mild hip-flexion contractures (5°), bilateral hamstring and rectus femoris contractures, bilateral femoral anteversion (40° right and 50° left), a mild left internal tibial torsion, and bilateral equinus contractures (right greater then left). Motor control is good and strength is rated 3–4/5 in general. Spasticity is felt to be mild at the hips and knees and moderate at the ankle-plantarflexors.

Kinematics of the transverse plane demonstrate excessive bilateral internal hip rotation, worse on the right, but with a more severe internal foot progression angle on the left (Fig. 20.12 a, b). These findings suggest contributions from excessive femoral anteversion bilaterally and internal tibial torsion on the left.

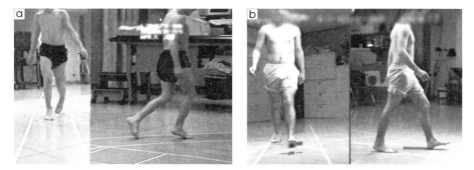

Fig. 20.12. Case study 1. Subject walking in gait laboratory prior to surgery (a) and following treatment, 6 years later (b). Kinematics of the left side (c) and right side (d) on three separate occasions: initial, 1994 (dotted line); 12 months after multiple lower-extremity reconstruction, 1995 (dashed line); and 6 years postoperatively at the end of the adolescent growth spurt, 2000 (solid line). (e, f) Corresponding kinetic data for the right and left sides. *See CD-Rom, Figure 20.12, for a dynamic illustration.*

Sagittal-plane kinematics are consistent with multilevel spasticity/contracture. He has a double-bump pelvic pattern, restriction of hip extension in terminal stance, excessive knee flexion at initial contact, diminished peak swing-phase knee flexion, mild genu recurvatum in mid-stance and equinus bilaterally (worse on the right than the left).

Coronal-plane findings are normal, with the exception of pelvic obliquity (right side elevated) and excessive adduction of the right hip. This is felt to be a compensation for the functional leg-length discrepancy caused by the asymmetric equinus deformity (again, worse on the right).

Sagittal-plane kinetics (Fig. 20.12 c, d) evaluation shows a lack of first rocker, a very abnormal and early ankle moment, lack of power generation for push-off at the ankle, excessive knee-flexion moments bilaterally (left worse than right), which is secondary to excessive PF/KE couples, and prolonged hip-extension moments in stance (hip-extensor dominance pattern). Walking speed is approximately 0.75 times normal.

Oxygen consumption is just outside the normal range (1.51 × normal).

This information suggested that spasticity was not severe enough to consider SDR. Motor control and strength were quite good making this patient a good candidate for rehabilitation following multiple lower-extremity surgery. There were multiple contractures and bone deformities. However, it was felt that the internal tibial torsion was not severe enough to warrant surgical correction. Based on this information, the surgeries included (1) bilateral intertrochanteric femoral derotational osteotomies, (2) bilateral psoas lengthenings at the pelvic brim, (3) bilateral medial hamstring lengthenings, (4) bilateral rectus femoris transfers to the gracilis, (5) bilateral Strayer gastrocnemius recessions, and (6) right soleus fascial striping.

Postoperative analysis was performed 10 months later. Preoperative to postoperative analysis showed correction of internal foot progression angle with normalization of hip rotation (Fig. 20.12 a, b). Anterior pelvic tilt and double bump pattern were improved. Knee extension in preparation for initial contact and at initial contact is improved. Knee hyperextension is resolved with normal knee extension at mid-stance with no evidence of crouch. Timing of

GILLETTE CHILDREN'S MOTION ANALYSIS LABORATORY

Joint Rotation Angles

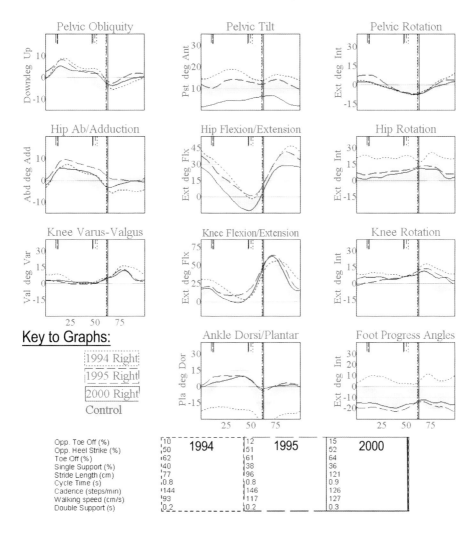

	1994	1995	2000
Opp. Toe Off (%)	10	12	15
Opp. Heel Strike (%)	50	51	52
Toe Off (%)	62	61	64
Single Support (%)	40	38	36
Stride Length (cm)	77	96	121
Cycle Time (s)	0.8	0.8	0.9
Cadence (steps/min)	144	146	126
Walking speed (cm/s)	93	117	127
Double Support (s)	0.2	0.2	0.3

Fig. 20.12, contd. See p.368 for caption

d

GILLETTE CHILDREN'S MOTION ANALYSIS LABORATORY

Joint Rotation Angles

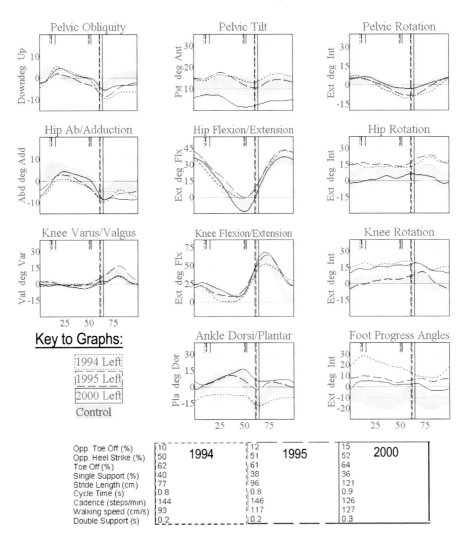

Fig. 20.12, contd. See p.368 for caption

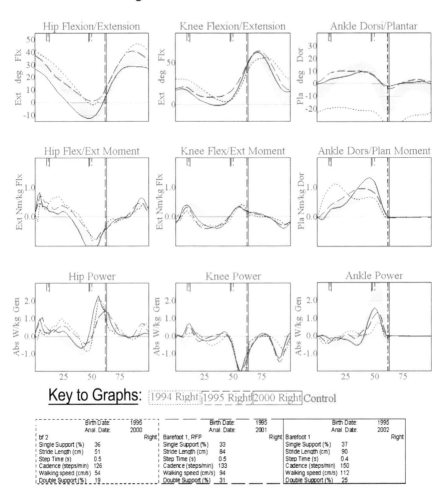

GILLETTE CHILDREN'S MOTION ANALYSIS LABORATORY

Sagittal Plane Moments and Powers

Key to Graphs: 1994 Right | 1995 Right | 2000 Right | Control

	Birth Date:	1995	
	Anal. Date:	2000	Right
bf 2			
Single Support (%)	36		
Stride Length (cm)	51		
Step Time (s)	0.5		
Cadence (steps/min)	126		
Walking speed (cm/s)	54		
Double Support (%)	19		

	Birth Date:	1995	
	Anal. Date:	2001	Right
Barefoot 1, RFP			
Single Support (%)	33		
Stride Length (cm)	84		
Step Time (s)	0.5		
Cadence (steps/min)	133		
Walking speed (cm/s)	94		
Double Support (%)	31		

	Birth Date:	1995	
	Anal. Date:	2002	Right
Barefoot 1			
Single Support (%)	37		
Stride Length (cm)	90		
Step Time (s)	0.4		
Cadence (steps/min)	150		
Walking speed (cm/s)	112		
Double Support (%)	25		

Fig. 20.12, contd. See p.368 for caption

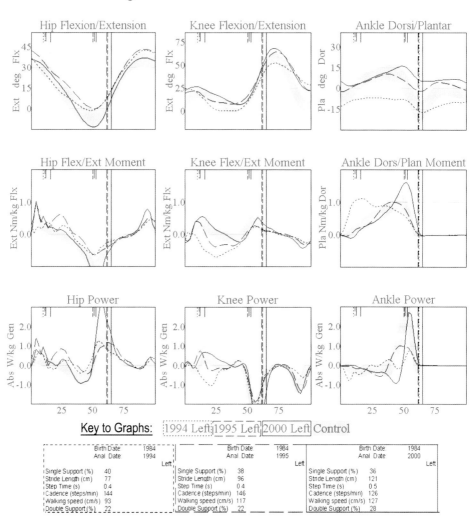

GILLETTE CHILDREN'S MOTION ANALYSIS LABORATORY

Sagittal Plane Moments and Powers

Fig. 20.12, contd. See p.368 for caption

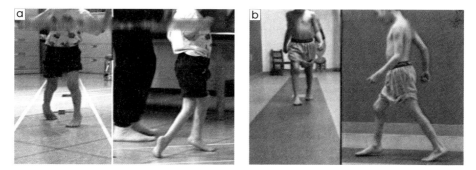

Fig. 20.13. Case study 2. Subject walking in gait laboratory before surgery (a) and after treatment, 2 years later (b). Kinematics of the right side (c) and left side (d) on three separate occasions: initial, 2000 (dotted line); 12 months after SDR, 2001 (dashed line); and 12 months after lower-extremity orthopaedic reconstruction, 2002 (solid line). (e, f) Corresponding kinetic data for the right and left sides for 2001 and 2002. *See CD-Rom, Figure 20.13, for a dynamic illustration.*

peak swing-phase knee flexion and magnitude are both improved due to rectus femoris transfer. The equinus contracture is resolved and pelvic obliquity is improved. Excessive hip adduction in stance remains secondary to persistent abductor weakness. On the left, there is a persistent internal foot-progression angle secondary to unresolved internal tibial torsion. Transverse-plane hip rotation does not appear to be improved, but in retrospect the knee alignment device may have been placed too internally rotated relative to the knee axis as there is an abnormal knee-varus wave in swing phase. Knee motion and equinus are similarly improved on the left side.

Ankle moment is improved bilaterally (Fig. 20.12c, d). The knee-flexion moment in stance on the left is normalized. Power generation at the ankle is maintained/improved. There is a persistence of hip-extensor dominance pattern. Oxygen consumption is now in the normal range (1.22 × normal), although self-selected walking speed for that test is slower than preoperatively. Femoral implants were removed as the femoral osteotomies were well healed.

Six years after surgery, at age 16, the patient was reexamined in the motion analysis laboratory to evaluate the effects of time, growth and therapy. Physical examination shows some hamstring contracture. The internal tibial torsion persists. There is mild gastrocnemius tightness.

Kinematics are in the normal range in the sagittal plane (Fig. 20.12 a, b). In particular, hip extension is normal in terminal stance, knee modulation is normal, there is no equinus, and hindfoot initial contact is normal. The internal foot-progression angle is persistent on the left as the internal tibial torsion has not resolved. Hip rotations are normal. Hip-abductor weakness is no longer evident either by kinematics or kinetics (typically these findings do improve following plate removal). The hip, knee and ankle moments are in the normal range (Fig. 20.12 c, d). Hip-flexor power-production at toe-off is increased, and ankle-plantarflexor power production is normal. This assessment shows no losses with growth despite having gone through the adolescent growth spurt (significant, because the natural history of untreated cerebral palsy is typically characterized by worsening). Oxygen consumption remains in the

373

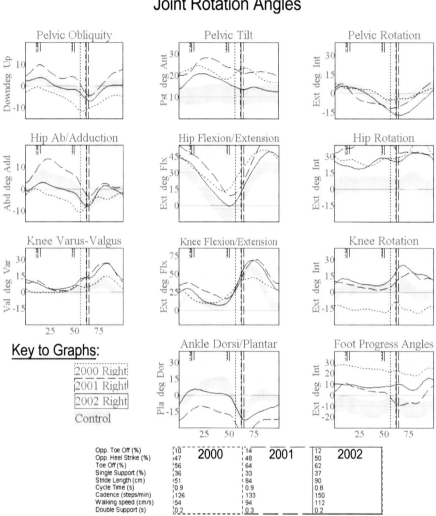

Fig. 20.13, contd. See p.373 for caption

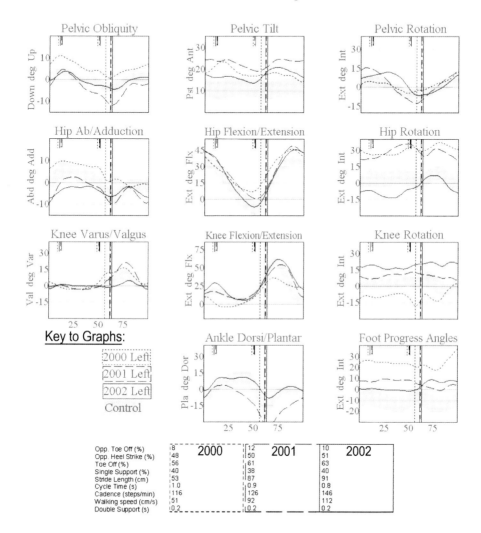

GILLETTE CHILDREN'S MOTION ANALYSIS LABORATORY

Joint Rotation Angles

Fig. 20.13, contd. See p.373 for caption

375

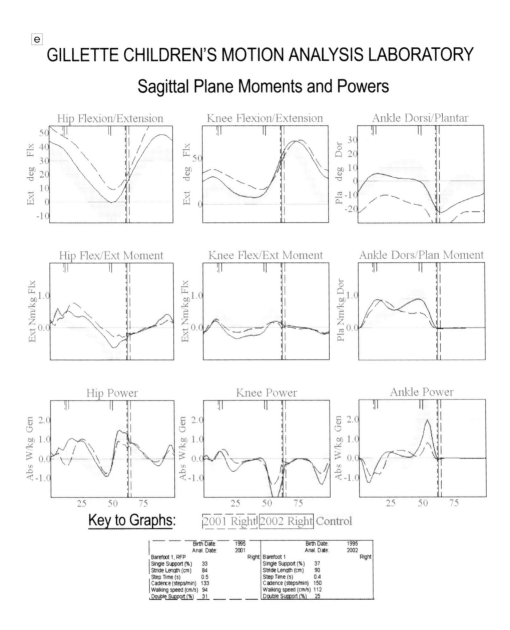

Fig. 20.13, contd. See p.373 for caption

GILLETTE CHILDREN'S MOTION ANALYSIS LABORATORY

Sagittal Plane Moments and Powers

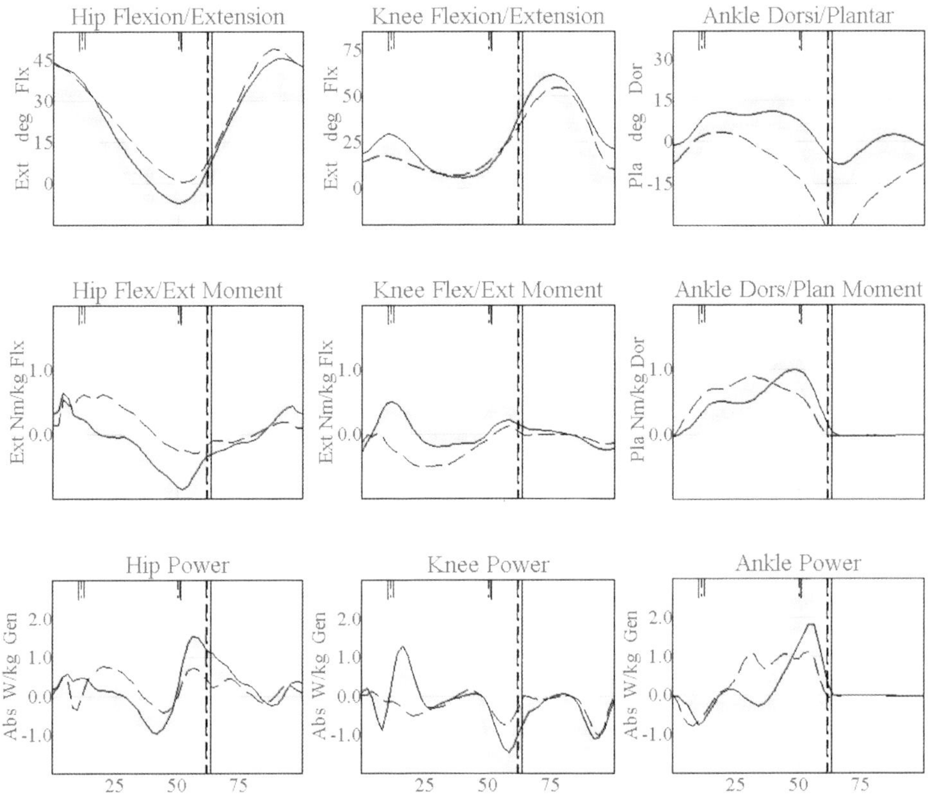

Hip Flexion/Extension
Ext deg Flx
45
30
15
0

Knee Flexion/Extension
Ext deg Flx
75
50
25
0

Ankle Dorsi/Plantar
Pla deg Dor
30
15
0
-15

Hip Flex/Ext Moment
Ext Nm/kg Flx
1.0
0.0

Knee Flex/Ext Moment
Ext Nm/kg Flx
1.0
0.0

Ankle Dors/Plan Moment
Pla Nm/kg Dor
1.0
0.0

Hip Power
Abs W/kg Gen
2.0
1.0
0.0
-1.0

Knee Power
Abs W/kg Gen
2.0
1.0
0.0
-1.0

Ankle Power
Abs W/kg Gen
2.0
1.0
0.0
-1.0

25   50   75   25   50   75   25   50   75

Key to Graphs: 2001 Left 2002 Left Control

	Birth Date:	1995		Birth Date:	1995
	Anal. Date:	2001		Anal. Date:	2002
		Left			Left
Single Support (%)	38		Single Support (%)	40	
Stride Length (cm)	87		Stride Length (cm)	91	
Step Time (s)	0.5		Step Time (s)	0.4	
Cadence (steps/min)	126		Cadence (steps/min)	146	
Walking speed (cm/s)	92		Walking speed (cm/s)	112	
Double Support (%)	22		Double Support (%)	22	

Fig. 20.13, contd. See p.373 for caption

normal range at a normal walking speed. Functionally, he is doing well (see Chapter 23).

PATIENT EXAMPLE NO. 2 (Fig. 20.13)

This 4½-year-old boy with diplegic cerebral palsy is a limited community ambulator with bilateral hinged AFOs. He was born 6 weeks before full term. Postnatal course included a three-week stay in the neonatal intensive-care unit, 1 day of ventilator assistance, apnea and jaundice. His birthweight was 4 lb 10 oz. He started walking at 15 months of age, on his toes. He uses a wheelchair for community distances and has ongoing physical therapy. He has had previous Botox injections to the hamstrings and gastrocnemius muscles.

Physical examination revealed bilateral excessive femoral anteversion and left pes valgus. There was multilevel spasticity including the hip-flexors and adductors, hamstrings, rectus femoris, and gastrocnemius bilaterally. Selective motor control and strength were felt to be acceptable to consider rhizotomy. Spasticity is rated moderate.

Kinematics (Fig. 20.13 a, b) showed bilateral severe internal foot-progression angles secondary to femoral anteversion (hip rotation severely internal). Sagittal-plane findings were consistent with multilevel spasticity with severe equinus, stiff knees, excessive hip flexion, and anterior pelvic tilt. Coronal-plane findings could be explained (as in the previous case) on the basis of functional leg-length discrepancy with a stiff hyperextended left knee and a flexed right knee.

It was not possible to collect force-plate data due to short step-lengths and clearance problems. EMG findings showed multilevel spasticity with co-contraction. However, even though the EMG signals were prolonged, there were some definite "off" times.

Oxygen consumption was 1.5 × normal at a slower than normal walking speed.

As a result of this assessment, it was felt that the patient was a good candidate for a SDR. A 42% right and 38% left rhizotomy was done. Evaluation 11 months post-surgery showed decreased spasticity, persistent equinus, persistent severe excessive femoral anteversion and pes valgus foot deformity.

Kinematics show persistent internal foot-progression angles with severe excessive internal hip rotation (Fig. 20.13 a, b). Sagittal-plane findings show improved hip extension, improved swing-phase knee flexion and improved equinus as a result of spasticity reduction. However, there is persistent equinus with a drop foot in swing phase. There is persistent crouch on the right with excessive knee flexion in stance, and there is significant anterior pelvic tilt. Walking-speed is significantly improved from less then 0.5 × normal prior to treatment to approximately 0.75 × normal after rhizotomy. Energy assessment shows improved walking speed with no change in oxygen consumption.

To correct lever arm dysfunction and residual contractures, the patient underwent (1) bilateral intertrochanteric femoral derotational osteotomies, (2) bilateral os calcis lengthenings, (3) bilateral triceps surae recessions, (4) bilateral medial hamstring Botox injections, and (5) right triceps surae Botox injection

Ten months later, assessment showed persistent internal hip rotation (Fig. 20.13 a, b) (although this may be because of incorrect marker placement due to abnormal knee varus in swing phase on the right). Anterior pelvic tilt, hip extension and intoeing are all improved bilaterally attributable to the correction of lever arm deformity via derotational femoral osteotomies. The knees are now nearly symmetric with resolution of crouch on the right and hyperextension on the left. Equinus is significantly improved. Self-selected walking-speed is now normal.

Oxygen consumption is measured as increased, although walking speed is also faster. Full assessment of his outcome will be presented in Chapter 23.

REFERENCES

Arnold AS, Delp SL. (2001) Rotational moment arms of the medial hamstrings and adductors vary with femoral geometry and limb position: implications for the treatment of internally rotated gait. *J Biomech* **34:** 437–447.

Arnold AS, Komattu AV, Delp SL. (1997) Internal rotation gait: a compensatory mechanism to restore abduction capacity decreased by bone deformity. *Dev Med Child Neurol* **39:** 40–44.

Baker LD. (1956) A rational approach to the surgical needs of the cerebral palsy patient. *J Bone Joint Surg Am* **38:** 313–323.

Barwood S, Baillieu C, Boyd R, Brereton K, Low J, Nattrass G, Graham HK. (2000) Analgesic effects of botulinum toxin A: a randomized, placebo-controlled clinical trial. *Dev Med Child Neurol* **42:** 116–121.

Blackburne JS, Peel TE. (1977) A new method of measuring patellar height. *J Bone Joint Surg Br* **59:** 241–242.

Bleck EE. (1971) Postural and gait abnormalities caused by hip-flexion deformity in spastic cerebral palsy. Treatment by iliopsoas recession. *J Bone Joint Surg Am* **53:** 1468–1488.

Bleck EE. (1987) *Orthopaedic Management in Cerebral Palsy*. London: Mac Keith Press. p 142–143.

Bottos M, Feliciangeli A, Sciuto L, Gericke C, Vianello A. (2001) Functional status of adults with cerebral palsy and implications for treatment of children. *Dev Med Child Neurol* **43:** 516–528.

Davids JR, Valadie AL, Ferguson RL, Bray EW 3rd, Allen BL Jr. (1997) Surgical management of ankle valgus in children: use of a transphyseal medial malleolar screw. *J Pediatr Orthop* **17:** 3–8.

Delp SL, Statler K, Carroll NC. (1995) Preserving plantar flexion strength after surgical treatment for contracture of the triceps surae: a computer simulation study. *J Orthop Res* **13:** 96–104.

Delp SL, Arnold AS, Speers RA, Moore CA. (1996) Hamstrings and psoas lengths during normal and crouch gait: implications for muscle-tendon surgery. *J Orthop Res* **14:** 144–151.

Delp SL, Hess WE, Hungerford DS, Jones LC. (1999) Variation of rotation moment arms with hip flexion. *J Biomech* **32:** 493–501.

Dennyson WG, Fulford GE. (1976) Subtalar arthrodesis by cancellous grafts and metallic internal fixation. *J Bone Joint Surg Br* **58:** 507–510.

Evans D. (1975) Calcaneo-valgus deformity. *J Bone Joint Surg Br* **57:** 270-278.

Feldkamp M (1990) Patella fragmentation in cerebral palsy. *Z Orthop Ihre Grenzgeb* **128:** 160–164. (German.)

Gage JR. (1990) Surgical treatment of knee dysfunction in cerebral palsy. *Clin Orthop* 45–54.

Gage JR. (2003) Editorial. Con: interobserver variability of gait analysis. *J Pediatr Orthop* **23:** 290–291.

Gage JR, Novacheck TF. (2001) An update on the treatment of gait problems in cerebral palsy. *J Pediatr Orthop B* **10:** 265–274.

Gage JR, Perry J, Hicks RR, Koop S, Werntz JR. (1987) Rectus femoris transfer to improve knee function of children with cerebral palsy. *Dev Med Child Neurol* **29:** 159–166.

Gage JR, Stout JL, Novacheck TF, Matsuo K. (2002) *Distal femoral extension osteotomy for treatment of persistent crouch gait*. Paper presented at meeting of the European Pediatric Orthopaedic Society.

Hoffinger SA, Rab GT, Abou-Ghaida H. (1993) Hamstrings in cerebral palsy crouch gait. *J Pediatr Orthop* **13:** 722–726.

Insall J, Salvati E. (1971) Patella position in the normal knee joint. *Radiology* **101:** 101–104.

Insall J, Goldberg V, Salvati E. (1972) Recurrent dislocation and the high-riding patella. *Clin Orthop* **88:** 67–69.

Kaye JJ, Freiberger RH. (1971) Fragmentation of the lower pole of the patella in spastic lower extremities. *Radiology* **101:** 97–100.

Koshino T, Sugimoto K. (1989) New measurement of patellar height in the knees of children using the epiphyseal line midpoint. *J Pediatr Orthop* **9:** 216–218.

Lloyd-Roberts GC, Jackson AM, Albert JS. (1985) Avulsion of the distal pole of the patella in cerebral palsy. A cause of deteriorating gait. *J Bone Joint Surg Br* **67:** 252–254.

Lotman DB. (1976) Knee flexion deformity and patella alta in spastic cerebral palsy. *Dev Med Child Neurol* **18:** 315–319.

McMulkin M, Barr KM, Ferguson R, Caskey P, Baird G. (2001) Outcomes of extensive rectus femoris release surgeries compared to transfers. *Gait Posture* **13:** 251. (Abstract.)

Mosca VS. (1995) Calcaneal lengthening for valgus deformity of the hindfoot. Results in children who had severe, symptomatic flatfoot and skewfoot. *J Bone Joint Surg Am* **77:** 500–512.

Mosca VS. (1996) Flexible flatfoot and skewfoot. *Instr Course Lect* **45:** 347–354.

Mosca VS. (1998) The child's foot: principles of management. *J Pediatr Orthop* **18:** 281–282.

Murphy KP, Molnar GE, Lankasky K. (1995) Medical and functional status of adults with cerebral palsy. *Dev Med Child Neurol* **37:** 1075–1084.

Noonan KJ, Halliday S, Browne R, O'Brien S, Kayes K, Feinberg J. (2003) Interobserver variability of gait analysis in patients with cerebral palsy. *J Pediatr Orthop* **23:** 279–287.

Novacheck TF. (1996) Surgical intervention in ambulatory cerebral palsy. In: Harris GF, Smith PA, editors. *Human Motion Analysis: Current Applications and Future Directions*. Piscataway, NJ: IEEE Press. p 231–254.

Novacheck TF, Trost JP, Schwartz MH. (2002) Intramuscular psoas lengthening improves dynamic hip function in children with cerebral palsy. *J Pediatr Orthop* **22:** 158–164.

Oeffinger DJ, Pectol RW Jr, Tylkowski CM. (2000) Foot pressure and radiographic outcome measures of lateral column lengthening for pes planovalgus deformity. *Gait Posture* **12:** 189–195.

Perry J. (1987) Distal rectus femoris transfer. *Dev Med Child Neurol* **29:** 153–158.

Pietu G, Hauet P. (1995) Stress fracture of the patella. *Acta Orthop Scand* **66:** 481–482.

Rosenthal RK, Levine DB. (1977) Fragmentation of the distal pole of the patella in spastic cerebral palsy. *J Bone Joint Surg Am* **59:** 934–939.

Saraph V, Zwick EB, Uitz C, Linhart W, Steinwender G. (2000) The Baumann procedure for fixed contracture of the gastrosoleus in cerebral palsy. Evaluation of function of the ankle after multilevel surgery. *J Bone Joint Surg Br* **82:** 535–540.

Schmidt DJ, Arnold AS, Carroll NC, Delp SL. (1999) Length changes of the hamstrings and adductors resulting from derotational osteotomies of the femur. *J Orthop Res* **17:** 279–285.

Schutte LM, Hayden SW, Gage JR. (1997) Lengths of hamstrings and psoas muscles during crouch gait: effects of femoral anteversion. *J Orthop Res* **15:** 615–621.

Schwartz M, Lakin G. (2003) The effect of tibial torsion on the dynamic function of the soleus during gait. *Gait Posture* **17:** 113–118.

Schwartz M, Novacheck T, Trost J. (2000) A tool for quantifying hip flexor function during gait. *Gait Posture* **12:** 122–127.

Schwartz MH, Viehweger E, Stout J, Novacheck T, Gage JR. (2003) Comprehensive treatment of ambulatory children with cerebral palsy: an outcome assessment. *J Pediatr Orthop*, in press.

Seil R, Muller B, Georg T, Kohn D, Rupp S. (2000) Reliability and interobserver variability in radiological patellar height ratios. *Knee Surg Sports Traumatol Arthrosc* **8:** 231–236.

Skaggs DL, Kaminsky CK, Eskander-Rickards E, Reynolds RA, Tolo VT, Bassett GS. (1997) Psoas over the brim lengthenings. Anatomic investigation and surgical technique. *Clin Orthop* 174–179.

Skaggs DL, Rethlefsen SA, Kay RM, Dennis SW, Reynolds RA, Tolo VT. (2000) Variability in gait analysis interpretation. *J Pediatr Orthop* **20:** 759–764.

Soejbjerg JO, Hvid I, Dalgaard E. (1986) The vertical position of the patella estimated by four radiographic measurements. *Eur J Radiol* **6:** 244–247.

Strayer LMJ. (1958) Gastrocnemius recession; five-year report of cases. *J Bone Joint Surg Am* **40:** 1019–1030.

Sutherland DH, Santi M, Abel MF. (1990) Treatment of stiff-knee gait in cerebral palsy: a comparison by gait analysis of distal rectus femoris transfer versus proximal rectus release. *J Pediatr Orthop* **10:** 433–441.

Sutherland DH, Zilberfarb JL, Kaufman KR, Wyatt MP, Chambers HG. (1997) Psoas release at the pelvic brim in ambulatory patients with cerebral palsy: operative technique and functional outcome. *J Pediatr Orthop* **17:** 563–570.

Sutherland DH, Kaufman KR, Wyatt MP, Chambers HG, Mubarak SJ. (1999) Double-blind study of botulinum A toxin injections into the gastrocnemius muscle in patients with cerebral palsy. *Gait Posture* **10:** 1–9.

Thompson NS, Baker RJ, Cosgrove AP, Corry IS, Graham HK. (1998) Musculoskeletal modelling in determining the effect of botulinum toxin on the hamstrings of patients with crouch gait. *Dev Med Child Neurol* **40:** 622–625.

Topoleski TA, Kurtz CA, Grogan DP. (2000) Radiographic abnormalities and clinical symptoms associated with patella alta in ambulatory children with cerebral palsy. *J Pediatr Orthop* **20:** 636–639.

Villani C, Billi A, Morico GF, Bonsignore D. (1988) A comparative study of the extensor force of the quadriceps between subjects with a normal patella and those with patella alta of neurological pathogenesis. *Ital J Orthop Traumatol* **14:** 401–406.

Walker P, Harris I, Leicester A. (1998) Patellar tendon-to-patella ratio in children. *J Pediatr Orthop* **18:** 129–131.

Waters RL, Perry J, McDaniels JM, House K. (1974) The relative strength of the hamstrings during hip extension. *J Bone Joint Surg Am* **56:** 1592–1597.

Winter DA. (1991) *The Biomechanics and Motor Control of Human Gait: Normal, Elderly, and Pathological*, 2nd edn. Waterloo, Ontario: University of Waterloo Press. p 75–85.

Zurcher AW, Molenaers G, Desloovere K, Fabry G. (2001) Kinematic and kinetic evaluation of the ankle after intramuscular injection of botulinum toxin A in children with cerebral palsy. *Acta Orthop Belg* **67:** 475–480.

21
TREATMENT PRINCIPLES FOR CROUCH GAIT

James R. Gage

In order to treat crouch gait intelligently, we must clarify what we know about the condition. Previous chapters have shown that during normal locomotion the skeleton provides the levers required for movement, muscles provide the power, and the joints serve as hinges. We also know that normal upright posture and locomotion depend upon adequate forces acting via rigid levers of appropriate length on stable joints.

There are three principal muscle groups that maintain erect posture (Õunpuu et al. 1991, Winter 1991) (Fig. 21.1): (1) hip-extensors, (2) vasti, and (3) the soleus. Hip-extensors (gluteus maximus and hamstrings) act during the first third of stance phase, and are thought to generate about 20%–30% of the force necessary to maintain erect posture. The vasti also act during the first third of stance phase, and are thought to generate about 20%–30% of the force necessary to maintain erect posture. The lowly soleus, meanwhile, produces about 40%–50% of the force needed to maintain erect stance. It accomplishes this by using the moment arm of the forefoot to harness the ground reaction force (GRF) such that it exerts a large extension moment on the knee, the so-called *plantarflexion/knee-extension* couple (see pages 63–4). This eliminates the need for action by other muscles that extend the hip and knee.

We should also bear in mind that biarticular muscles such as the rectus femoris do not provide much antigravity support, but rather function as energy transfer straps to move kinetic energy from one body segment to another.

As we saw in Chapter 12, a child with cerebral palsy has primary problems that relate directly to the neurological injury. These include abnormal tone, poor distal selective motor control and difficulty with balance. These primary problems produce abnormal growth forces, which in turn give rise to the secondary problems that occur during the years of growth. These primary and secondary abnormalities of gait act in concert to interfere with upright posture and locomotion. Chapter 12 also explained how the secondary abnormalities include abnormal muscle growth (disproportionate muscle lengths between agonists and antagonists) and lever-arm dysfunction or LAD (bony deformities of the hip and foot plus long-bone torsions). Disproportionate agonist and antagonist muscle lengths implies that some muscle groups are contracted (too short) whereas others are too long. For example, the adolescent child with spastic diplegia and crouch gait typically presents with LAD (usually a combination of femoral anteversion, external tibial torsion and pes valgus) plus abnormal muscle lengths. With respect to the muscles, the soleus, vasti and gluteus maximus are generally too long, whereas the gastrocnemius and hip-flexors are too short. The relative lengths of the

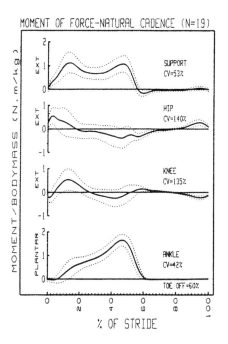

MOMENT OF FORCE–NATURAL CADENCE (N=19)

SUPPORT
CV=53%

HIP
CV=140%

KNEE
CV=135%

ANKLE
CV=42%

TOE OFF=60%

% OF STRIDE

Fig. 21.1. Winter's support moment. The algebraic summation of the sagittal-plane moments about the ankle, knee and hip is referred to by Winter (1991) as the "support moment". Winter points out that the ankle provides a fairly constant extension moment, which is roughly 50% of the total necessary for erect posture. The vasti and hip-extensors supply the remainder of the necessary support, but with a large variance in contribution between the two joints from stride to stride and at different speeds.

hamstrings and rectus femoris, however, are variable and depend a great deal on the pelvic position. As such, they may be long, short or of appropriate length (Hoffinger et al. 1993, Delp et al. 1996, Schutte et al. 1997, Arnold 1999, Arnold et al. 2001, Thompson et al. 2001).

In Chapter 12, we defined LAD as a condition in which internal and/or external lever arms become distorted due to bony or positional deformities. We then discussed five distinct types of LAD: (1) short lever arm, (2) flexible lever arm, (3) malrotated lever arm, (4) abnormal fulcrum or action-point, and (5) positional LAD. Since all five types of LAD and their sequelae occur in crouch gait, if the principles of LAD do not readily come to mind, it would be a good idea to go back to Chapter 12 now and spend a few minutes reviewing these concepts.

The child known as C.D. (Fig. 21.2) provides a beautiful demonstration of the natural history of LAD. At about 4 years of age she had a selective dorsal rhizotomy, which was the appropriate and correct procedure to do at the time. Serial videos taken over the next several years initially showed improvement. However, 2–3 years following rhizotomy a crouch-gait pattern was evident. This progressed steadily over the next few years. Finally the crouch-gait pattern became so severe that she developed bilateral patellar stress-fractures with resultant knee pain that made walking impossible.

Elements of crouch gait

If we study this case and others like it, the elements of crouch gait quickly become apparent. For example, crouch gait usually occurs during the adolescent growth spurt. In addition, the precipitating factors almost always include LAD and/or previous weakening of the soleus. Soleus weakening is usually iatrogenic and comes about either by means of a tendo-

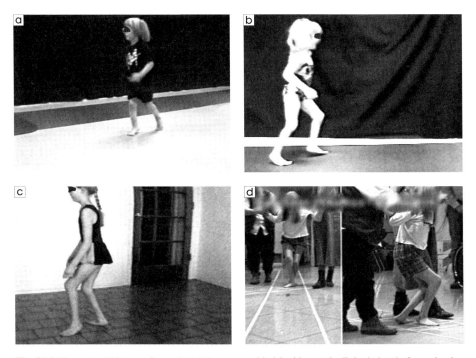

Fig. 21.2. The natural history of crouch. (a) Four-year-old girl with spastic diplegia just before selective dorsal rhizotomy (SDR). (b) The same child 1 year after SDR. Her gait has improved significantly. (c) Five years after SDR, at age 9, there is a noticeable increase in LAD (femoral anteversion, tibial torsion and pes valgus) as well as progression of crouch gait. (d) At age 11, nearly 7 years after SDR, her crouch has progressed to the point that she now has bilateral patellar stress fractures and pain, and can no longer walk without assistance. *See CD-Rom, Figure 21.2, for a dynamic illustration.*

Achilles lengthening and/or a selective dorsal rhizotomy, particularly one in which a fair number of dorsal rootlets were sectioned at the S1 and S2 levels. Because soleus weakening and/or LAD both act to diminish the internal moment that restrains forward motion of the tibia, the ankle dorsiflexes excessively during second rocker. This allows the GRF to move behind the knee so that instead of exerting an extension force, it now exerts a flexion force on the knee. In other words, the PF/KE couple no longer exists (Fig. 21.3). Kinetics of the knee verifies what is occurring in crouch gait (Fig. 21.4). An individual who is walking in crouch always will demonstrate a continuous knee-extensor moment throughout stance phase. By definition, this means that in order to prevent the knee from collapsing into flexion, the quadriceps must act continuously throughout stance phase and the PF/KE couple, which normally maintains knee extension during the second half of stance, is absent.

Because of the "law of magnitude", the adolescent growth spurt is an important contributor to crouch. To refresh your memory regarding the law of magnitude, return to Figure 4.5 and the text that describes it. Basically, the law of magnitude states that as we grow our strength increases in proportion to the cross-sectional area of our muscles (πR^2), but since weight or mass represents volume, it increases by the cube (R^3). The implication

384

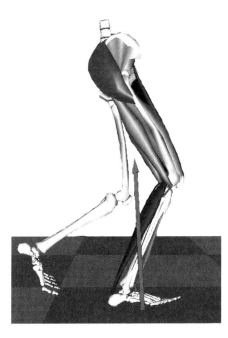

Fig. 21.3. In normal gait, the GRF is in front of the knee during mid-stance and so provides a strong extension force. In crouch gait, however, the GRF falls behind the knee and generates a flexion force at both the hip and knee. Consequently the hip- and knee-extensors must be active continuously to prevent these joints from collapsing into flexion.

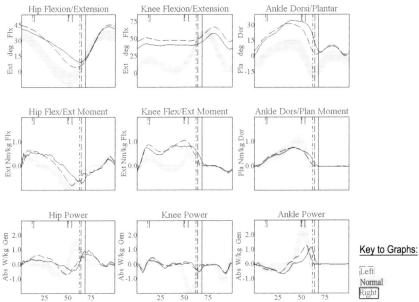

Fig. 21.4. Sagittal-plane kinetics of a patient with crouch gait. Normal values ± 1 S.D. are included for comparison. Note that there is a continuous extension moment at the knee throughout stance (middle graph of middle column), which indicates that the quadriceps must remain active to prevent the knee from collapsing. In addition, notice the "late cross-over" on the hip moment graph and the large hip-extension power that is required until the point of the moment cross-over to prevent collapse of the hip into flexion.

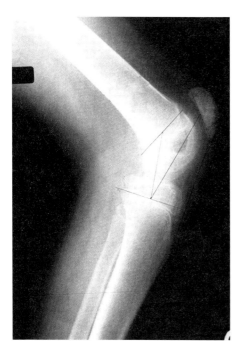

Fig. 21.5. A lateral X-ray of the child's knee shown in Figure 21.2 at the time she presented to Gillette Children's Specialty Healthcare. Note the stress fracture in the inferior pole of the patella. Stress fracture of the patella is an extremely common finding in crouch gait and will usually cause enough pain to severely limit walking.

of this is that our strength to mass ratio declines in inverse proportion to the rate of growth. A child who has lost the PF/KE couple will have lost about half of the force required to maintain erect posture. What is worse, however, is that once the GRF moves behind the knee it actually contributes to the flexion moments at the knee and hip. At that point it has, so to speak, "joined the enemy" as an active contributor to crouch. Prior to the adolescent growth spurt, the power-to-mass ratio is large enough that s/he can still maintain erect posture using only the hip- and knee-extensors. However as the adolescent growth spurt begins, body mass increases much more rapidly than muscle power and the ratio of power to mass falls precipitously. Consequently, the hip- and knee-extensors, acting alone without the benefit of the PF/KE couple, soon become inadequate to prevent crouch. Once this threshold is crossed, crouch gait increases rapidly as does the strain on the patellar mechanism. Over time, the stress on the patellar mechanism causes excessive elongation of the patellar tendon with resultant patellar alta in virtually all cases. In our experience with children with crouch gait, this will eventually lead to failure of the patellar mechanism with resultant fracture of either of patella itself or the tibial tubercle to which it attaches in about half the cases (Fig. 21.5) (Gage et al. 2002). The incidence may well be higher, however; Topoleski et al. (2000) noted an overall incidence of radiographic abnormalities within either the patella or the proximal tibia in 21% (41 knees) of the 193 affected knees in 117 randomly selected, skeletally immature, ambulatory children with spastic cerebral palsy. Stress fracture of the patella, when it occurs, is characteristically in the distal pole of the patella, since that is where the forces are highest (Rosenthal and Levine 1977, Villani et al. 1988, Lengsfeld et al. 1990).

Problems associated with contracture of the knee joint

In stance the reduction of extension joint moments produced by the LAD plus the elongated soleus, vasti and gluteus maximus muscles, allow the ankle to dorsiflex excessively and the hip and knee to drop into flexion. The GRF, which is now posterior to the knee, plus the abnormal action of the biarticular hamstrings, rectus femoris and gastrocnemius, all act to increase the flexion moments at the hip, knee and ankle. If hip and knee flexion are to be prevented, the gluteus maximus and hamstrings must act as hip-extensors and the three vasti as knee-extensors throughout stance. Unfortunately, the moment arm of the hamstrings at the knee increases in direct proportion to knee flexion, such that the hamstrings now become more powerful knee-flexors than hip-extensors (see the section on positional LAD in Chapter 12). Recall too that the gastrocnemius crosses both the knee and the ankle. Nevertheless, as long as the PF/KE couple maintains knee stability in terminal stance, the gastrocnemius acts only as an ankle-plantarflexor. Regrettably, however, the knee is now in flexion and PF/KE couple is gone, so the gastrocnemius, which crosses both the knee and the ankle, now acts primarily as a knee-flexor during its time of peak activity in terminal stance. Finally, the demand for an adequate extensor force to prevent collapse at the knee requires that the rectus femoris be recruited as an accessory knee-extensor in stance (a role it never plays in normal gait). Sadly, since it takes its origin from the pelvis, it will act as a hip-flexor as well.

The result of all of this is that the muscle-extensor moments, which are acting exclusively at the hip and knee, may increase by several orders of magnitude. Furthermore, whereas the extensor moments at both of these joints normally act only during the first half of stance phase, they are now obliged to work throughout the entire period of stance. The end result is excessive energy consumption, great inefficiency of gait, and excessive stress and strain on the joints themselves. Patella alta and failure of the patellar mechanism have already been discussed. However, long-term patellar femoral arthritis usually occurs as well (Bleck 1987).

Treatment of crouch gait

Now that we have a good picture of how crouch gait occurs, and the long- and short-term problems produced by it, we can set about fixing the problem. Since this is a condition that will produce chronic pain and eventually take most affected individuals off their feet entirely, it should be obvious to the reader that it is worth the significant effort and morbidity that are required to correct the condition. In principle, crouch gait is fairly easy to correct. In the simplest terms we must restore the extension moments and weaken the flexion moments. In order to accomplish the former, we must reestablish the PF/KE couple. In addition, the simple act of bringing the individual up into a more erect posture will do much to reduce the flexion forces on the hip, knee and ankle. To accomplish this, we merely have to (1) correct LAD, (2) lengthen muscles that are contracted, (3) correct fixed joint-flexion contractures (usually only the knee), (4) shorten muscles that are excessively long, and (5) deal appropriately with the affected biarticular muscles. With respect to the latter point, I mean that we may need to come up with some other strategies to correct the problems of the confounded biarticular muscles, particularly the rectus femoris and perhaps the hamstrings.

(I use the term "confounded" to mean bewildered or confused, as the affected biarticular muscles have lost their normal function and been recruited to a different task.)

In devising a specific treatment protocol, it would clearly be best not to let the condition occur in the first place. In order to prevent this tragedy from happening, May I suggest the following. (1) Do your best to *never* lengthen a heel-cord in a child with spastic diplegia or quadriplegia. At the time of surgery, a simple Silfverskiöld test (see Chapter 5) done under anesthesia will confirm that the soleus is almost always of normal length or longer. A simple Strayer or Baumann procedure is usually all that is required (Strayer 1958, Baumann and Koch 1989, Saraph et al. 2000). (2) If a selective dorsal rhizotomy is done, avoid excessive sectioning of rootlets at the S1–S2 levels (Buckon et al. 2002). (3) Correct all LAD (femoral anteversion, tibial torsion, foot deformities, and/or hip subluxation) prior to the onset of the adolescent growth spurt. (4) If crouch gait is occurring despite these measures, use Saltiel-type floor-reaction AFOs (see Chapter 17) to prevent excessive growth lengthening/weakening of the soleus.

Unfortunately I have seldom been in the position of being able to prevent crouch, since by the time many of my patients are referred to me, in the midst of the adolescent growth spurt, crouch is already firmly established. In many cases heel-cord lengthening or selective dorsal rhizotomy was done many years previously, often with a good initial result. Subsequently, however, the child insidiously started to go down into crouch: slowly at first, but then rapidly once the growth spurt began (see Fig. 21.2).

If the child still has enough growth remaining (Fig. 21.6), we can do the following. (1) Correct all LAD (femoral anteversion, tibial torsion, foot deformities, and/or hip subluxation). (2) Lengthen muscles that are contracted. The biarticular muscles are a problem here, because depending upon the pelvic position the psoas or hamstrings may be of normal length or contracted. In fact, as noted previously, in crouch gait the hamstrings may actually be long (Hoffinger et al. 1993, Delp et al. 1996, Schutte et al. 1997). Because of this, as part of our gait analysis, we have developed a special software program that prints out a comparison of the lengths of the child's hamstrings and psoas to a normal range (Figs 20.5, 20.6). (3) Fixed joint contractures, if present, must be corrected. (4) Following recovery from surgery, use bilateral floor-reaction AFOs to maintain erect posture. The floor-reaction AFOs are required to restore the PF/KE couple and to keep the child erect until such time as the soleus recovers its strength. Muscle growth is driven by stretch (see Chapter 12). If the patient is maintained in an erect posture, the soleus will not be stretched and so will not grow significantly in length. Meanwhile, growth of the long bones will "take up the slack" and re-tension the muscles that were excessively long (soleus, vasti and gluteus maximus). (5) Deal appropriately with the affected biarticular muscles.

The principles upon which the surgery was based are listed above. The specific surgeries that were done are listed in the figure captions. The outcome is demonstrated on the CD-Rom (Fig. 21.6).

In assessing what can be done for an individual with severe crouch who presents herself for treatment after the conclusion of the adolescent growth spurt (Fig. 21.7), we must refer back to our original treatment list: (1) correct the LAD, (2) lengthen muscles that are contracted, (3) correct fixed joint-flexion contractures (usually only the knee), (4) shorten

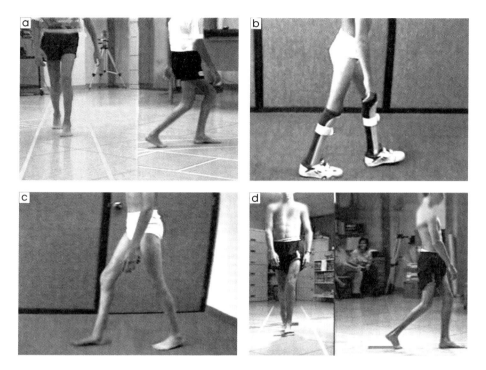

Fig. 21.6. Correction of crouch prior to adolescence. (a) Nine-year-old boy with severe crouch and stiff-knee gait. His only previous surgery was a tendo-Achilles lengthening at 4 years of age. This boy provides an excellent demonstration as to why soleus lengthening should not be done in spastic diplegia. (b) The same child at 10 years of age, 6 months following multiple lower-extremity surgery (MLEP), which consisted of bilateral femoral and right tibial osteotomies plus bilateral intramuscular hamstring and psoas lengthenings, plus rectus femoris transfers. Floor-reaction type AFOs are being used to control the excessively long and weak soleus muscles. (c) Nine months after surgery at age 11, he is now in the midst of his adolescent growth spurt and the tibias have grown enough to re-tension the soleus muscles. Consequently, he is now able to maintain erect posture without the use of floor-reaction AFOs. (d) Seven years after MLEP surgery at age 18. He is now fully grown, and enough growth has taken place to re-tension his muscles. Consequently he no longer uses orthotics. *See CD-Rom, Figure 21.6, for a dynamic illustration.*

muscles that are excessively long, and (5) deal appropriately with the affected biarticular muscles.

In determining the treatment for the boy who had a pre-adolescent growth spurt, we utilized points 1, 2, 4 and 5. He did not have fixed joint contractures, so point 3 was unnecessary. In addition, we were able to use Saltiel AFOs together with his future growth to accomplish point 4. In the case of the girl with severe crouch gait, however, things are different. She does have fixed knee-flexion contractures, more severe on the left than the right. In addition, her growth is complete, so we cannot use growth to accomplish the re-tensioning of the muscle groups that are long. However, since the gastrocnemius crosses the knee and the knee is in flexion, if we could bring the knee back into full extension during

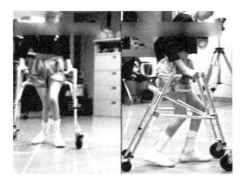

Fig. 21.7. Correction of crouch after puberty. A young woman, age 15, with severe crouch, LAD and stiff-kneed gait. Her only previous surgical procedure was a selective dorsal rhizotomy at 5 years of age. As in the case of the girl shown in Figure 21.2, with the onset of the adolescent growth spurt, SDR without concomitant correction of LAD will almost always lead to crouch. *See CD-Rom, Figure 21.11, for a dynamic illustration.*

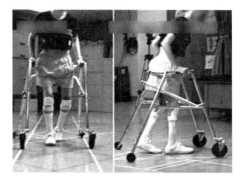

Fig. 21.8. The same girl at age 17, 16 months following MLEP, which consisted of bilateral femoral osteotomies, os calcis lengthenings with subtalar arthrodeses plus bilateral transfer of semitendinosis to adductor magus insertion, and rectus femoris transfers. Floor-reaction type AFOs are being used to control the excessively long and weak soleus muscles. Note that the right knee comes into full extension, but she still has a fixed knee-flexion contracture of 25° on the left. *See CD-Rom, Figure 21.11, for a dynamic illustration.*

mid- and terminal stance, we would at least partially re-tension the triceps surae. By that I mean that even though the solei may be excessively long, because the gastrocnemius crosses the knee and given the degree of her knee flexion in stance, the gastrocnemii are likely to be of normal length or even slightly short.

Furthermore, if we could get her knees back into full extension, the vasti would be long, but they could be re-tensioned by transferring the tibial tubercles distally on a block of bone. The rectus femori are spastic and, as I stated earlier, "confounded". Consequently, distal rectus femoris transfer would perhaps be the best way to deal with them (Gage et al. 1987, Perry 1987, Sutherland et al. 1990, Õunpuu et al. 1993a, b, Rethlefsen et al. 1999, Yngve et al. 2002). Therefore we merely have to accomplish points 1, 2 and 5 and reevaluate her

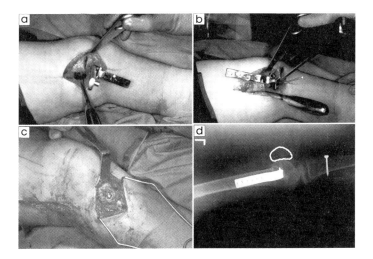

Fig. 21.9. Technique of distal femoral extension osteotomy and tibial tubercle advancement. (a) The femoral shaft has been exposed through a lateral approach and an inverted AO chisel driven into the bone at the level of the distal femoral physis. With the knee in maximum extension, the chisel guide is aligned to the long axis of the tibia. Two saw cuts that intersect at the posterior cortex have been made proximal to the chisel. In order to remove a wedge of bone equal to the flexion contracture (in this case about 25°), the proximal cut is at an exact right angle to the long axis of the femur and the distal is parallel to the chisel blade. (b) The chisel has been removed and replaced with an inverted AO hip spline. The guide pin, which was placed prior to the insertion of the chisel, can be seen distal to the blade plate. (c) Following correction of the knee-flexion contracture, the tibial tubercle has been advanced and fixed with a cancellous bone screw. (d) Lateral X-ray following the completion of the procedure. Note that the knee is now in complete extension and the patella (circled) has been advanced to the point where its proximal edge is about at the level of the distal femoral physis.

following recovery (Fig. 21.8). Since her vasti and soleus muscles were long and her gastrocnemii weak, she still needed to go into floor-reaction AFOs until we could fully correct her knee-flexion contractures and re-tension her vasti. Following that, once she had adequately strengthened and was fully rehabilitated, the AFOs could be discontinued. Again, I have tried to set out in the text the surgical principles by which she was treated, but the specific surgeries that were required are listed in the figure caption and the result demonstrated on the CD-Rom.

Before finishing with this case, however, it would be well to spend a bit of time discussing the techniques we use to restore full knee extension and re-tension the vasti.

EXTENSION OSTEOTOMY AND PATELLAR TENDON ADVANCEMENT
We came to extension osteotomy of the distal femur about 8 years ago when we were confronted with a young adult patient who came to us in severe crouch. In accord with the protocol we were using at the time, we performed the multiple lower-extremity procedure (MLEP) and then put the young man into bilateral Saltiel-type floor-reaction AFOs. Following rehabilitation, however, neither he nor his father was satisfied with the end result. The young man still had fixed knee-flexion contractures of 25° on the right and 15°

on the left and could not walk long distances without his Saltiel AFOs. Consequently, at the time of hardware removal, I elected to do an extension osteotomy on his more severe side. In order to minimize the deformity of the distal femur, I wanted to make the osteotomy as far distally as possible. To accomplish this, I decided to use an inverted 90° AO hip spline and insert the blade at the level the distal femoral physeal scar (Fig. 21.9). The osteotomy and the internal fixation went well, although several technical points became apparent that will be discussed. At the time of surgery, however, two things became apparent. First, because this boy had a severe patella alta, following the osteotomy the patella came to rest directly over the osteotomy site, and I was concerned that this might become a source of patellar–femoral pain. Secondly, the patellar mechanism was now extremely loose—"like a sail out of the wind". Accordingly, there seemed to be little choice but to re-tension the patellar mechanism. Since the young man was skeletally mature, I accomplished this by moving the tibial tubercle distally on a block of bone. Because the fixation was solid, I could start knee motion in a continuous passive motion (CPM) machine 3 days after surgery. As was our custom with osteotomies, I then started partial weightbearing 3 weeks after surgery using a Bledsoe brace with knee flexion limited to 45° to protect the osteotomy and tibial tubercle advancement. He recovered quickly, and to my surprise was soon able to maintain his right knee fully extended in stance without the aid of his Saltiel brace. A short time later he asked me to perform the identical surgery on the opposite side. Six months after having the second side done, he walked without braces with his knees fully extended, although he still used Lofstrand crutches for balance.

Over the next few years, Dr Novacheck and I started to use the extension osteotomy procedure more and more. In the younger patients who still had open growth plates, we did the osteotomy at a slightly higher level, inserting the blade of the AO hip spline just proximal to the distal femoral physis. Because prior to skeletal maturity the patellar tendon inserts directly into the proximal tibial epiphysis, we initially did not re-tension the quadriceps in the younger patients. This meant that we soon had two groups of patients who had had extension osteotomy: an older group that had had the quadriceps re-tensioned via tibial tubercle advancement, and a younger group that had not. When enough of these individuals had come back for postoperative analysis, we were surprised to see that the two groups had very different outcomes (Fig. 21.10).

On clinical examination, both groups had full passive knee extension. During ambulation, however, only the group with tibial tubercle advancement had complete knee extension in stance phase of gait. There were two other interesting findings as well. First, we found that the group which had had tibial tubercle advancement had increased lumbar lordosis, whereas the other group did not. Apparently this was because the psoas contracture had been ignored in both groups at the time of the MLEP surgery. This was done because most of the individuals in both groups used walking aides (crutches or walkers), and at the time we had been concerned about excessive weakening of the hip-flexors. We now know, however, that that concern was unnecessary (Novacheck et al. 2002). Consequently, we have now returned to do intramuscular psoas lengthening in a few of these individuals, although we still do not have enough data to know whether or not we have solved the lordosis problem.

Our second finding was that, even though both groups had had distal rectus femoris

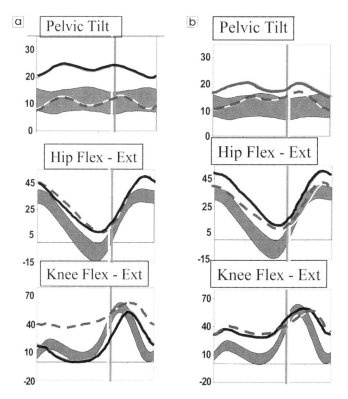

Fig. 21.10. Sagittal-plane kinematics of extension osteotomy with and without patellar tendon advancement. (a) Preoperative (dashed line) and postoperative (solid line) means of the kinematics of 12 knees before and after distal femoral extension osteotomy with tibial tubercle advancement. Note that the hip-flexion/extension graph is unchanged, kinematics of the knee are markedly improved, and pelvic lordosis has increased. Normal values ± 1 S.D. are included for comparison. (b) Preoperative (dashed line) and postoperative (solid line) means of the kinematics of seven knees before and after distal femoral extension osteotomy without tibial tubercle advancement. Note none of the parameters is significantly changed. Normal values ± 1 S.D. are included for comparison. On the basis of these two sets of kinematic graphs, we became convinced that tibial tubercle advancement should be combined with distal femoral extension osteotomy in almost all cases.

transfer as part of their first MLEP, the group with quadriceps re-tensioning now had nearly normal knee kinematics whereas the group with extension osteotomy had no significant change in knee kinematics preoperatively to postoperatively. In other words the rectus femoris transfer that had done very little to improve knee function after the initial surgery in both groups, now started to work superbly in the group with tibial tubercle advancement.

RESULTS

Figures 21.11 and 22.12 (a, b) demonstrate the results, following the completion of treatment, of the two young women presented in the first part of the chapter. The videos of their gaits before and after treatment can be seen on the CD-Rom. In both cases the end-result was good in that they were walking independently without the use of AFOs. However, both required

393

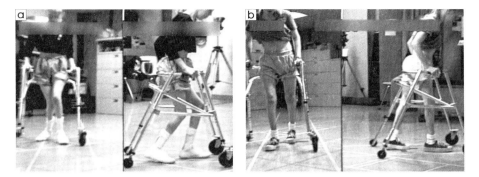

Fig. 21.11. Final result of the woman shown in Figure 21.7. (a) The young woman, age 15, shown in Figure 21.7 before her treatment at Gillette. (b) The same woman, 7 months following distal femoral extension osteotomy and tibial tubercle advancement on the left side and 23 months following bilateral MLEP. She is now able to maintain erect posture without the use of floor-reaction AFOs. *See CD-Rom, Figure 21.11, for a dynamic illustration.*

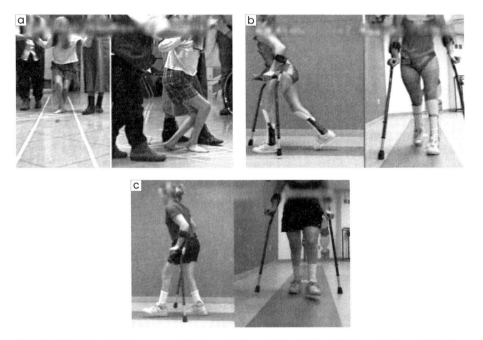

Fig. 21.12. Final result of the young girl shown in Figure 21.2. (a) The girl shown in Figure 21.2 (d) at age 11 just prior to the onset of her treatment at Gillette Children's Specialty Healthcare. (b) The same young woman 5 years later at age 16, following correction of her LAD (bilateral femoral and tibial torsion and pes valgus), appropriate bilateral muscle lengthenings and rectus femoris transfers. She is now able to maintain erect posture with the use of floor-reaction AFOs (FROs) and is back to full community ambulation with Lofstrand crutches. (c) About 18 months later, following bilateral tibial tubercle advancements (done on one side at a time so that we would not have to take her off her feet and could minimize her rehabilitation time), her quadriceps lag is now gone, and she can maintain erect posture without the use of FROs. However, she still requires crutches for community ambulation. *See CD-Rom, Figure 21.12, for a dynamic illustration.*

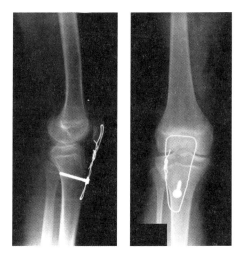

Fig. 21.13. AP and lateral roentgenograms of patellar advancement after cerclage wiring. After having to reoperate on several children when the patella tendon pulled loose, we finally settled on a cerclage wire to stabilize the repair. The wire is drilled through the waist of the patella and then back through the tibia just distal to the point of anchorage of the tendon. It is then tied back upon itself so that it encircles the repair. Knee motion is started on a continuous passive motion (CPM) machine about 3 days following surgery, and most children have about 60°–70° of knee flexion by the time the wire is removed 6–8 weeks after surgery. The wire needs to be removed under general anesthesia as a day-patient surgery, but it has totally solved the "pull-off problem".

balance assists (walker or Lofstrand crutches), which would probably not have been necessary if their LAD had been corrected in a timely manner before puberty.

MOST PROBLEMS ARE CAUSED BY SOLUTIONS

It now seemed clear that whenever we did an extension osteotomy of the distal femur, we also needed to re-tension the quadriceps mechanism. Accordingly, in the patients who were not skeletally mature, we carefully shaved the patellar tendon off the proximal tibial epiphysis and anchored it distally with screws and/or Sta-Tac sutures. Unfortunately, within a few months we had at least five postoperative "pull-offs" from the anchorage site and the hospital care committee was requesting that we discontinue the procedure. After several attempts at better internal fixation, we finally settled on a cerclage wire drilled through the waist of the patella and the tibia just distal to the point of anchorage. It is then tied back upon itself so that it encircles the repair (Fig. 21.13). The wire needs to be removed as a day-patient surgery 6–8 weeks later, but it has totally solved the "pull-off" problem.

SURGICAL PEARLS LEARNED THE HARD WAY

When doing the extension osteotomy of the distal femur it is easy to make technical errors, including the following.

Creating knee varus/valgus deformities. There is little or no room for error here. If the guide chisel is not placed precisely at the correct angle to the long axis of the femur, noticeable varus or valgus deformities will be created.

Losing rotational control of the distal segment. In my own first procedures, I did not pay sufficient attention to rotation. I now place a percutaneous pin in the femoral neck and a second one as far distally as possible in the axis of the condyles. I then readjust the anteversion into the correct range. If necessary about 25° of rotation can be introduced with no apparent detriment to function, even though it produces some "wrapping" of the quadriceps around the femur.

Putting the sciatic nerve at risk. Since there is trumpeting of the metaphysis, it is easy to place the guide chisel too far anteriorly, which results in a large posterior "step-off deformity". Minimize this by placing the guide chisel fairly far posteriorly. Examine the posterior femoral cortex prior to closure and if a step off deformity is present smooth it with an osteotome or saw. If a large wedge must be removed, slight shortening of the femur is probably prudent. After surgery, sciatic nerve function must be monitored carefully and, if problems arise, instruct nurses to turn the patient prone and flex knee to about 45° immediately to take the tension off the nerve.

Removing an improperly sized wedge. An appropriately sized wedge is easily ascertained at surgery by extending the knee maximally and then measuring the residual contracture. When driving the chisel, align the chisel guide with the long axis of the tibia. The first cut (made 15 mm proximal to the chisel insertion site) is parallel to the chisel in all planes. The second cut (which intersects the first at the posterior femoral cortex) is made at 90° to the long axis of the femur.

Properly tensioning the patellar mechanism. When advancing the patella, with the knee in full extension we attempt to get the proximal pole of the patella to the level of the distal femoral physis. After the repair has been secured, this should allow at least 60° of knee flexion under anesthesia without undue tension.

Conclusions
Finally, it is worth repeating the aims of treatment as stated by Dr Cary in a personal communication: (1) define the end product in terms of long-range treatment objectives; (2) identify the patient's problems, both immediate and future, with precision; (3) analyze the effects of growth on the problems, with and without the proposed treatment; (4) consider valid treatment alternatives, including non-treatment; and (5) treat the whole child, not just his motor-skeletal parts.

REFERENCES

Arnold AS. (1999) *Quantitative descriptions of musculoskeletal geometry in persons with cerebral palsy: guidelines for the evaluation and treatment of crouch gait.* PhD thesis, Northwestern University, Evanston, Illinois.
Arnold AS, Blemker SS, Delp SL. (2001) Evaluation of a deformable musculoskeletal model for estimating muscle-tendon lengths during crouch gait. *Ann Biomed Eng* **29:** 263–274.
Baumann JU, Koch HG. (1989) Ventrale aponeurotische Verlängerung des Musculus gastrocnemius. *Operat Orthop Traumatol* **1:** 254–258.
Bleck EE. (1987) *Orthopaedic Management in Cerebral Palsy.* London: Mac Keith Press. p 133.
Buckon CE, Thomas SS, Harris GE, Piatt JH Jr, Aiona MD, Sussman MD. (2002) Objective measurement of muscle strength in children with spastic diplegia after selective dorsal rhizotomy. *Arch Phys Med Rehabil* **83:** 454–460.
Delp SL, Arnold AS, Speers RA, Moore CA. (1996) Hamstrings and psoas lengths during normal and crouch gait: implications for muscle-tendon surgery. *J Orthop Res* **14:** 144–151.
Gage JR, Perry J, Hicks RR, Koop S, Werntz JR. (1987) Rectus femoris transfer to improve knee function of children with cerebral palsy. *Dev Med Child Neurol* **29:** 159–166.
Gage JR, Stout JL, Novacheck TF, Matsuo K. (2002) *Distal femoral extension osteotomy for treatment of persistent crouch gait.* Paper presented at meeting of the European Pediatric Orthopaedic Society, Istanbul, Turkey.
Hoffinger SA, Rab GT, Abou-Ghaida H. (1993) Hamstrings in cerebral palsy crouch gait. *J Pediatr Orthop*

13: 722–726.

Lengsfeld M, Ahlers J, Ritter G. (1990) Kinematics of the patellofemoral joint. Investigations on a computer model with reference to patellar fractures. *Arch Orthop Trauma Surg* **109:** 280–283.

Novacheck T, Trost J, Schwartz M. (2002) Intramuscular psoas lengthening improves dynamic hip function in children with cerebral palsy. *J Pediatr Orthop* **22:** 158–164.

Õunpuu S, Gage JR, Davis RB. (1991) Three-dimensional lower extremity joint kinetics in normal pediatric gait. *J Pediatr Orthop* **11:** 341–349.

Õunpuu S, Muik E, Davis RB 3rd, Gage JR, DeLuca PA. (1993a) Rectus femoris surgery in children with cerebral palsy. Part I: the effect of rectus femoris transfer location on knee motion. *J Pediatr Orthop* **13:** 325–330.

Õunpuu S, Muik E, Davis RB 3rd, Gage JR, DeLuca PA. (1993b) Rectus femoris surgery in children with cerebral palsy. Part II: a comparison between the effect of transfer and release of the distal rectus femoris on knee motion. *J Pediatr Orthop* **13:** 331–335.

Perry J. (1987) Distal rectus femoris transfer. *Dev Med Child Neurol* **29:** 153–158.

Rethlefsen S, Tolo VT, Reynolds RA, Kay R. (1999) Outcome of hamstring lengthening and distal rectus femoris transfer surgery. *J Pediatr Orthop B* **8:** 75–79.

Rosenthal RK, Levine DB. (1977) Fragmentation of the distal pole of the patella in spastic cerebral palsy. *J Bone Joint Surg Am* **59:** 934–939.

Saraph V, Zwick EB, Uitz C, Linhart W, Steinwender G. (2000) The Baumann procedure for fixed contracture of the gastrosoleus in cerebral palsy. Evaluation of function of the ankle after multilevel surgery. *J Bone Joint Surg Br* **82:** 535–540.

Schutte LM, Hayden SW, Gage JR. (1997) Lengths of hamstrings and psoas muscles during crouch gait: effects of femoral anteversion. *J Orthop Res* **15:** 615–621.

Strayer LMJ. (1958) Gastrocnemius recession; five-year report of cases. *J Bone Joint Surg Am* **40:** 1019–1030.

Sutherland DH, Santi M, Abel MF. (1990) Treatment of stiff-knee gait in cerebral palsy: a comparison by gait analysis of distal rectus femoris transfer versus proximal rectus release. *J Pediatr Orthop* **10:** 433–441.

Thompson NS, Baker RJ, Cosgrove AP, Saunders JL, Taylor TC. (2001) Relevance of the popliteal angle to hamstring length in cerebral palsy crouch gait. *J Pediatr Orthop* **21:** 383–387.

Topoleski TA, Kurtz CA, Grogan DP. (2000) Radiographic abnormalities and clinical symptoms associated with patella alta in ambulatory children with cerebral palsy. *J Pediatr Orthop* **20:** 636–639.

Villani C, Billi A, Morico GF, Bonsignore D. (1988) A comparative study of the extensor force of the quadriceps between subjects with a normal patella and those with patella alta of neurological pathogenesis. *Ital J Orthop Traumatol* **14:** 401–406.

Winter DA. (1991) *The Biomechanics and Motor Control of Human Gait: Normal, Elderly and Pathological.* Waterloo, Ontario: University of Waterloo Press.

Yngve DA, Scarborough N, Goode B, Haynes R. (2002) Rectus and hamstring surgery in cerebral palsy: a gait analysis study of results by functional ambulation level. *J Pediatr Orthop* **22:** 672–676.

22
POSTOPERATIVE CARE AND REHABILITATION

Lynn Christianson and Sue Murr

Pre-surgical preparation

Postoperative care begins with preoperative planning. Surgical decision-making to improve ambulation can be accomplished only after a comprehensive evaluation, which normally includes a good history, physical examination, appropriate roentgenograms and gait analysis. These have been discussed in detail in Section 2 of this book (Chapters 5–11), which dealt with patient assessment. Following the completion of this assessment, and after giving careful thought to specific surgical procedures, further preoperative planning includes a discussion of the goals of treatment, the patient's readiness for surgery, pain management in the immediate postoperative phase, and the program for long-term recovery that will be required to maximize outcome. In order to accomplish this, an adequate amount of time must be spent with the family to discuss the specifics of their child's problem and what, if anything can be done to improve his/her functional abilities. This includes a discussion of the risks involved as well as the probability of successful achievement of the goals outlined. In most textbooks this would be termed "informed consent", but the type of discussion of which we are speaking is more comprehensive than that. For example, in addition to discussing in great detail the specifics of the surgery, aftercare and recovery, we try to show the family preoperative and postoperative videos of a child with similar involvement, to give an idea of what they can expect. We also often put families in contact with families of children who have already gone through the procedures. Depending upon the patient's age and level of understanding, these discussions should include both the patient and the caregivers.

Other team-members may need to be consulted and/or included in this discussion: e.g. the neurologist, if the child has a seizure history; a pediatrician, if there are concerns about baseline nutritional status needed for surgery and healing; and the hospital social-worker, who can provide valuable input regarding the family dynamics and circumstances. For example, the social-worker is often needed in procuring caregiver assistance such as a home health aide. The social-worker also may assist a family in informing the child's school or the young adult's work-site of postoperative restrictions and necessary accommodations. Finally, we depend on our social-service department to assist the family in obtaining the temporary equipment that will be needed after the surgery is performed. This might include items such as a hospital bed, bedside commode, and reclining wheelchair.

A consultation with physical therapy in advance of surgery often is extremely useful.

If it is known, for example, that a child will require crutches or a walker post-surgery, the therapist can recommend the specific equipment that will be required. In addition, it is much easier to teach the child how to use crutches or a walker in advance of surgery when s/he can do so with relative ease, as opposed to after surgery when the child is uncomfortable and fearful. At our institution, we also use child-life specialists in advance of the hospital admission to explain, in terms the child can understand, the process of surgery and what to expect in the immediate postoperative period. This does a great deal to allay the anxiety of both the child and the parents. To help the child understand anesthesia, intravenous lines and pain management, the child-life specialist often uses medical play with dolls.

Post-surgical pain management

The plan for postoperative pain management also begins preoperatively. Useful information may be learned concerning the child's response to previous surgeries and subsequent care. An interview with the family and a review of the chart may suggest which approaches were more effective in relieving postoperative pain and anxiety. The response of the respiratory system to anesthesia and postoperative medications may be predicted, in part, through interviews with the family and a review of the medical records.

The primary focus of immediate postoperative care is relief of pain and anxiety. The ongoing monitoring of vital signs, which includes pulse oximetry and cardiorespiratory monitoring, helps to assess the safety and effectiveness of analgesia. The input from one of the visual analogue pain scales supplements the assessment by parents and regular caregivers, since many of our patients have impaired or non-existent verbal skills. It is also important to make as clear a distinction as possible between a child's ability to speak and/or sign, and the ability to understand verbal communication from others. This usually requires input from the parents and regular caregivers.

EPIDURAL ANALGESIA

Epidural analgesia has proven to be a safe and effective method of postoperative analgesia in the majority of patients who have multiple lower-extremity procedures (Fig. 22.1). Over the past few years, an increasing number of patients have come to surgery following previous surgeries on the lower back. These include selective dorsal rhizotomies, placement of intrathecal baclofen pump catheters, or occasionally spinal fusions. In these patients the caudal approach is a necessary alternative to the lumbar approach to the epidural space. Despite the disruption of normal lumbar anatomy from earlier surgeries, if an epidural catheter can be placed into the sacral canal, the majority of patients will have effective analgesia.

In infants and small children the caudal approach to catheter placement is easier, and in some respects safer, than the lumbar approach for the following reasons. (1) The anatomy is easier to feel by palpation than in older children and adults. (2) The catheter is more easily passed cephalad and in the midline than with the lumbar approach (Bosenberg et al. 1988, 2002, Bosenberg 1998). (3) The risk of dural puncture and spinal cord trauma is lessened by the fact that the dural sac terminates cephalad to the sacral hiatus or entry site.

The anatomy of the sacrum changes in ways that make the caudal approach more

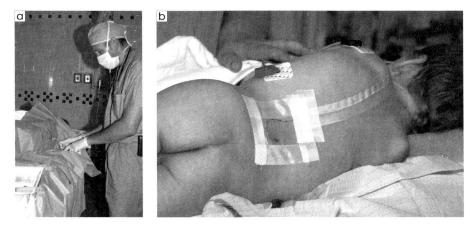

Fig. 22.1. (a) After the patient is anesthetized, the anesthesiologist places the epidural catheter. (b) The insertion needle has been withdrawn and the catheter taped into place. We routinely use continuous epidural anesthesia with clonidine 2 μg/cc in conjunction with a 0.1% solution of ropivacaine delivered at a rate of 0.2–0.3 ml per kg per hour for 72 hours after surgery.

difficult as patients age. These include asymmetry of bone growth and increased thickness of overlying fibrous and fatty tissue. These changes are discussed in detail by Willis (1998). Despite these changes, experience and careful technique are the keys to success.

Some anesthesiologists are reluctant to place an epidural catheter via the caudal approach because of the perceived increased risk of soiling with stool and urine. As with any lumbar or thoracic site, the skin must be meticulously prepared with antiseptic and draped with attention to sterile technique. After catheter placement, a sterile, clear, adhesive dressing such as Tegaderm™ is applied over the catheter with the help of tincture of benzoin. This clear dressing is very durable and allows for regular inspection of the catheter and entry site. All patients receiving continuous epidural infusion have an in-dwelling bladder catheter and stooling is infrequent until significant oral intake is resumed. The removal of catheters from patients with spica casts is usually easier from the caudal site than the lumbar.

EPIDURAL AGENTS

The intraoperative use of epidural catheters with bupivacaine, 0.1%–0.25%, allows reduction in the intravenous or inhalation anesthetic. This allows for more rapid emergence from anesthesia after surgeries that last 4–6 hours. This more rapid emergence in turn allows shorter times spent in post-anesthesia recovery units, and earlier assessment of sensory and motor block and analgesia. In most patients the local anesthetic, bupivacaine or ropivacaine, is used in higher concentrations, up to 0.25% intraoperatively, to allow greater reduction in anesthetic agents. Near the end of surgery and postoperatively, lower concentrations of 0.1% bupivacaine or ropivacaine are used as a continuous infusion. The goal is to achieve analgesia at rest with sensation to light touch intact and minimal reduction of motor tone.

CHOICE OF LOCAL ANESTHETIC

Bupivacaine (Marcaine, Sensorcaine) is widely used for epidural analgesia due to its long duration and ability to provide more sensory than a motor block. However, equipotent doses of bupivacaine are more cardiotoxic than lidocaine. This toxicity from bupivacaine is difficult to treat and is exacerbated by acidosis, hypoxemia and hypercarbia. Careful placement of catheters and small incremental doses of bupivacaine, however, will reduce the incidence and severity of toxic blood levels of bupivacaine.

A newer amide local anesthetic agent, ropivacaine (Naropin), was developed as an S-enantiomer to have less cardiotoxicity than bupivacaine (Cederholm 1997, Bosenberg et al. 2002). Equipotent doses are reported to spare motor block even more than bupivacaine, and equal doses are slightly less potent than bupivacaine (Anonymous 1997). For continuous infusions via epidural catheters, a 0.1% solution of ropivacaine or bupivacaine is delivered at a rate of 0.2–0.3 ml per kilogram per hour.

ANESTHESIA ADJUNCTS

For many years at Gillette Children's Specialty Healthcare the local anesthetic was supplemented with fentanyl, 1–2 µg per ml of epidural solution. For the past 2 years we have eliminated the fentanyl component and replaced it with clonidine (Nishina et al. 1999). This change has virtually eliminated itching and greatly reduced nausea and vomiting without sacrificing effectiveness of analgesia. Although clonidine does sedate patients mildly, it is less potent in its effect on respiratory effort than fentanyl in epidural solutions. Blood pressure is reduced by clonidine, but for reasons that are not clear, this effect is much less in children than in adults and teenagers (J. Eisenach, personal communication). Clonidine can also produce significant bradycardia in teenagers and adults and, if it occurs, may require either a reduction in the concentration of the epidural solution or elimination of the clonidine from it.

For those patients who are not candidates for epidural delivery of analgesics, or those who do not consent to epidural placement of a catheter, a continuous infusion of narcotic medication is a good alternative. If the patient is alert and physically able to press a button, this infusion can be set up on a patient-controlled analgesia (PCA) pump. If the patient is not capable, the nurse at the bedside can give supplemental bolus doses as needed. Many different narcotics are effective in PCA systems, but for an individual patient one may need to try several to find the narcotic with the fewest side-effects.

OTHER MEDICATIONS

Even a perfectly placed epidural catheter with appropriate doses of medication delivery to the epidural space will not result in a patient who is 100% pain-free. The most common causes of intermittent or new onset pain in a previously comfortable patient are muscle spasms, changing position in bed or chair, and casts or wrapped dressings which exert too much pressure due to postoperative swelling. Muscle spasms are impossible to eliminate 100%, but both baclofen (Lioresal) and diazepam (Valium) can be helpful in reducing their severity. Tight casts and wrapped dressings can be split or loosened to reduce pressure on swollen tissue. Pain, which is increasing in intensity and not relieved by medication or reducing external pressure, may indicate compartment syndrome, which is a surgical emergency. In order to minimize the chance of compartment syndrome, it is our policy not to apply closed casts in the operating room. Instead a splinted Robert-Jones type dressing is applied. This is usually changed to a closed short leg cast on the third postoperative day just prior to removing the epidural catheter. If the child is fearful or anxious, an appropriate dose (usually 0.1mg/kg) of intravenous midazolam (Versed) can be used as an adjunct.

Ketorolac (Toradol) is a non-steroidal anti-inflammatory drug that may be given intravenously or intramuscularly. Due to its potential for gastric ulceration, it should not be given for more than 5 days. If there is any question about hemostasis, platelet count or function, ketorolac should not be used. Although widely used in orthopaedics, because it is known to inhibit bone-healing, most surgeons prefer to avoid ketorolac in surgeries involving spinal fusion or repair of non-unions.

Stages of surgical recovery
It is always helpful for the child and family to understand the stages of recovery typical to the postoperative period (Gage 1991). These stages include (1) healing of the soft tissues and bone (approximately 6 weeks), (2) strengthening (approximately 12–16 weeks) and (3) retraining and refining of gait (up to 12 months).

Although we make every attempt to minimize it, postoperatively there is generally some form of immobilization. As mentioned earlier, when femoral derotation osteotomies are performed along with procedures in the lower leg, Robert-Jones dressings are applied in the operating room. These are then replaced with a pair of fiberglass short leg casts after 72 hours to ensure that swelling has gone down and the casts fit more securely. A removable Denis-Browne bar is then applied to the dorsal surface of the casts to prohibit rotation of the lower extremities while still allowing flexion and extension mobility at the hips and knees. Knee-immobilizers are often used once the patient has had casts applied. They assist with comfort and help to maintain the knee in extension, especially when hamstring or gastrocnemius recessions have been performed.

Even if a pelvic osteotomy has been performed, we try to avoid casting in the operating room. However, on rare occasions, if a pelvic osteotomy is unstable and/or the hip must be maintained in a particular position referable to the pelvic, a plaster hip spica cast may need to be applied. Even if a spica cast is applied, however, we have found that in nearly all cases it can be removed and gentle passive motion started 3 weeks after surgery.

Physical therapy goals (Fig. 22.2)
THE FIRST THREE WEEKS
The goals for the first 3 weeks postoperatively include safe transfers, positioning and passive range of motion to prevent stiffness and/or muscle contractures during the period of immobilization. When supine, the patient should be positioned in extension without pillows under the knees. When prone, the child should lie flat without pillows under the hips. This is particularly important if intramuscular psoas lengthening has been done. The child will be more comfortable with hips in flexion, but if the hips are not maintained in extension most of the time (particularly during the first few weeks after surgery), intramuscular

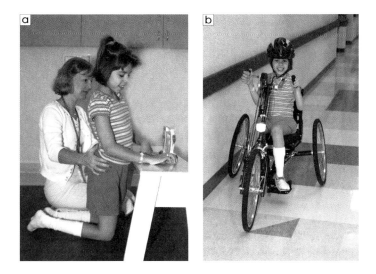

Fig. 22.2. (a) Good therapy is imperative to the end-result. We start passive range-of-motion to the lower extremities on the third postoperative day. The child usually goes home in short leg-casts tied together with a Denis-Browne bar. At the time of discharge the parents are taught to transfer the child and given a program for passive range-of-motion. Three weeks after surgery the child returns to the outpatient department for X-rays, brace-molding and application of walking-casts. Formal physical therapy 2–3 times weekly starts at this point and stresses range-of-motion and strengthening as well as gait and balance training. (b) A good program of rehabilitation stresses the trunk and upper extremities as well as the lower limbs. Since most of these children require a walker or crutches initially, it is important to maintain good upper-extremity strength.

scar may render the muscle shorter after surgery than it was before intervention.

At the time of discharge from the hospital, a reclining wheelchair is provided. This can be used during part of the day as an alternative to the bed. Toward the end of the hospital stay, the child goes to physical therapy. There, caregivers are shown how to transfer their child and instructed in passive range of motion exercises, which are to be performed several times daily. Depending upon the procedures performed and/or the postoperative fixation, restrictions to the postoperative therapy program may be imposed by the physician. Otherwise passive range-of-motion is done to the patient's tolerance. In order to maintain mobility of the tendon transfer, patients who have distal femoral extension ostestomies or transfer of the distal end of the rectus femoris (generally to the gracilis or sartorius) usually receive a continuous passive motion (CPM) machine for use in the first 3 weeks following surgery. This is used for 30 minutes three times daily. It is set to allow 45° of knee flexion initially, and increased within the range of the child's comfort during the first 3 weeks. The goal is to have 90° of knee flexion 6 weeks after surgery.

THREE TO SIX WEEKS
When bony procedures have been performed, the patient is generally kept non-weightbearing for the first 3 weeks. Three weeks after surgery, the child returns to the hospital as an

outpatient. At that time his/her casts are removed, roentgenograms of the osteotomies are obtained, braces are molded, and short-leg walking-casts are applied. Once the X-rays are checked, the child goes to physical therapy to begin weightbearing. Ambulation is initiated with an assistive device, generally a reverse walker since studies have offered support that reverse-walkers led to decreased hip and trunk flexion and a more upright posture in children with cerebral palsy (Logan et al. 1990). Even patients, who were walking independently before surgery, begin walking with a walker or crutches as they are learning new balance and alignment. Re-education and the learning of a new gait pattern can be aided by verbal cueing by caregivers and physical therapists as well as by the patient's visual assessment as s/he walks toward a long mirror.

Range-of-motion exercises continue with the addition of active exercise. The overall goal is full range at all joints including hip internal and external rotation, abduction and adduction. A goal of strengthening is added and, if s/he has isolated motor control, the patient can work on gaining strength by isolated exercise. In the absence of good motor control, strengthening can be accomplished through transitional movements and mat mobility. Cycling, or the equivalent reciprocal motion, may be initiated using a tricycle, stationary bike or restorator.

In order to increase knee flexion and improve toe clearance in walking, both on level surfaces and in stair-climbing, muscle re-education can begin by practising single-limb stance, stepping up on to a low bench and/or over low obstacles (without compensating with circumduction). This is particularly important if rectus femoris transfer has been performed.

At this point in the patient's postoperative rehabilitation phase, it is beneficial to receive physical therapy on an outpatient basis 2–3 times per week. In addition to this therapy, however, the patient needs to be involved in a daily home program of stretching and strengthening (as demonstrated by the 2001 physical therapy protocols from Gillette Children's Specialty Healthcare).

SIX TO TWELVE WEEKS

When lower-leg procedures have been performed, the second set of casts is removed when the osteotomies have healed (generally 6 weeks post-surgery), and orthoses are donned. As was discussed in Chapter 17, the type of orthosis chosen is dependent upon the specific procedures completed and the need for prolonged support. Strengthening and the selective motor control that the patient achieves postoperatively largely determine the length of time that the orthosis is worn. For example, a patient who was walking with a crouch gait preoperatively will probably start in Saltiel-type floor-reaction ankle–foot othoses (AFOs). However, as s/he gains strength and the ability to stay upright, we might wean the child into dynamic ankle–foot orthoses (DAFOs) or even foot orthotics. In general, any orthosis that is worn post-surgery is provided to improve function, and it is our policy to brace the limb as minimally as possible. Usually the wearing time of the orthosis can be gradually reduced once the gait pattern has stabilized as this serves to encourage strengthening and functional use of the calf muscles. Strengthening should continue 2–3 times per week, and can progress to resistance training. In the appropriate patient, neuromuscular electrical stimulation and biofeedback (surface electromyography) can be of assistance in muscle re-education and generation of strong muscular contractions. Since all casts are removed at this point in rehabilitation, activities can expand to include swimming, therapeutic horse-riding and cycling without AFOs.

Ambulation should continue to progress by increasing distance as the patient's endurance improves. With respect to reducing the assistive device recommended, each patient is an individual. Some may wean directly from the walker to independent walking and some may transition to Lofstrand crutches or a single cane. When a femoral derotation osteotomy has been performed, some degree of Trendelenburg gait will usually persist until the femoral hardware is removed.

After 12 weeks from the date of surgery, therapy may either continue at the same frequency as preoperatively, or be discontinued when the patient has demonstrated sufficient strength and a good gait pattern. Regular stretching programs and periodic strengthening programs, in addition to some form of regular aerobic exercise are recommended to maintain fitness, but—as demonstrated by the 2001 physical therapy protocols from Gillette Children's Specialty Healthcare—vary substantially from one patient to another.

REFERENCES

Anonymous. (1997) Ropivacaine—a new local anesthetic. *Med Lett Drugs Ther* **39:** 80.

Bosenberg AT. (1998) Epidural analgesia for major neonatal surgery. *Paediatr Anaesth* **8:** 479–483. (Comment.)

Bosenberg AT, Bland BA, Schulte-Steinberg O, Downing JW. (1988) Thoracic epidural anesthesia via caudal route in infants. *Anesthesiology* **69:** 265–269.

Bosenberg A, Thomas J, Lopez T, Lybeck A, Huizar K, Larsson LE. (2002) The efficacy of caudal ropivacaine 1, 2 and 3 mg x l(-1) for postoperative analgesia in children. *Paediatr Anaesth* **12:** 53–58.

Cederholm I. (1997) Preliminary risk-benefit analysis of ropivacaine in labour and following surgery. *Drug Saf* **16:** 391–402.

Gage JR. (1991) *Gait Analysis in Cerebral Palsy.* London: Mac Keith Press. p 173–183.

Logan L, Byers-Hinkley K, Ciccone C. (1990) Anterior versus posterior walkers: a gait analysis study. *Dev Med Child Neurol* **32:** 1044–1048.

Nishina K, Mikawa K, Shiga M, Obara H. (1999) Clonidine in paediatric anaesthesia. *Paediatr Anaesth* **9:** 187–202.

Willis RJ. (1998) Caudal epidural blockage. In: Cousins MJ, editor. *Neural Blockade in Clinical Anesthesia and Management of Pain*, 2nd edn. Philadelphia: Lippincott–Raven. p 323–327.

23
FUNCTIONAL ASSESSMENT OF OUTCOMES

Tom F. Novacheck and Michael Schwartz

At least three factors necessitate outcome studies. First, the only reliable way of optimizing treatment methods is through a careful and objective study of outcome. Outcome studies help to expose underlying principles, confirm existing clinical beliefs, and occasionally to debunk persistent and pervasive myths. Making a universal link between crouch gait and hamstring contracture, for example, has led many surgeons to recommend hamstring-lengthening procedures. Gait analysis and musculoskeletal modeling, however, reveal that the hamstrings are not contracted in all cases of crouch gait, but that other causes such as lever-arm dysfunction may be present. Elsewhere in this book we have discussed the underlying principles of correction of lever-arm dysfunction and spasticity management, and we now want to focus on the role outcome studies continue to play in the improvement of treatment methods.

Outcome analysis provides the evidence of positive treatment outcomes third-party payers require in this era of cost containment. Utilization of services and treatments varies widely by geographic region, as health-care expenditure for a relatively common diagnosis such as cerebral palsy (CP) can be high. Payers must decide which treatments they will or will not support. Without satisfying outcome data, they will make their decision based on the only other available piece of data, the cost of intervention.

More importantly, the families of children with CP—a complex and chronic condition—face difficult decisions about the best treatment for their children and want the answers that outcome studies provide. Families must sort through the many different options offered by standard medical care, and discern among the varying opinions regarding recommended management advocated by different practitioners and institutions. Additionally, they must consider the many alternative types of care available such as hyperbaric oxygen, chiropractic management and conductive education. How is a family to decide among these treatments? How much improvement should they expect? What types of changes will they see? Properly performed outcome analysis helps to address these questions.

Finally, outcome studies serve to disarm skeptics fond of arguing that the environment for gait assessment is artificial, so children do not walk in their typical fashion and the information obtained is inaccurate and possibly even useless. Wishing to dispute the value and insight of the tool, some claim that the technical information gathered in the laboratory does not correlate with gross motor ability or daily community functional ability, or that the postoperative improvements measured in the gait laboratory do not translate to improved daily function for the child.

TABLE 23.1

TABLE 23.1
NCMRR definitions

Level	Definition
Pathophysiology	The interruption of, or interference with, normal physiological and developmental processes or structures
Impairment	A loss or abnormality at the organ or organ system level of the body
Functional limitation	Restriction or lack of ability to perform an action in the manner or within the range consistent with the purpose of an organ or organ system
Disability	A limitation in performing tasks, activities, and roles to levels expected within physical and social contexts
Societal limitation	Restrictions attributable to social policy or barriers (structural or attitudinal) which limit fulfilment of roles or deny access to services and opportunities associated with full participation in society

It was in response to these types of concerns that we at the Gillette Center for Gait and Motion Analysis took three major steps. In 1987 the center's founder, Dr Steve Koop, proposed that oxygen consumption testing be a standard procedure for all patients (Koop et al. 1989). We have continuously gathered this data since that time (Stout et al. 2003). Then, in 1992 and 1993, we developed the Functional Assessment Questionnaire (FAQ), which has been used routinely for all patients seen in the laboratory since the start of January 1994 (Novacheck et al. 2000). The third major step was the development of a global gait pathology index, known as the Normalcy Index (NI) (Schutte et al. 2000). Together, these three global measures—oxygen consumption, functional assessment and NI—give a comprehensive picture of outcome on levels spanning from highly technical and objective to highly functional and subjective.

Some of the challenges to completing good outcomes analysis are knowing where to start and having the proper tools to assess the results meaningfully (Goldberg 1991, Butler et al. 1999). In this chapter we aim (1) to describe the NCMRR model for understanding of outcome analysis, (2) to discuss several outcome assessment tools utilized at Gillette Children's Specialty Healthcare, and provide evidence of their utility, and (3) to delineate the improvements in function that appropriate diagnosis and intervention based on information derived from computerized gait analysis can achieve.

We hope that this chapter's discussion of outcome assessment will help in the assessment of treatment results, and in the critical evaluation of the tools for outcome measurement currently employed in other laboratories.

Shortcomings of univariate analysis

Rehabilitation research, and therefore outcome studies, can be conducted at many levels. The National Center for Medical Rehabilitation Research (NCMRR), a division of the US National Institutes of Health, developed a framework to describe the multiple dimensions of disability (Table 23.1) (NCMRR 1993). The primary aim of this chapter is to focus on three of their criteria: impairment, functional limitation and disability. Their other criteria (pathophysiology and societal limitations) are important topics, but generally fall outside the realm of gait analysis—even though fundamental changes in the pathophysiology of

TABLE 23.2
Data available for outcome analysis

Group	Example	Accuracy	Objectivity	Reliability	Specificity	Level of applicability
Physical exam	Contractures, bony torsion	Fair/poor	Fair/poor	Fair/poor	Specific	1°: Impairment 2°: Functional limitation
Functional questionnaires	FAQ MODEMS	Fair	Poor	Fair/poor	General	1°: Functional limitation 2°: Disability
Satisfaction questionnaires		Good	Poor	Fair	General	1°: Functional limitation 2°: Disability 2°: Societal limitation
Quantitative gait data	Knee flexion, hip rotation	Fair/good	Good	Good	Specific	1°: Functional limitation 2°: Impairment
Oxygen assessment	Oxygen cost	Fair/good	Good	Fair/good	General	1°: Functional limitation 2°: Impairment 2°: Pathophys.
MVA	NI	Good	Good	Good	General	1°: Functional limitation 2°: Impairment

CP produced (e.g. by botulinum toxin or intrathecal baclofen) can alter gait, and a change in gait can have an impact on societal limitations.

An outcome study measures the impact of a treatment or lack of treatment on a patient's gait. At our disposal in this task are data derived from the physical exam, energy assessment, quantitative gait analysis, patient/parent report functional questionnaires and patient satisfaction surveys. To be useful, the measures we select as indicators of outcome must be accurate, objective, and reliable (Table 23.2). They must also be reflective of the system being studied, whether it is an individual joint, the lower extremity or the entire body. Countless articles have addressed the effects of individual surgical procedures on isolated joints or body segments. These focused studies are of great value, and we do not mean to dismiss this branch of research. However, the emphasis here is on a more comprehensive assessment of outcome for children with CP. The latter (comprehensive assessment), particularly from the perspective of quantitative, objective, technical outcome measures, has received much less attention than the former.

Focused outcome studies have generally relied on the use of univariate measures (e.g. peak knee flexion), whose appeal is clear as these variables generally have direct clinical significance, are simple to acquire, store and process. Finally, they lend themselves to reasonably well-understood statistical tests. However, the univariate approach has at least two significant shortcomings: specificity and interdependence. Variables that are specific give information about an isolated aspect of gait, but fail to adequately capture the overall picture. Mean stance-phase knee flexion, for example, may be a good indicator of sagittal-plane crouch gait, but it is a poor indicator of transverse-plane torsional anomalies. Aware of the complexities of gait, researchers often employ multiple and simultaneous univariate measures. While this approach has a natural appeal, interdependence (correlation) among

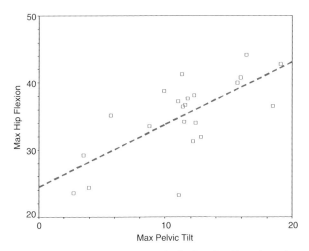

Fig. 23.1. Linear correlation between maximum hip flexion (MHF) and maximum pelvic tilt (MPT). For a group of able-bodied subjects, these two variables are strongly correlated, which is largely due to the definition of hip flexion (i.e. position of the thigh relative to the pelvis). The strong correlation means that a researcher who uses both MHF and MPT as outcome measures is essentially counting the same thing twice.

gait variables can obfuscate potentially important features and mislead the interpreter of the data.

There are two primary means by which variables can be correlated to one another: by definition and by function (it is also possible for variables to exhibit both types of correlations). Consider the variables maximum pelvic tilt and maximum hip flexion/extension. These variables often are cited as indicators of sagittal-plane hip function. By definition, hip-flexion/extension measures the position of the thigh relative to the pelvis, thereby correlating the variables to one another. For a group of able-bodied individuals, the Pearson's correlation coefficient between maximum pelvic tilt and maximum hip flexion is $r = 0.70$ ($P<0.01$) (Fig. 23.1). Thus a study that uses both maximum pelvic tilt and maximum hip flexion as outcome measures essentially counts the same variable twice, resulting in a "double-jeopardy" (or "double-bonus") effect that artificially enhances their apparent strength.

Variables can also be functionally correlated. Functional correlation means that underlying anatomical or physiological factors result in interdependence of variables. The influence of walking-speed on the kinematics and kinetics of gait provides an important example. Walking-speed affects kinematics and kinetics by increasing the segmental inertia contributions to the equations of dynamic equilibrium. Stansfield and colleagues (2001) proved that many effects traditionally attributed to age, size or natural variability can actually be explained by differences in walking speed. Other examples of functional correlation include the plantarflexion/knee-extension couple described in earlier chapters.

Clearly you should be very careful when including univariate measures in outcome studies. Lack of understanding of the correlation structure among the variables virtually guarantees their erroneous interpretation.

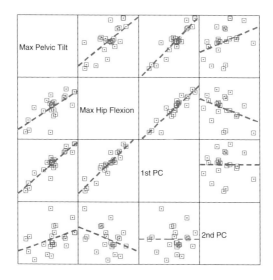

Fig. 23.2. Decoupling of variables via principal component analysis.

Multivariate analysis and the Normalcy Index

The above examples, among countless others, demonstrate the necessity for multivariate analysis (MVA). MVA is a general term for a collection of methods that may be used to examine correlated univariate measures in a rational way. The field of MVA is quite complex; those interested in details of the foundation of MVA can find references readily available, many of these stemming from the pioneering work of Kendall (1975).

Principal component analysis (PCA), one of MVA's most useful techniques, is a method for transforming correlated (interdependent) variables into uncorrelated (independent) variables in such a manner that the greatest amount of variation can be explained by the smallest number of variables. An additional benefit of PCA transformation is that it occurs without supervision, thereby removing subjective and potentially biased decisions regarding the relative weighting of different variables.

In the pelvic tilt/maximum hip-flexion (PT/MHF) example described above, two uncorrelated variables can be computed by transforming the strongly correlated PT and MHF (Fig. 23.2). Further examination shows that the first transformed variable accounts for 85% of the variation contained in both of the original variables. This indicates that rather than measuring the two variables PT and MHF, a researcher can simply measure the first principal component, thereby reducing the complexity of the system by 50%. This example highlights the two basic uses for PCA: decoupling and reducing complexity of variable sets.

The PCA methodology can also serve in more elaborate systems of variables. The NI is an example of this process. It uses a single number to measure the deviation of a patient's gait from the average gait of subjects without pathology. The deviation is based on a PCA transformation of 16 clinically relevant kinematic variables. The fact that these variables are correlated implies that a simple distance calculation, such as the sum of the squares of

TABLE 23.3
Variables included in the NI

Parameter	Mean value	Standard deviation
Time of toe off (% gait cycle)	61.87	2.67
Walking speed/leg length	1.43	0.21
Cadence (step/sec)	1.94	0.11
Mean pelvic tilt (°)	9.26	4.26
Range of pelvic tilt (°)	3.57	1.60
Mean pelvic rotation (°)	0.15	2.51
Minimum hip flexion (°)	−11.14	6.75
Range of hip flexion (°)	45.00	5.15
Peak abduction in swing (°)	−0.30	3.27
Mean hip rotation in stance (°)	10.91	7.33
Knee flexion at initial contact (°)	6.83	4.69
Time of peak flexion (% gait cycle)	71.40	2.70
Range of knee flexion (°)	54.44	10.59
Peak dorsiflexion in stance (°)	13.31	6.45
Peak dorsiflexion in swing (°)	3.21	4.88
Mean foot progression angle in stance (°)	−9.76	6.46

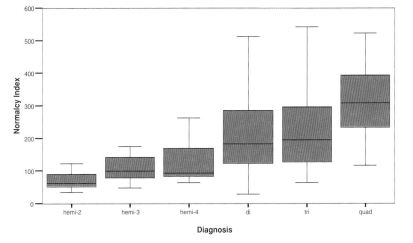

Fig. 23.3. Normalcy Index by diagnosis. Boxes denote the 25th–75th centiles; whiskers show the 10th–90th centiles. Note that increase of NI correlates with severity of involvement.

the deviations of each variable, would not accurately represent the degree of gait abnormality. Standard techniques from MVA decouple and weight the discrete variables, resulting in a more meaningful measure of gait pathology. Although details of the NI calculation can be found elsewhere, the variables that make up the NI are listed here for reference (Table 23.3).

The NI has several attributes which make it well suited to comprehensive outcome studies.

1. Robustness. The NI can measure a wide range of pathology: from mild conditions, such as idiopathic toe-walking, to severe impairments such as quadriplegia. The NI measures these pathologies in a manner that corresponds with clinical impressions (Fig. 23.3).

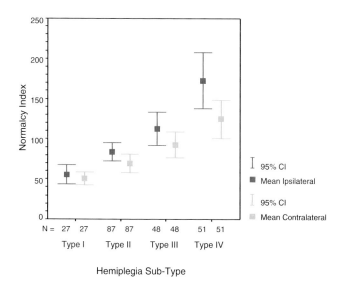

Fig. 23.4. Normalcy Index for hemiplegia types: affected (ipsilateral) versus unaffected (contralateral) limb. Gait compressions required for walking may account for some of the increase in NI on the unaffected (contralateral) side.

2. Sensitivity. The NI can measure subtle gradations of pathology, such as the difference between the affected and unaffected sides of subjects with hemiplegia (Fig. 23.4). Further, the difference between the affected and unaffected sides increases as the level of hemiplegia increases, correlating once again with clinically meaningful definitions.

3. Reliability. As a consequence of the MVA methods used in the NI's development, the variability in the NI is less than that of many of its component variables (Schwartz et al. 2003). Specifically, the NI component variables are automatically weighted to reduce the influence of less consistent variables.

4. Objectivity (Fig. 23.5). Each laboratory uses its own control data as a reference, thereby eliminating any biasing effects of model differences or differences in experimental procedures, the NI is largely independent of the laboratory in which it is computed.

Other comprehensive measures

The NI provides a valuable measure for overall gait pathology based on quantitative gait data. Kinematics tells just a part, albeit an important part, of the outcome story. The other comprehensive outcome measures include oxygen consumption, functional questionnaires and patient satisfaction. Table 23.2 shows that an outcome assessment based on only one subset of the data (e.g. oxygen assessment) will not give a comprehensive picture of the patient's functional and technical outcome. This chapter, however, does not include patient satisfaction as a clinical outcome measure. While patient satisfaction is important, it often reflects many things unrelated to the clinical outcome of the patient: e.g. hospital rooms, difficulties with scheduling, and bedside manner of the physician.

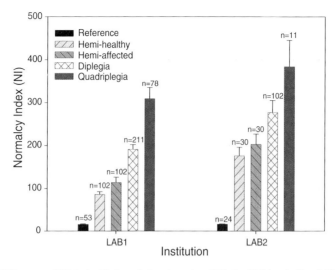

Fig. 23.5. Indifference of NI to institution. Laboratory 1 = Gillette Children's Speciality Healthcare Motion Analysis Laboratory. Laboratory 2 = "L. Divieti" Posture and Movement Analysis Laboratory, Department of Bioengineering, Milan Polytechnic, Italy.

ENERGY CONSUMPTION

Normal gait depends on an efficient use of energy, something that quantitative gait data cannot directly measure. Energy (oxygen) consumption gives an objective picture of the overall efficiency of the patient's gait. Many factors influence energy consumption, including spasticity, bony deformity, strength and selective motor control. Thus energy efficiency reflects the cumulative effect of many factors (Koop et al. 1989, Stout et al. 1993, 2003, Waters and Mulroy 1999).

In the Gillette Center for Gait and Motion Analysis, we measure oxygen consumption during steady-state walking (MedGraphics CPX-D system, MedGraphics Corporation, St Paul, MN, USA). To compare individuals, normalized oxygen consumption is calculated for each subject as the ratio of patient's O_2 consumption/able-bodied O_2 consumption at matched velocity. The denominator in this ratio is drawn from the oxygen consumption-velocity data of an able-bodied reference population (Koop et al. 1989, Stout et al. 2003).

FUNCTIONAL QUESTIONNAIRES AND THE FAQ

Functional questionnaires give insight into the community function of the patient, information that, again, data from the controlled environment of the gait laboratory does not directly reflect. In the early 1990s, when adequate tools for assessing mobility and community function were lacking, popularly available tools were the WeeFIM (Msall et al. 1994, WeeFIM 1995, McAuliffe et al. 1998), the Gross Motor Function Measure (GMFM) (Russell et al. 1993), and the Pediatric Disability Inventory (PEDI) (Haley et al. 1992). For a variety of reasons, we have discovered these to be too limited in their scope or to have ceiling effects. The WeeFIM, for example, with a scale limited to the ability to ambulate

TABLE 23.4
FAQ defined

Level	Definition
1	Cannot take any steps at all
2	Can do some stepping on his/her own with the help of another person. Does not take full weight on feet; does not walk on a routine basis
3	Walks for exercise in therapy and/or less than typical household distances.
4	Walks for household distances, but makes slow progress. Does not use walking at home as preferred mobility (primarily walks in therapy or as exercise)
5	Walks for 5–50 feet outside the home, but usually uses a wheelchair or stroller for community distances or in congested areas
6	Walks outside for community distances, but only on level surfaces (cannot perform curbs, uneven terrain, or stairs without assistance of another person)
7	Walks outside the home for community distances, is able to get around on curbs and uneven terrain in addition to level surfaces, but usually requires minimal assistance or supervision for safety
8	Walks outside the home for community distances, easily gets around on level ground, over curbs and on uneven terrain, but has difficulty or requires minimal assistance or supervision for safety
9	Walks outside the home for community distances, easily gets around on level ground, over curbs and on uneven terrain but has difficulty or requires minimal assistance or supervision with running, climbing, and/or stairs. Has some difficulty keeping up with peers
10	Walks, runs, and climbs on level and uneven terrain and does stairs without difficulty or assistance. Is typically able to keep up with peers

TABLE 23.5
Validation of FAQ: Pearson correlation coefficients between the FAQ and other outcome instruments indicate that they are all related.

	FAQ	WeeFIM	NI	O2	POSNA	POSNA (G)
FAQ	-	0.635	-0.456	-0.424	0.764	0.686

150 feet, is an illustration of a ceiling effect. We felt we needed a functional walking scale that was able to stratify across the spectrum of community mobility. In 1992 and 1993, a dedicated group of Gillette Children's Hospital medical professionals (physicians, nurses, physical therapists and health information specialists) developed the FAQ, a 10-level parent-report scale that encompasses a range of walking abilities from non-ambulatory to ambulatory in a variety of community settings and terrains (Novacheck et al. 2000). We have routinely administered the Gillette FAQ to all individuals who have undergone gait and motion analysis since January 1994. There have already been published reports of its reliability and validity (Novacheck et al. 2000, Tervo et al. 2002). The POSNA Modems scale, another appropriate tool for measuring motor function, was developed soon after we put the FAQ into regular clinical use (Daltroy et al. 1998).

The 10 levels of walking function in the FAQ cover a wide range of abilities (Table 23.4). Comparison of the FAQ to the established tools of the WeeFIM, NI, energy data and the subsequently developed POSNA modems questionnaire have confirmed its content and concurrent validity (Tervo et al. 2002). The Pearson correlation coefficients between these measures indicate that they are all related (Table 23.5). Observation of trends for FAQ levels

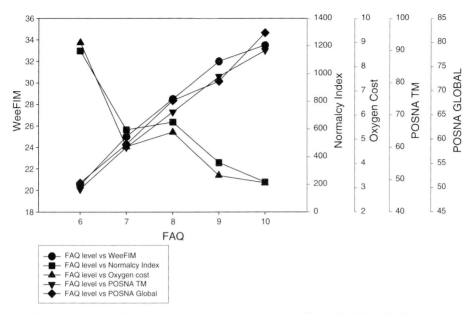

Fig. 23.6. Comparison of FAQ with other functional measures. Higher FAQ level indicates greater mobility (higher level of functional walking). FAQ correlates positively with both POSNA scores (transfers/mobility and global) and with WeeFIM. FAQ is inversely related to both oxygen cost and Normalcy Index (higher values indicate lower level of function).

6–10 appropriate to the other measures offers further support for the validity of the FAQ scale (Fig. 23.6).

To maintain validity, an instrument must produce consistent results within and between observers. The potential reliability of a parent report scale (i.e. would a parent rate his/her child the same on two independent occasions and would another person familiar with the child rate him/her the same) has been a source of concern. Because of this uncertainty, some have recommended the use of an administered performance tool such as the WeeFIM. To assess reliability of the FAQ, we compared the results of an FAQ completed by a classroom, physical education, or adaptive physical education teacher, and a second parent FAQ done 1 month after original completion. The interrater and intrarater reliability was found to be very good with interclass correlation coefficients of 0.92. The Cronbach alpha statistic also indicated good internal consistency among the items in the scale, further supporting good construct validity; the tool is able to measure an abstract concept (walking ability) over the range of possible functional abilities (Novacheck et al. 2000).

Subsequent to the initial report on the validity and reliability testing 3 years ago, other retrospective clinical reports have used the Gillette FAQ. An evaluation of the safety and efficacy of intramuscular psoas lengthening showed that children who underwent psoas lengthening had no loss of clinical mobility (Novacheck et al. 2002).

Like the Normalcy Index, the FAQ can discriminate between individuals with different CP diagnosis subtypes (Fig. 23.7) (Tervo et al. 2002). The greater the level of disability as

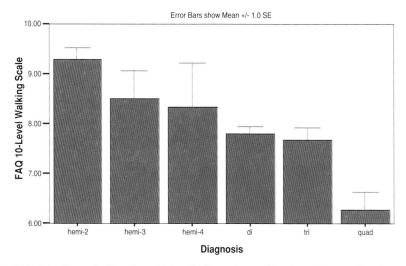

Fig. 23.7. FAQ by diagnosis. Note that a higher FAQ correlates with a lesser degree of involvement.

evidenced by increasing severity of neurologic damage, the lower the functional walking level as indicated by the FAQ. Also, individuals with milder forms of hemiplegia have higher FAQ walking-scale scores.

The second FAQ measure evaluates 22 specific higher-level skills (Table 23.6). These skills were included to offset concerns that the 10-level walking scale would not be sensitive enough to detect changes over time, or following intervention. Changes in skills (preoperative to postoperative) can be categorized as "added", "improved", "lost", "decreased", "unchanged" or "not able to perform".

Group outcome data: ambulatory subjects with diplegia
Examination of outcome data for a group of diplegic patients provides our institution with a concrete measure of the effectiveness of our treatment. In a recently completed retrospective outcome study of independently ambulatory children with spastic diplegic CP (Schwartz et al. 2003). One hundred and thirty-five children who underwent assessment and surgical treatment between January 1994 and January 2002 were analyzed according to the treatment they received during this time interval: orthopaedic surgery only (ORTHO), orthopaedic surgery and rhizotomy (ORTHO+RHIZO), and rhizotomy only (RHIZO). Eighty-two percent (111/135) of the subjects showed an improved Normalcy Index. Changes in NI were statistically significant for the entire sample of subjects as well as for each treatment group (Fig. 23.8) (Table 23.7). All three groups exhibited improvements (reduction) in oxygen consumption (Fig. 23.9). Both the ORTHO group (9%) and the RHIZO group improved (10%), while the ORTHO+RHIZO group, with its 25% decrease in oxygen consumption, demonstrated the largest improvement due to the additive benefits of spasticity reduction and correction of lever-arm dysfunction these individuals received (Table 23.8). Each of the groups showed modest improvement in the FAQ 10-level walking score, although they

416

TABLE 23.6
FAQ 22 higher-level skills defined

	Easy	A little hard	Very hard	Cannot do at all	Too young for activity
Walks carrying an object					
Walks carrying an fragile object or glass of liquid					
Walks up and down stairs using the railing					
Walks up and down stairs without using the railing					
Steps up and down curb independently					
Runs					
Runs well including around a corner with good control					
Can take steps backwards					
Can maneuver in tight areas					
Gets on and off a bus by him/herself					
Jumps rope					
Jumps off a single step					
Hops on right foot					
Hops on left foot					
Steps over an object, right foot first					
Steps over an object, left foot first					
Kicks a ball with right foot					
Kicks a ball with left foot					
Rides 2-wheel bike					
Rides 3-wheel bike					
Ice-skates or roller-skates					
Rides an escalator, can step on/off without help					

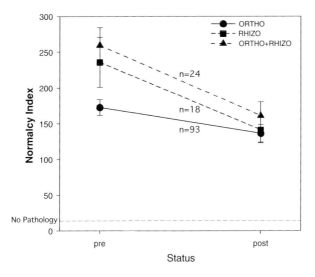

Fig. 23.8. Normalcy Index before and after treatment for each of the three groups. Normal function is equivalent to the "No Pathology" line (NI=15). S.E.M. is indicated for each group. All three groups demonstrated significant changes before and after treatment ($P < 0.05$).

417

TABLE 23.7
Average Normalcy Index decrease following surgical intervention in all three groups

Group	Number of subjects	Pre-surgery	Post-surgery	% change
ORTHO	9	172.5	136.3	21%
RHIZO	18	235.7	140.9	40%
ORTHO+RHIZO	24	259.2	160.7	38%
ENTIRE STUDY GROUP	135	196.3	141.3	27%

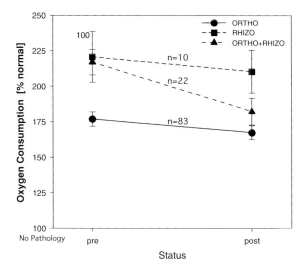

Fig. 23.9. Oxygen outcome before and after treatment for each of the three groups, expressed as a percentage of normal. Normal function is at 100% by definition; S.E.M. is indicated for each group. The improvements for both the ORTHO and ORTHO + RHIZO groups reached statistical significance (P < 0.05).

TABLE 23.8
Average percentage oxygen consumption decrease for all three groups following surgical intervention

	% change
ORTHO	9*
RHIZO	10
ORTHO+RHIZO	25*

were significant only for the entire study population (+0.4 levels) and for the ORTHO group (+0.3 levels) (Fig. 23.10). Of the 22 higher-level skills measured on the second part of the FAQ, which are acquired at different stages of development in a healthy population, 18 were selected as age-appropriate to the subjects in this study group. All treatment groups demonstrated a net addition of skills post-operatively. The RHIZO and the ORTHO + RHIZO groups had a higher percentage of added skills than the ORTHO group. The ORTHO group had a higher percentage of skills in the unchanged category (25%) than either of the other groups. The RHIZO group had the lowest percentage of lost skills.

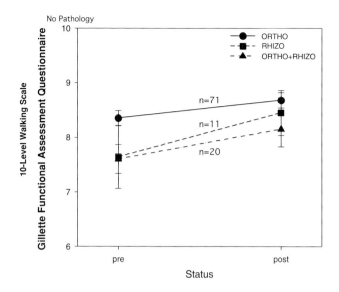

Fig. 23.10. FAQ 10-level walking scale before and after treatment for each of the three groups; S.E.M. is indicated for each group. While all three groups improved, only the changes for ORTHO group reached statistical significance (P < 0.05).

In summary, patients who underwent a combination of orthopaedic surgery and rhizotomy made the greatest gains: 38% in overall gait pathology; 25% reduction in oxygen consumption; one-third of a level in overall functional mobility; and 60% with added or improved higher-level functional skills. These results are not surprising, since this group benefited from both spasticity reduction and lever-arm deformity correction. Improvements among the ORTHO group were significant and consistent. While the rhizotomy-only group also improved, the group size was relatively small. In addition, since individuals in this group are typically candidates for later lower-extremity surgery to correct lever-arm dysfunction, they represent an intermediate result.

When contemplating treatment decisions, families and patients are interested in both efficacy and risk. To analyze the question of safety, it is important to consider individual outcomes. Seventy-seven percent (71/91) of subjects showed clinically relevant improvement on a predominance of outcome measures. Of these individuals, 11 improved on 4/4 measures and 28 improved on 3/4 measures. Of the seven subjects who registered losses, only two showed a decline on 3/4 measures and none worsened on 4/4 measures. This low rate of iatrogenic worsening shows that decision-making based on gait analysis results in a favorable risk/benefit ratio and a high level of safety.

The significant improvements in gait (NI), energy efficiency (O2) and overall function (on the FAQ) demonstrate that an approach using computerized gait analysis to guide operative decision making and subsequent surgical intervention leads to improved outcomes. The design of this study also demonstrates the value of a comprehensive approach to outcome assessment that includes both global technical and functional measures.

419

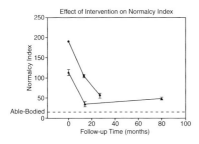

Fig. 23.11. Normalcy Index outcome for our selected case studies.

Selected case examples

Two clinical case examples were presented in Chapter 20 ("Diplegia and Quadriplegia: Pathology and Treatment"). In the first case the patient underwent orthopaedic surgery alone while in the second, the patient had both a selective dorsal rhizotomy and orthopaedic intervention to correct lever-arm dysfunction. The technical and functional outcome data for each is as follows.

Subject 1 underwent orthopaedic surgery at age 9. The preoperative Normalcy Index was 114, FAQ walking level 7 (indicating that the child walks outside the home for community distances, can get around on curbs and uneven terrain in addition to level surfaces, but usually requires minimal assistance or supervision for safety), and was able to perform 18/22 higher-level skills. The postoperative Normalcy Index (14 months later) showed significant improvement to 35 (a 70% change). His functional ambulation improved to level 8 (indicating that he walks outside the home for community distances, easily gets around on level ground, over curbs and on uneven terrain, but requires some minimal assistance or supervision for safety). While he made no gains in the number of higher-level skills that he was able to accomplish, his ability to do them improved in 16 of the 18. The family felt that he had improved strength and endurance, and was better able to keep up with peers. The family also observed that he had better balance, achieved reciprocal stair-climbing, fell less frequently, walked faster, and had a more natural gait.

Following his adolescent growth spurt at age 16, the patient came in for another gait study to be sure that no new problems had developed over the years of growth. He had not received any surgical or botulinum toxin treatments in the intervening years. The NI showed only slight deterioration to 49 (Fig. 23.11). This patient still maintained a 57% improvement in gait function compared to his preoperative status seven years earlier, despite the growth encountered during adolescence. With an FAQ level of 10, an increase of two more levels above the one-level increase seen postoperatively, his ambulatory function rating had actually improved. Gait efficiency remained within 1 S.D. of normal (1.2 times average normal) at a normal walking speed. (See Fig. 20.12 on the CD-Rom for a dynamic illustration.)

Subject 2 underwent selective dorsal rhizotomy at age 4 years 2 months. The child's preoperative NI was 191 and FAQ walking level was 6 (indicating that the patient walks more than 15–50 feet outside the home but usually uses a wheelchair or stroller for community distances or in congested areas.). He could perform only five of the higher-level skills.

Post-rhizotomy assessment, performed 13 months later, showed a 46% improvement in Normalcy Index, to 105. His FAQ walking level was unchanged, but there had been a gain of 13 higher-level skills. The family noted easier running and swimming as well as increased jumping and bike riding. The patient then underwent orthopaedic surgery to correct lever-arm dysfunction. This second intervention resulted in further improvements in the NI, which then fell to a level of 56 for a total improvement in NI of 71% (Fig. 23.11). The family now reported an FAQ walking level of 9 (indicating that the child walks outside the home for community distances, easily gets around on level ground, over curbs and on uneven terrain but has difficulty or requires minimal assistance or supervision with running, climbing, and /or stairs, and has some difficulty keeping up with peers). He was now able to perform 19 of the 22 higher level skills. Once again, the family reported improved walking, running, and balance, and fewer tripping episodes. Walking speed was maintained at a normal level, but oxygen consumption measured somewhat higher (1.9 times normal) possibly related to further need for strengthening following the orthopaedic reconstruction. (See Fig. 20.13 on the CD-Rom for a dynamic illustration.)

Conclusion

Meaningful assessment of outcome of intervention, a challenging enterprise, must be comprehensive. Essential to it are the use of valid and reliable scales such as the Normalcy Index to quantify gait dysfunction, normalized oxygen consumption to measure global gait efficiency, and functional assessment scales to measure community function. Preoperatively, the evaluation of status these measures provide guide sound clinical decision-making. Postoperatively, they serve as a means to thoroughly assess surgical outcome. A multifaceted approach for outcome assessment can produce valid outcomes analysis and the use of gait analysis to guide operative decision-making can ensure effective and safe surgical intervention for the vast majority of children with cerebral palsy.

REFERENCES

Butler C, Chambers H, Goldstein M, Harris S, Leach J, Campbell S, Adams R, Darrah J. (1999) Evaluating research in developmental disabilities: a conceptual framework for reviewing treatment outcomes. *Dev Med Child Neurol* **41:** 55–59.

Daltroy LH, Liang MH, Fossel AH, Goldberg MJ. (1998) The POSNA pediatric musculoskeletal functional health questionnaire: report on reliability, validity, and sensitivity to change. Pediatric Outcomes Instrument Development Group. Pediatric Orthopaedic Society of North America. *J Pediatr Orthop* **18:** 561–571.

Goldberg MJ. (1991) Measuring outcomes in cerebral palsy. *J Pediatr Orthop* **11:** 682–685.

Haley S, Coster W, Ludlow LH, Haltiwanger JT, Andrellos PJ. (1992) *Pediatric Evaluation of Disability Inventory (PEDI), Version 1.0.* Boston: New England Medical Center Hospitals.

Kendall MG. (1975) *Multivariate Analysis.* London: Charles Griffin.

Koop S, Stout J, Starr R, Drinken W. (1989) Oxygen consumption during walking in normal children and children with cerebral palsy. *Dev Med Child Neurol* **31** (suppl. 59): 6. (Abstract.)

McAuliffe C, Wenger R, Schneider J, Gaebler-Spira DJ. (1998) Usefulness of the Wee-Functional Independence Measure to detect functional change in children with cerebral palsy. *Pediatr Phys Ther* **10:** 23–28.

Msall ME, DiGaudio K, Duffy LC, LaForest S, Braun S, Granger CV, Campbell J, Wilczenski F, Rogers BT, Catanzaro NL. (1994) WeeFIM. Normative sample of an instrument for tracking functional independence in children. *Clin Pediatr (Phila)* **33:** 431–438.

NCMRR. (1993) *National Institutes of Health Research Plan for the National Center for Medical Rehabilitation Research (93-3509).* Bethesda, MD: National Institutes of Health.

Novacheck TF, Stout JL, Tervo R. (2000) Reliability and validity of the Gillette Functional Assessment Questionnaire as an outcome measure in children with walking disabilities. *J Pediatr Orthop* **20:** 75–81.

Novacheck TF, Trost JP, Schwartz MH. (2002) Intramuscular psoas lengthening improves dynamic hip function in children with cerebral palsy. *J Pediatr Orthop* **22:** 158–164.

Russell D, Gowland C, Hardy S, Lane W, Plews N, McGavin H, Cadman D, Jarvic S. (1993) *Gross Motor Function Measure Manual*, 2nd edn. Toronto: Easter Seals Research Institute.

Schutte LM, Narayanan U, Stout JL, Selber P, Gage JR, Schwartz MH. (2000) An index for quantifying deviations from normal gait. *Gait Posture* **11:** 25–31.

Schwartz M, Viehweger E, Stout J, Novacheck T, Gage JR. (2003) Comprehensive treatment of ambulatory children with cerebral palsy: an outcome assessment. *J Pediatr Orthop*, in press.

Stansfield BW, Hillman SJ, Hazlewood ME, Lawson AA, Mann AM, Loudon IR, Robb JE. (2001) Sagittal joint kinematics, moments, and powers are predominantly characterized by speed of progression, not age, in normal children. *J Pediatr Orthop* **21:** 403–411.

Stout JL, Gage JR, Koop SE. (1993) A comparison of metabolic energy expenditure after surgery or selective dorsal rhizotomy. *Proceedings of the Eighth Annual East Coast Gait Laboratories Conference, Rochester, Minnesota, 101.* (Abstract.)

Stout J, Koop S, Luxenberg M. (2003) Oxygen consumption and cost in cerebral palsy. *Gait Posture*, in press.

Tervo RC, Azuma S, Stout J, Novacheck T. (2002) Correlation between physical functioning and gait measures in children with cerebral palsy. *Dev Med Child Neurol* **44:** 185–190.

Waters RL, Mulroy S. (1999) The energy expenditure of normal and pathologic gait. *Gait Posture* **9:** 207–231.

WeeFIM. (1995) *Uniform Data Systems for Medical Rehabilitation: FIMware User Guide and Self Guided Training Manual for the Functional Independence Measure for Children (WeeFIM), Version 4.31.* Buffalo, NY: State University of New York at Buffalo.

EPILOGUE

This book represents an overview of the progress in the treatment of gait problems in cerebral palsy over the course of 25 years I have been working in the field. Until recently, this progress was due to the work of the relatively few individuals who recognized that treatment of cerebral palsy was a poorly practiced art, littered with iatrogenic complications, and passed on without question through generations of pediatric orthopaedists. Now, however, with better understanding of gait in general, and the neuropathology of cerebral palsy in particular, there are hints that what has been a "poor art" may soon become a better science. New methods of treatment to reduce spasticity and avoid unnecessary surgical muscle lengthenings have appeared. Technology has improved to the point that, in the near future, computer modeling may become a reality in clinical decision-making. Finally, genuine outcome studies based on objective and reproducible criteria are starting to appear.

I have always told my residents that, in the surgical treatment of cerebral palsy, the approaches to problems relating to spinal deformity and those relating to ambulation are very different. In the former the situation is static; in the latter it is dynamic. In the former the surgical decision-making is straightforward; in the latter it is complex. In the former the surgery is technically difficult and carries a significant risk of long-term morbidity; in the latter the surgery is relatively easy and carries a low risk of morbidity (except, of course, in the case of long-term, iatrogenic morbidity resulting from the choice of the wrong procedure). However, the significant technical challenges and the operative risks of scoliosis surgery are precisely why only those with adequate training and experience attempt it. On the other hand, the relative ease and low risk of surgical procedures performed on the lower extremities, with the aim of improving ambulation, have fostered a tendency among many orthopaedists to skip the difficult analysis and decision-making we have discussed in these chapters, in favor of some relatively simple but often very harmful surgeries. Cases in point are the lengthening of heelcords and/or hamstrings; neither procedure offers much by way of technical challenges, but both contribute significantly to incidences of severe iatrogenic long-term morbidity unless done for very specific indications. This book was written in the hope that it might help to provide a scientific basis to the treatment of gait disorders in cerebral palsy and so turn the "traditional treatment primacy" tide in orthopaedics. If you have absorbed all that has been written by those whom I consider to be experts in this field, you now have an adequate knowledge-base both to treat these children and to carry the science forward. I wish you well – both for your sake and for the sake of the children you will treat.

JAMES R. GAGE, M.D.
Medical Director Emeritus, Gillette Children's Specialty Healthcare
Professor of Orthopaedics, University of Minnesota

INDEX

425

427

kinetic, 50, 57
production, 43
source
    muscles, 43, 147
    normal gait, 43
"stretch", muscles, 50
energy expenditure, in CP, 146, 153
    see also energy, consumption
    assessment, as outcome tool, 146
    assessment methods, 146–150
        calorimetry, 146–147
        heart rate and speed, 147–149
        inverse dynamic method, 149, 174
        mathematical/mechanical, 149–150
        work-energy theorem, 149–150
    clinical metabolic energy data, 156–157
    contractures effect, 153
    efficiency, 146, 150
    as guide for treatment planning, 161
    hemiplegia subtypes, 157–158
    increased by spasticity, 286, 297
    metabolic, measurement, 156–157
    muscle stiffness and, 156
    orthoses effect, 161, 275
    physiologic reasons, 153–156
        anerobic power and muscle fibers, 155
        co-contraction and mechanical power,
            155–156
        muscle mechanics, 155–156
        VO_2 max alterations, 153–155
    subtypes of CP, 157–158
        based on function and contractures, 158–160
    walking, 150
        children *vs* adults/teenagers, 150, 151
        developing children (normal), 150–153
    walking speed, 50–51, 57, 150–153
Energy Expenditure Index (EEI), 147–149
engineers, motion analysis laboratory, 96
"engram", 251
epidural analgesia, 399–400
    agents, 400
epilepsy, 22, 27
epiphyseal plates, 186
equilibrium responses, 84
    see also balance
    improvement by training, 184
    standing, testing, 184
    testing, 183
equinovalgus foot *see* talipes equinovalgus
equinus contractures, 241
equinus foot deformity
    ankle, management, 316
    botulinum toxin A therapy, 261
    leaf-spring ankle–foot orthosis for, 279
equinus gait, 166, 171
    anterior pelvic tilt and, 221, 222
    causes, 171
    musculoskeletal simulation of cause/therapy,

        171–173
Euler angles, 102, 104
excitatory synapses, 12
exercise scientist, motion analysis laboratory, 97
extension osteotomy of distal femur *see under*
        crouch gait treatment
extensor carpi ulnaris, transfer, 336
extensor digitorum communis (EDC), transfer, 337
extensor hallicis longus (EHL), type I lower
        extremity hemiplegia, 316–317
extrapyramidal system, 33, 36
    disorders, 252
    dyskinesias associated, 75
extrapyramidal tone, 288
extrapyramidal tract *see* corticobulbospinal tracts

F
"fear of falling", 284
femoral anteversion, 79–80
    causes, 187
    excessive, internally rotated gait and, 169–170
    hip rotation angle and, 117
    malignant malalignment syndrome and, 198–199
    remodeling failure, 187, 198, 212
femoral derotational osteotomy, 362–363, 405
femoral extension osteotomy *see under* crouch gait
        treatment
femoral nerve, 359
femur
    anatomical coordinate system, 93–94
    distal, extension osteotomy *see under* crouch gait
        treatment
    torsion, bilateral, 206
fentanyl, 401
'final common pathway', motor control, 11
fine movements
    control, 134
    upper extremity hemiplegia, 333
finger(s)
    assessment in wrist flexion deformity treatment,
        337
    examination, 329–330
finger deformity in hemiplegia, 335, 337–338
    spastic flexion deformity, 337
    swan-neck deformity, 337–338
first-ray mobility, assessment, 82
fitness programs, 248
flexion deformities *see specific flexion deformities*
    (e.g. wrist, flexion deformity)
flexion reflex, 12
flexor carpi ulnaris, transfer, 336, 337
flexor digitorum longus, transfer, 317
flexor digitorum superficialis, release, 338
flexor hallicis longus
    transfer, 317
    type I lower extremity hemiplegia, 316
flexor muscles, 12
    see also specific muscles/tendons

431

438